Handbook of
Experimental Pharmacology

Volume 156

Springer

Berlin
Heidelberg
New York
Hong Kong
London
Milan
Paris
Tokyo

Mechanisms in Carcinogenesis and Cancer Prevention

Contributors

J.U. Ali, F.X. Bosch, N. Frank,
C. Gerhäuser, C.A. Gonzáles, E. Gormally,
P. Hainaut, K. Hemminki, E. Hietanen[†],
L.M. Howells, E.A. Hudson, R. Kaaks, G. Kelloff,
F. Lyko, M. Manson, H. Ohgaki, H. Ohshima,
O. Pelkonen, P. Peltomäki, H. Raunio, J. Ribes,
S. De Sanjosé, C.C. Sigman, B. Stewart, M. Tatemichi,
K. Vähäkangas, H. Vainio, Z.-Q. Wang, C. Wild,
W. Yasui, J. Yokota

Editors

HARRI U. VAINIO and EINO K. HIETANEN[†]

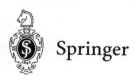 Springer

H. Vainio
Unit of Chemoprevention
International Agency for Research on Cancer
150, cours Albert-Thomas
69372 Lyon
France
e-mail: vainio@iarc.fr

E. Hietanen[†]

With 30 Figures and 24 Tables

ISBN 3-540-43837-8 Springer-Verlag Berlin Heidelberg New York

Cataloging-in-Publication Data applied for
Bibliographic information published by Die Deutsche Bibliothek
Die Deutsche Bibliothek lists this publication in the Nationalbibliografie;
detailed bibliographic data is available in the Internet at
<http://dnb.ddb.de>.

Springer-Verlag Berlin Heidelberg New York
a member of BertelsmannSpringer Science+Business Media GmbH

© Springer-Verlag Berlin Heidelberg 2003
Printed in Germany

Cover design: design & production GmbH, Heidelberg
Typesetting: SNP Best-set Typesetter Ltd., Hong Kong

27/3020/kk – 5 4 3 2 1 0 – printed on acid-free paper

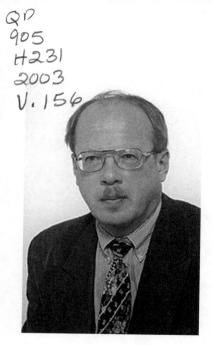

Eino Hietanen (13.10.1947–16.09.2002)

This book is dedicated to my long-time friend, Eino Hietanen, MD, PhD, who passed away unexpectedly on September 16th, 2002. Eino was a compassionate physician and a steadfast and innovative toxicologist with deep understanding of research and commitment to better protect people from environmental insults and to advance public health. Eino's abilities are dearly missed.

Harri Vainio

Preface

Overall, cancer is a preventable disease. Modifiable external factors, discovered by epidemiological studies during the last 50 years, account for a majority of all cancer deaths. Tobacco smoking remains the largest etiological contributor to cancer, while the contribution of inadequate diet and obesity may be equally important, but much more difficult to quantify. Most of the biological agents with established carcinogenic potential are rare in high-resource countries, but important in low-income countries. The association of human papillomaviruses (HPVs) with cervical neoplasia is very strong. Persistent infections with HPV types that carry a high oncogenic risk lead to invasive cervical neoplasia. After 20 years of intensive research, a point has been reached at which prevention of cervical cancer by vaccination against HPV infection will be possible in the foreseeable future.

Implementation of cancer prevention takes place slowly and incrementally, rather than through major breakthroughs. Avoidance of tobacco smoke, including environmental tobacco smoke, is a first priority in prevention. With respect to diet, increased consumption of fruits and vegetables and reduced consumption of refined carbohydrates, salt, red meat and animal fat are likely to contribute substantially to the primary prevention of cancer. Increased physical activity, avoidance of excessive alcohol intake, avoidance of obesity and overweight throughout life are also desirable. Vaccination against hepatitis B and control of transmission of hepatitis C virus and some of the HPVs will have a modest impact in developed countries, but a major impact in developing countries. Avoidance of exposure to sunlight, strict control of occupational exposures and a sound environmental policy can also contribute to the avoidance of a small fraction of the cancer burden.

Carcinogenesis is a multiyear, multistep, multipath disease of progressive genetic and associated tissue damage. The past two decades have been golden years for the genetics of cancer. It has become clear through the work of several research groups that both inherited and sporadic cancers arise through defects of misregulations of their genomes. The cartography of the order, accumulation and interactions of genetic lesions during tumor initiation and progression is reasonably detailed for many human tumor types. Such information is proving to be tremendously valuable in grouping patients into prognostic categories, and also in opening new avenues for mechanism-based cancer prevention.

The good news is that basic research into molecular genetics and biology of cancer is delivering better diagnoses and smarter drugs. However, despite increasing research and development efforts in cancer prevention, new drug approvals for preventive indications have been slow to emerge. New preventive strategies with earlier endpoints, such as intraepithelial neoplasia, may provide practical and feasible approaches to the rapid development of new tools to treat and prevent precancer rather than full-blown invasive cancer. Most of these approaches still need to be fully tested before they can be more widely adopted. The ultimate prize, which could be available within the next 10–15 years, would be a preventive tool that works on the particular genes in a particular sequence of events. Genetic tests may one day accurately identify those precancers that are likely to become invasive and spread. The tests may also tell physicians to which drugs a given precancer is most vulnerable.

HARRI VAINIO, EINO HIETANEN
Lyon, June 2002

List of Contributors

ALI, I.U., Division of Cancer Prevention, National Cancer Institute,
Bethesda, MD 20892-7332, USA
e-mail: ialt@nih.gov

BOSCH, F.X., Epidemiology and Cancer Registry Unit, Catalan Institute of
Oncology (ICO), Hospital Duran I Reynals, Avda. Gran Via,
L'Hospitalet de Llobregat, 08907 Barcelona, Spain
e-mail: x.bosch@ico.scs.es

FRANK, N., Deutsches Krebsforschungszentrum, Im Neuenheimer Feld 242,
69120 Heidelberg, Germany
e-mail: n.frank@dkfz.de

GERHÄUSER, C., Deutsches Krebsforschungszentrum, Im Neuenheimer
Feld 242, 69120 Heidelberg, Germany
e-mail: c.gerhauser@dkfz-heidelberg.de

GONZÁLEZ, C.A., Epidemiology and Cancer Registry Unit, Catalan Institute
of Oncology (ICO), Hospital Duran I Reynals, Avda. Gran Via,
L'Hospitalet de Llobregat, 08907 Barcelona, Spain

GORMALLY, E., Molecular Carcinogenesis, International Agency for Research
on Cancer, 150 Cours Albert-Thomas, 69372 Lyon, France

HAINAUT, P., Molecular Carcinogenesis, International Agency for Research
on Cancer, 150 Cours Albert-Thomas, 69372 Lyon, France
e-mail: Hainaut@iarc.fr

HEMMINKI, K., Department of Biosciences at Novum, Karolinska Institutet,
Novum, 14157 Huddinge, Sweden
e-mail: Kari.hemminki@cnt.ki.se

HIETANEN, E., †

HOWELLS, L., Cancer Biomarkers and Prevention Group, Biocentre,
    University of Leicester, University Rd, Leicester, LE1 7RH, UK

HUDSON, E., Cancer Biomarkers and Prevention Group, Biocentre,
    University of Leicester, University Rd, Leicester, LE1 7RH, UK

KAAKS, R., Unit of Nutrition and Cancer, International Agency for Research
    on Cancer, 150 Cours Albert-Thomas, 69372 Lyon, France
    e-mail: kaaks@iarc.fr

KELLOFF, G.J., National Cancer Institute, Division of Cancer Treatment and
    Diagnosis, Biomedical Imaging Program, Executive Plaza North, Room
    6058, 6130 Executive Boulevard, Rockville, MA 20852, USA
    e-mail: kelloffg@mail.nih.gov

LYKO, F., Research Group Epigenetics, Deutches Krebsforschungszentrum,
    Im Neuenheimer Feld 28, 69120 Heidelberg, Germany
    e-mail: f.lyko@dkfz-heldelberg.de

MANSON, M., Cancer Biomarkers and Prevention Group, Biocentre,
    University of Leicester, University Rd, Leicester, LE1 7RH, UK
    e-mail: Mmm2@le.ac.uk

OHGAKI, H., Unit of Molecular Pathology, International Agency for
    Research on Cancer, 150 Cours Albert-Thomas, 69372 Lyon, France
    e-mail: Ohgaki@iarc.fr

OHSHIMA, H., Endogenous Cancer Risk Factors, International Agency for
    Research on Cancer, 150 Cours Albert-Thomas, 69372 Lyon, France
    e-mail: ohshima@iarc.fr

PELKONEN, O., Department of Pharmacology and Toxicology, PO Box 5000,
    University of Oulu, 90014, Finland
    e-mail: Olavi.pelkonen@oulu.fi

PELTOMÄKI, P., Division of Human Cancer Genetics, Biomedicum Helsinki,
    Department of Medical Genetics, PO Box 63 (Haartmaninkatu 8),
    University of Helsinki, 00014 Finland
    e-mail: Paivi.Peltomaki@Helsinki.fi

RAUNIO, H., Department of Pharmacology and Toxicology, PO Box 5000,
    University of Oulu, 90014, Finland

RIBES, J., Epidemiology and Cancer Registry Unit, Catalan Institute of
    Oncology (ICO), Hospital Duran I Reynals, Avda. Gran Via,
    L'Hospitalet de Llobregat, 08907 Barcelona, Spain

DE SANJOSÉ, S., Epidemiology and Cancer Registry Unit, Catalan Institute of Oncology (ICO), Hospital Duran I Reynals, Avda. Gran Via, L'Hospitalet de Llobregat, 08907 Barcelona, Spain

SIGMAN, C.C., CCS Associates, 2005 Landings Drive, Mountain View, CA 94303, USA

STEWART, B.W., Cancer Control Program, South Eastern Sydney Area Health Service, Locked Bag 88, Randwick, Australia
e-mail: StewartB@sesahs.nsw.gov.au

TATEMICHCI, M., Unit of Endogenous Cancer Risk Factors, International Agency for Research on Cancer, 150 Cours Albert-Thomas, 69372 Lyon, France

VÄHÄKANGAS, K., Department of Pharmacology and Toxicology, PO Box 5000, University of Oulu, 90014, Finland

VAINIO, H., Unit of Chemoprevention, International Agency for Research on Cancer, 150 Cours Albert-Thomas, 69372 Lyon, France
e-mail: vainio@iarc.fr

WANG, Z.-H., Gene Environment Interactions, International Agency for Research on Cancer, 150 Cours Albert-Thomas, 69372 Lyon, France
e-mail: zqwang@iarc.fr

WILD, C., Molecular Epidemiology Unit, Academic Unit of Epidemiology and Health Services Research, School of Medicine, University of Leeds, LS2 9JT, UK
e-mail: c.p.wild@leeds.ac.uk

YASUI, W., Department of Pathology, Hiroshima University School of Medicine, Hiroshima 734-8551, Japan

YOKOTA, J., Biology Division, National Cancer Center Research Institute, Tokyo 104-0045, Japan

Contents

CHAPTER 6

Apoptosis
B.W. STEWART. With 2 Figures   83

CHAPTER 7

Deficient DNA Mismatch Repair in Carcinogenesis
P. PELTOMÄKI   107

CHAPTER 11

Arachidonic Acid Pathway in Cancer Prevention
G.J. KELLOFF and C.C. SIGMAN 187

CHAPTER 12

**Infections, Inflammation and Cancer: Roles of Reactive Oxygen and
Nitrogen Species**

CHAPTER 13

**Infections and the Etiology of Human Cancer: Epidemiological Evidence
and Opportunities for Prevention**

CHAPTER 14

Xenobiotic Metabolism and Cancer Susceptibility

CHAPTER 17

Molecular Epidemiology in Cancer Prevention

CHAPTER 1
Causes of Cancer and Opportunities for Prevention

H. Vainio and E. Hietanen

A. Cancer Burden and Health Challenge by Cancer

The global incidence of cancer is soaring due to the rapidly aging populations in most countries. In 2000, there were ten million new cancer cases, six million cancer deaths, and 22 million people living with cancer (Parkin 2001). By the year 2020, there will be an estimated 20 million new cancer patients each year. Almost three quarters of them will be living in countries that between them have less than 5% of the resources of cancer control (Sikora 1999).

Lung cancer was the most common cancer worldwide in 2000, both in terms of incidence, with 1.2 million new cases, or 12% of the world total, and mortality (1.1 million deaths or 18% of the total) (Fig. 1). This is by far the most frequent cancer of men, with the highest rates in North America and Europe (especially eastern Europe). Moderately high rates are also seen in temperate South America, Oceania, and in parts of Asia (Singapore, Hong Kong, the Philippines). In women, the incidence rates were lower (overall, the rate of 11 per 10^5 women, compared with 35 per 10^5 in men). The major cause of lung cancer is tobacco smoking, and in general, incidence rates in a country closely reflect the past history of tobacco smoking (Doll and Peto 1981). Heavy smoking increases the risk by around 30-fold, and smoking causes over 80% of lung cancers in Western countries.

Breast cancer is by far the most common cancer of women (22% of all new cancers) and ranks overall second (with 1.05 million cases) when both sexes are considered together. Breast cancer is the most prevalent cancer in the world today; there are an estimated 3.9 million women alive who have had breast cancer diagnosed within past 5 years (Pisani et al. 2001). Incidence rates are about five times higher in Western countries than in the developing countries and in Japan. Incidence rates of breast cancer are increasing in most countries, but especially in those countries where the rates have previously been low.

The major influences on breast cancer are environmental and lifestyle related (reproductive factors, diet, physical activity, energy balance). Much of the international variation is due to differences in established reproductive risk factors such as age at menarche, parity and age at births, and breastfeeding, but differences in dietary habits and physical activity may also contribute.

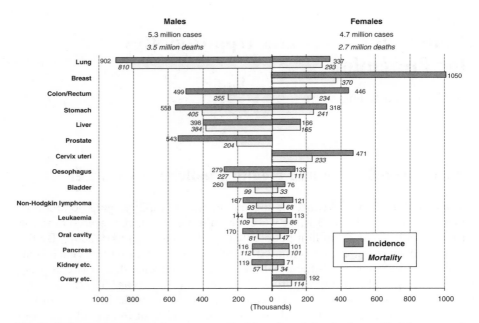

Fig. 1. Estimated number of new cases (*incidence*) and deaths (*mortality*) by sex and site. (Data from Globocan 2000)

Colorectal cancer accounted for about 9.4% of new cases in 2000, and ranked third in frequency of incidence (Parkin 2000). Numbers were similar in males and females. The highest incidence rates are in "developed" parts of the world; they are about tenfold higher in developed than in developing countries. Rates in Africa are very low (except in South Africa). Incidence rates have been increasing in countries where they were previously low. The relatively good prognosis means that colorectal cancer is the second most prevalent cancer in the world, with estimated 2.4 million people alive with the disease diagnosed in the previous 5 years.

Dietary exposures are the main risk factors. The best established dietary-related factor is overweight/obesity. Physical activity has been consistently associated with decreased risk (IARC 2002). Consumption of diet rich in fruits and vegetables has shown protective effects in numerous observational epidemiological studies; however, results from recent large prospective studies have been inconsistent.

Stomach cancer is the fourth in rank overall incidence (about 9% of the total). Almost two-thirds occurred in developing countries. Until about 20 years ago, stomach cancer was the most common cancer in the world; mortality rates have been falling in all Western countries and stomach cancer is now much more common in Asia than in Europe and North America. Stomach cancer incidence was highest in Japan in 2000. High incidence was also found in eastern Asia and Central and South America. Migrant studies have demonstrated that there is a strong environmental component in stomach cancer etiology. Infection with *Helicobacter pylori* is an established risk factor. Stomach cancer has been shown to develop in patients with *H. pylori* infection but not in uninfected patients (UEMURA et al. 2001). According to Japanese data, stomach cancer develops in 5% of *H. pylori*-positive persons over 10 years. The introduction of refrigeration has been associated with decreased risk, probably through reducing intakes of salted foods and facilitating year-round fruit and vegetable availability.

Liver cancer was the fifth most common cancer in the world in 2000. It is primarily a problem of developing countries, where over 75% of cases occur. Most liver cancers are hepatocellular carcinomas. The major risk factors for this type of cancer are chronic infection with hepatitis viruses (HBV and HCV) and, in tropical parts of Asia and Africa, where contamination of food grains with the fungus *Aspergillus flavus* is common, exposure to mycotoxins (aflatoxin B1). Chronic infections with hepatitis viruses carry a substantial increase in risk (more than 20-fold); furthermore, there is a clear (multiplicative) interaction with concomitant exposure to aflatoxins and hepatitis B virus. Excessive alcohol consumption is the main diet-related risk factor for liver cancer in Western countries, probably via cirrhosis and alcoholic hepatitis.

Cholangiocarcinoma, a tumor of the epithelium of the intrahepatic bile ducts, is particularly high in some locations where infection with liver flukes is common, such as northeast Thailand.

Prostate cancer is the third in importance in men overall (10.2% of all new cancer cases). Incidence rates are influenced by screening asymptomatic individuals, so that where this practice is common, the "incidence" may be very high (104 per 10^5 in the USA, for example). Incidence is also high in Europe and Australia/New Zealand. The estimated prevalence in 2000 was 1.6 million. There has been a rapid increase in incidence of prostate cancer over the past 20 years, also in low-incidence countries such as in Japan and China.

Little is known about the etiology of prostate cancer, although ecological studies suggest that it is positively associated with a Western-style diet. Hormones control the growth of the prostate, and interventions that lower androgen levels are moderately effective in treating prostate cancer. Prospective epidemiological studies suggest that the risk may be increased by high levels of bioavailable androgens and of insulin-like growth factor-1 (CHAN et al. 1998; STATTIN et al. 2000).

Cervical cancer is second in frequency in women worldwide; almost 80% of cases occur in less developed parts of the world. The geographical pattern is a complete contrast to breast cancer; the highest incidence is observed in parts of Africa, Asia and Latin America. In developed countries, the incidence rates are generally low.

The major etiological agents are the oncogenic subtypes of human papilloma viruses (HPV); indeed, it may be that the disease does not occur in the absence or infection. Other cofactors, such as parity and oral contraceptives, may modify the risk in women infected with HPV.

Esophageal cancer is the eighth most common cancer worldwide (4% of the total number of new cases). It is mainly a cancer of developing countries. Tobacco and alcohol are the main cause of the squamous cell cancer of the esophagus; in Europe and North America, over 90% of cases can be attributed to these causes. Chewing of tobacco and betel quid is an important risk factor in India. Hot beverages have been shown to increase the risk. Nutritional deficiencies are thought to underline the high risk in central Asia, China and southern Africa. Overweight and obesity are associated with increased risk specifically for adenocarcinoma (but not squamous cell carcinoma) of the esophagus.

Bladder cancer, the seventh most frequent cancer in men, is considerably less common in women (15th rank). Tobacco smoking is the main cause of bladder cancer. In regions in Africa, high endemic urinary schistosomiasis is known to be associated with risk of squamous cell cancer of the bladder.

Kidney cancer was estimated to account over 336,000 cases in 2000. The geographic variation in incidence is moderate, with the highest incidence in Scandinavia and among the Inuit. Overweight/obesity is an established risk factor for cancer of the kidney, and may account for up to one third of kidney cancers in both men and women (IARC 2002).

B. Main External Causes and Cancer Control

The identification of chemical, physical, and biological agents and factors with potential for cancer causation, the potential of gene–environment interaction, increasing knowledge of the pathways of carcinogenesis on the path to cancer, increased knowledge from the human genome projects – all of these present difficult challenges for prevention (see Fig. 2).

I. Tobacco Smoking

Tobacco smoking is the largest preventable risk factor for morbidity and mortality worldwide. It has central importance in the etiology of cancers of the lung, head and neck, urinary tract, pancreas, and esophagus. More recent evidence indicates that several other types of cancers, of which the most important worldwide are stomach, liver and probably cervix, are also increased by smoking. The relative importance of different smoking-related diseases varies between populations, as smoking usually multiplies the background rate due to other factors (Peto 2001). The prevalence of smoking among adults in Europe is currently around 30% or more. China, with 20% of the world's population, produces and consumes about 30% of the world's cigarettes. The overall proportion of male cancer deaths caused by smoking in China in 1990

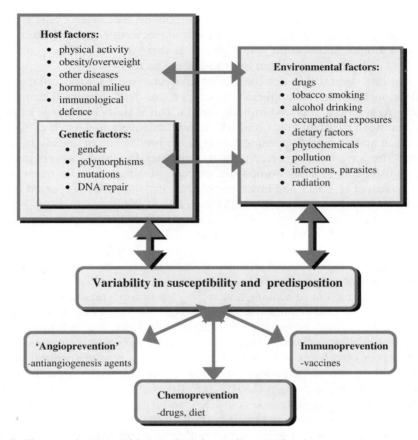

Fig. 2. Host–environmental interactions in carcinogenesis

was 22% and rising (LIU et al. 1998). Chronic obstructive pulmonary disease causes more deaths due to tobacco than lung cancer in China. Smoking also causes more premature deaths from liver cancer than from heart disease in China.

II. The Effect of Diet and Overweight

Diet and nutrition is an important life-style factor modulating carcinogenesis. Dietary factors include both genotoxic compounds and those having promotional effects. Genotoxic dietary compounds include heterocyclic amines produced upon heating processes and producing cancers in breast, colon, and prostate although epidemiological evidence is not always evident (SUGIMURA 2000). Although many micronutrients and flavonoids may be protective, even their role is not always clear. The microcomponents like heterocyclic amines are major genotoxic compounds in the diet but macronutrients may exert due to promotional modification major effects as there always will be genotoxic events in cells "exposing" them to promotional factors.

The last several decades have been characterized by major changes in lifestyle, in both the economically developed and less developed countries, leading to a general increase in body weight. This is particularly true of populations living in urban areas, and which have relatively low levels of formal education and income. Increasing trends in the prevalence of obesity in adult populations have been reported in many countries. In Europe, approximately half of men and 35% of women are currently estimated to be overweight (Bergstrom et al. 2001), and levels up to 30%–35% have been reported in the Middle East and Latin America (Martorell et al. 2000).

These high values for prevalence of obesity and changes over time seem to be related mainly to a lifestyle characterized by over-consumption of energy and physical inactivity. A diminished physical activity is the result of economical, social, and technological changes. These environmental factors have led to an increase of automation and computerization in workplace and in domestic chores, a reduction of walking and cycling for transportation, a decrease of recreational exercising and a rise in sedentary occupations such as watching television and use of computers. Overweight and obesity are well-known risk factors for cardiovascular disease and diabetes. There is now a consensus that several types of cancers, such as cancer of the colon, postmenopausal breast cancer, kidney cancer, and adenocarcinoma of the esophagus, are commoner in people who are overweight (IARC 2002; Bianchini et al. 2002). It has been estimated that among nonsmokers in USA, about 10% of all cancer deaths in nonsmokers are caused by overweight (Peto 2001).

Radical changes in dietary habits within a population are not easy to achieve. Dietary supplements such as vitamins and other micronutrients seem an attractive alternative, but they may not have the same effects as the foods that contain them, and some may even be harmful. The only reliable way to assess their effectiveness is in large randomized intervention trials that continue for many years. For example, there is substantial evidence from nutritional epidemiology that consumption of foods containing beta-carotene correlates with reduced risk of lung cancer. However, two large-scale intervention trials showed no benefit, and suggested that supplemental beta-carotene might even increase the risk of lung cancer and the overall mortality (IARC 1998) possibly due to the co-carcinogenic effects (Paolini et al. 1999). Aspirin and other nonsteroidal anti-inflammatory drugs probably reduce colorectal cancer incidence but may take a decade or more to do so, and with significant toxic side effects (IARC 1997).

Although flavonoids are known to be even protective against cancers acting as free radical scavengers, they are not equal in chemoprevention or may be harmful (Bear and Teel 2000; Hammons et al. 1999; Hatch et al. 2000).

III. Reproductive and Hormonal Factors

The effects of reproductive factors on breast and ovarian cancer have long been assumed to reflect the underlying hormonal processes, and this is confirmed by the effects of both endogenous and exogenous hormones. Breast cancer incidence is increased by oral contraceptives or by hormonal replacement therapy (containing estrogens), and is permanently decreased by menarche, early menopause, early first childbirth and high parity (IARC 1999). Endometrial cancer incidence is also increased by hormone replacement therapy. The development of cancers of the testis and prostate may also depend on hormonal effects, but apart from the increased risk in the undescended testis, no behavioral or reproductive correlate is strongly predictive of these diseases.

IV. Viruses, Bacteria and Parasites

The most important discoveries of the past two decades relate to the carcinogenic effects of infectious pathogens that had not been characterized 20 years ago. *Helicobacter pylori*, a chronic gastric bacterial infection that can cause gastric ulcers, is a major factor in the development of stomach cancer (IARC 1994b). More than 100 human papillomaviruses (HPVs) have been sequenced and some of them have been shown to be necessary factors in the causation of cervical cancers (IARC 1995). The contribution of hepatitis-B virus (HBV) to liver cancer in high-incidence regions has long been recognized (IARC 1994). The hepatitis-C virus infection is similarly carcinogenic (IARC 1994).

Other pathogens that cause a substantial cancer risk in certain populations include Epstein-Barr virus (EBV), human T-cell lymphotropic virus type 1, HIV, human herpesvirus 8, schistosomiasis and liver flukes. These are discussed in more detail in Chap. 13 by X. Bosch et al. (this volume).

V. Occupational and Environmental Carcinogens

In the past, at least in the industrialized countries, occupational exposures and occupational cancers used to be easily detected due to the massive exposure and clearly define target organs, e.g., pleura, bladder, or liver (caused by such agents as asbestos, arylamines or vinyl chloride). The occupational exposures were orders of magnitude higher than the exposures among general public. Also in the occupational surroundings, multiple exposures at fairly high doses are common.

The uncontrolled asbestos use had been widespread in the European construction industry from the 1950s to the mid-1970s, when public concern lead to a rapid reduction. The resulting epidemic of mesothelioma in construction workers and other workers born after 1940 did not become apparent until 1990s owing to the long latency of the disease. Incidence rates are still rising, and asbestos exposure prior to 1980 may eventually cause a quarter of million mesotheliomas and a similar number of lung cancers in the western Europe. There will be many more cases in the developing countries where asbestos use is still continuing. The carcinogenic effects of asbestos were known by 1960, and much of asbestos-related cancer epidemic could have been avoidable. The increase in cancer incidence caused by exposure to asbestos fibers can only be observed in humans several decades after first exposure – emphasizing the limitations of epidemiology as an early warning system.

The role of environment in carcinogenesis in the general public is often a controversial subject as the exposures are often very small; the total burden may still be of significance (FIDZGERALD et al. 1998). Air pollution may lead to considerable exposure due to the large quantities of air breathed daily that contains many biologically very active substances such as ozone, aromatic hydrocarbons, nitrogen oxides, etc. The indoor air is an issue of importance as well, since, depending on the site of building, there may be, for example, radon exposure. Passive smoking is also an important cancer risk-increasing factor. Drinking water undergoes many purification processes such as chlorination, which may yield to reactive compounds when reacting with organic products in water. Nitrates may also be common in water.

Epidemiological evidence on human cancer rates still suggests that the cancer risks caused by living near an oil refinery or a high-voltage power line are not large. Apart from skin cancers due to sunlight (IARC 2001), the only substantial and widespread cancer risk known to be caused by an avoidable environmental factor in developed countries is the further increase in lung cancer among smokers caused by indoor radon escaping from the ground or building materials, although both indoor and outdoor air pollution from fossil fuels may also contribute to the risk in smokers.

VI. Radiation

Sunlight (ultraviolet radiation) is an important cause of skin cancer (basal cell cancer, squamous cell cancer and melanoma) (IARC 2001). Information on the health effects of ionizing radiation has been accumulating from atomic bombing, nuclear power plant accidents, therapeutic and diagnostic uses of radiation. With ionizing radiation, the risk for leukemia and other cancers is dose-related. The ionizing radiation is a potent causative agent to cancer without any observable threshold (IARC 2000). Both gamma- and x-rays are known to cause cancers.

VII. Genetic and Familial Risks

Highly penetrant hereditary conditions such polyposis coli, Li-Fraumeni syndrome, and familial retinoblastoma cause at most a few per cent of the majority of cancers. *BRCA1* and *BRCA2* genes may have genetic mutations which lead to increased risk for breast cancer (STAFF et al. 2001; SWISHER 2001). In families with multiple breast cancers most of the cancer risk, but only about 2% of all cases, is due to the mutations in *BRCA1* or *BRCA2* (PETO et al. 1999).

The hereditary breast cancer may occur in various phenotypes and may also be associated with some other cancers as with ovarian cancer. In hereditary polyposis coli mutations in the APC/beta-catenin/Tcf-4 pathway may lead to changes increasing cancer risk (TEJPAR et al. 2001). Prostate and melanoma and nonmelanoma skin cancers appear to have genetic background (IKONEN et al. 2001, TSAO 2001). For more discussion, see Chap. 2 by K. HEMMINKI (this volume).

C. Potential of Cancer Prevention in the Future

The "war" on cancer, after 30 years of effort, is only partially won. After a quarter of century of rapid advances, cancer research is developing into a logical science, where complexities of the disease, described in the laboratory, clinic, as well as in populations, will become understandable in terms of a handful of underlying principles. We are starting to understand the intricate workings of the human genome – ultimately responsible for controlling all biological processes in health and disease. Gene chips will detect minute code changes of considerable relevance. Novel screening technologies will allow us to detect just a few cancer cells in a patient.

Because of the knowledge we have gained of the carcinogenesis process, and the role of various etiological and protective factors, it is now a widely accepted concept that cancer is mostly a preventable disease. A new paradigm of cancer prevention includes modulation of DNA damage and repair mechanisms, DNA methylation pathways influencing gene expression and cellular phenotypes, antioxidant rearranging and oxidative stress modulation, target receptors and signaling pathways, cell cycle controls and check points, and antiangiogenic properties. This knowledge allows us to set the framework for cancer prevention research that includes biomarkers of early responses, research on biological mechanisms underlying putative cancer relationships, and identification of the molecular targets of cancer prevention.

The future of cancer prevention will benefit from technological advances in the field of molecular biology and genetics. But as technology becomes more complex, the gap between the global rich and poor will widen. The export of unhealthy lifestyles – cigarette smoking, "fast food" with high energy content and high glycemic index, sedentary occupations – will disproportionally increase cancer and other chronic diseases such as cardiovascular diseases and diabetes in many developing countries, which can least afford the treatment costs.

The key success in cancer prevention is careful targeting. In developed countries, cancer prevention programs will lead towards individualized prevention – a combination of genetic environmental and lifestyle data will be used to construct very specific personalized messages.

Countries with limited resources should not continue reinventing the wheel. In developing countries, tobacco control is the most urgent need. With forceful "anti-smoking" programs, which are not "high-tech," to stop people from taking up the habit, and helping those who have already started to quit smoking, we could have a major effect on future disease trends. Infections are important causes of cancer especially in developing world, where an estimated 22% of cancer has an infectious cause (PISANI et al. 1997). Hepatitis B immunization in children has significantly reduced the incidence of infection in China, Korea and West Africa. Prophylactic vaccines are becoming available against oncogenic papillomaviruses.

After the sequencing of the human genome, and with the advancing technologies, it is likely that genetic polymorphisms of various sorts will be identified that will begin to make it possible to get a better handle on an individual's susceptibility to various cancers. Research on environment (nutrient)-gene interactions will provide pathophysiological mechanisms of cancer causation and prevention, and improve our ability to identify at-risk populations. Whether this will then result in an improvement in our ability to control cancer generally is unclear. If particular subgroups that are at increased risk of a specific cancer can be identified, it may be worthwhile to use certain drugs or other agents to prevent cancer in them, or to concentrate screening on them. That may make certain types of cancer control actions more cost-effective, but may not necessarily result in a greater impact in the population.

References

Bear WL, Teel RW (2000) Effects of citrus flavonoids on the mutagenicity of hetero-cyclic amines and oncytochrome P450 1A2 activity. Anticancer Res 20:3609–3614

Bergström A, Hsieh CC, Lindblad P, Lu CM, Cook NR, Wolk A (2001) Obesity and renal cell cancer – a quantitative review. Br J Cancer 85(7):984–90

Bianchini F, Kaaks R, Vainio H (2002) Weight control and physical activity in cancer prevention. Obesity Review 3:5–8

Chan JM, Stampfer MJ, Giovannucci E, Gann PH, Ma J, Wilkinson P, Hennekens CH, Pollak M (1998) Plasma insulin-like growth factor-I and prostate cancer risk: a prospective study. Science 279:563–566

Doll R, Peto R (1981) The causes of cancer: quantitative estimates of avoidable risks of cancer in the United States today. J Natl Cancer Inst 66(6):1191–308

Fitzgerald EF, Schell LM, Marshall EG, Carpenter DO, Suk WA (1998) Environmental pollution and child health in central and eastern Europe. Environ Health: Perspec 106:307–311

Hammons GJ, Fletcher JV, Ste:s KR, Smith EA, Balentine DA, Harbowy ME, Kadlubar FF (1999) Effects of chemoprotective agents on the metabolic activation of the carcinogenic arylamines PhIP and 4-aminobiphenyl in human and rat microsomes. Nutr Cancer 33:46–52

Hatch FT, Lightstone FC, Colvin ME (2000) Quantitative structure-activity relationship of flavonoids for inhibition of heterocyclic amine mutagenicity. Environ Mol Mutagen 35:279–299.

IARC Handbooks of Cancer Prevention (2002) Weight Control and Physical Activity Vol. 6. pp 1–315

IARC Handbooks of Cancer Prevention (2001) Sunscreens. Vol. 5, pp 1–193
IARC Monographs on the Evaluation of Carcinogenic Risks to Humans (2000) Ionizing radiation. Part I: X- and Gamma (γ)-Radiation, and Neutrons. Vol. 75 pp 1–491
IARC Monographs on the Evaluation of Carcinogenic Risks to Humans (1999) Hormonal Contraception and Post-menopausal Hormonal Therapy. Vol. 72 pp 1–629
IARC Monographs on the Evaluation of Carcinogenic Risks to Humans (1997) Some Pharmaceutical Drugs. Vol. 66 pp 1–514
IARC Monographs on the Evaluation of Carcinogenic Risks to Humans (1995) Human papillomaviruses . Vol. 64 pp 1–409
IARC Monographs on the Evaluation of Carcinogenic Risks to Humans (1994) Hepatitis Viruses. Vol. 59 pp 1–284
IARC Monographs on the Evaluation of Carcinogenic Risks to Humans (1994b) Schistosomes, Liver Flukes and Helicobacter pylori. Vol. 61 pp 1–270
IARC Monographs on the Evaluation of Carcinogenic Risks to Humans Tobacco smoking (1986) Vol. 38 pp 1–421
Ikonen T, Matikainen M, Mononen N, Hyytinen ER, Helin HJ, Tommola S, Tammela TL, Pukkala E, Schleutker J, Kallioniemi OP, Koivisto PA (2001) Association of e-cadherin germ-line alterations with prostate cancer. Clin cancer Res 7:3465–3471
Liu BQ, Peto R, Chen ZM, Boreham J, Wu YP, Li JY (1998) Emerging tobacco hazards in China: Retrospective proportional mortality study of one million deaths. BMJ 317(7140):1411–22
Martorell R, Khan LK, Hughes ML, Grummer-Strawn LM (2000), Obesity in women from developing countries Eur J Clin Nutr 54(3):247–52
Parkin D.M. (2001) Global cancer statistics in the year 2000. Lancet Oncology 2:533–43
Paolini M, Cantelli-Forti G, Perocco P, Pedulli GF, Abdel-Rahman SZ, Legator MS (1999) Co-carcinogenic effect of β-carotene. Nature 398:760–761
Peto R, Lopez AD (2000) Future world-wide health effects of current smoking patterns. Critical Issues in Global Health. Koop, C.E.; Pearson,C.E.; Schwarz, M.R. pp 154–161
Peto J, Collins N, Barfoot R, Seal S, Warren W, Rahman N, Easton DF, Evans C, Deacon J, Stratton MR (1999) Prevalence of BRCA1 and BRCA2 gene mutations in patients with early-onset breast cancer. J Nat Cancer Inst 9:943–949
Pisani P, Bray F, Ferlay J, Parkin DM, (2001) Estimates of the world-wide prevalence of cancer for 25 sites in the adult population. Int J 94 (in press)
Pisani P, Parkin DM, Munoz N, Ferlay J (1997) Infection and Cancer burden, Cancer and Infection: estimates of the attributable fraction in 1990 Cancer Epidemiol Biomarkers Prev 6:387–400
Staff S, Isola JJ, Johannsson O, Borg AA, Tanner MM (2001) Frequent somatic loss of BRCA1 in breast tumors from BRCA2 germ-line mutation carriers and vice versa. Br J Cancer 19:1201–1205
Stattin P, Bylund A, Rinaldi S, Biessy C, Dechaud H, Stenman UH, Egevad L, Riboli E, Hallmans G, Kaaks R (2000) Plasma insulin-like growth factor-I, insulin-like growth factor-binding proteins, and prostate cancer risk: a prospective study. J Natl Cancer Inst 92:1910–1917
Sugimura T (2000) Nutrition and dietary carcinogens. Carcinogenesis 21:387–395
Swisher E (2001) Hereditary cancers in obstetrics and gynecology. Clin Obstet Gynecol 44:450–463
Tejpar S, Cassiman JJ, Van Cutsem E (2001) The molecular basis of colorectal cancer. Acta Gastroenterol Belg 64:249–254
Tsao H (2001) Genetics of non melanoma skin cancer. Arch Dermatol 137:1486–1492
Uemura N, Okamoto S, Yamamoto S, Matsumura N, Yamaguchi S, Yamakido M, Taniyama K, Sasaki N, Schlemper T (2001) Helicobacter-pylori Infection and the development of gastric. Cancer N Engl J Med 345:784–789

CHAPTER 2

Genetic and Environmental Factors in Carcinogenesis[1]

K. Hemminki

A. Introduction

Cancer is a genetic disease in which the malignant cells have undergone mutations and chromosomal alterations that maintain the transformed phenotype
even when cultured or when injected in immunologically tolerant experimental animals (Hanahan and Weinberg 2000; Vogelstein and Kinzler 1998).
Yet, the views about the environmental (somatic) and inherited origin of the
genetic alterations in human cancer have been debated and any reasonable
agreement can be reached only when the causation appears clear, i.e., in case
of a hereditary cancer syndrome or an overwhelming environmental cause,
such as tobacco smoking or human papilloma virus. Even in such cases, one
type of causation may not be pure, and when interactions exist, it may be impos-
sible to apportion causation (Rothman and Greenland 1998). In the present
chapter I will discuss causes of cancer, keeping in mind that, due to interactions,
some of the quantitative measures may be imprecise and even arbitrary. Even
so, an understanding of these causes will be helpful for scientific, clinical, and
cancer preventive measures. A certain notion of cancer causation, often
implicit, underlies many science and health policy decisions.

John Higginson, then the director of the International Agency for
Research on Cancer, shook the prevailing view on the heritable etiology of
cancer in 1968 by stating that between 80% and 90% of all cancers were
causally related to environmental factors (Higginson 1968). Higginson based
his argument on the large differences in the incidence of cancer between populations and on the disappearance of these differences upon migration. These
findings have later been used as the proof for the importance of environmental etiology in cancer (Doll 1998; Doll and Peto 1981; IARC 1990; Parkin
and Khlat 1996). The earlier misconceptions about predominant heritable
causes were likely to be due to the biases from clinical and case-control studies,
some of which have shown very high familial risks (Houlston and Peto 1996).
Also the distinction between the terms "genetic" and "heritable" has not
always been clear because "genetic" is often used to denote both somatic and
heritable events. In the present review, I will revisit the above arguments and

---

[1] To the memory of Eino Hietaneu, a colleague and friend.

assess how the current data on familial risks and immigrants weight between the environmental and heritable causation of cancer. Four types of evidence are considered: familial clustering of cancer, cancer in twins, multiple cancers in the same individual, and migrant studies. For an introduction, it is necessary to consider cancer models. Most of the discussion will be on the estimation of heritable effects, and then, by elimination, estimates are also derived for environmental effects. Thus the term "environmental" denotes here anything that is not inherited.

B. Cancer Models

Cancer syndromes, such as retinoblastoma, *BRCA*-linked breast cancer and hereditary nonpolyposis colorectal cancer (HNPCC), follow a dominant mendelian pattern of inheritance, the penetrance is high and close to 50% of the offspring of an affected parent present with the disease (Connor and Ferguson-Smith 1997). Because of the high risk, these syndromes are rare; the frequency of the mutant gene is of the order of 1/1000 or less; the most common cancer syndromes BRCA1 and BRCA2 and HNPCC are thought to account for 1%–3% of all breast and colorectal cancers, respectively (Aarnio et al. 1999; Peto et al. 1999; Syrjäkoski et al. 2000). Bloom syndrome, ataxia telangiectasia and xeroderma pigmentosum are examples of mendelian recessive syndromes, in which cancer is a manifestation. About 25% of the offspring of two heterozygote parents display symptoms, including neoplasms. It is relatively easy to estimate the proportion of all cancer due to such monogenic syndromes of high risk, and 1% appears to be a good estimate (Fearon 1997).

However, most common cancers are caused by alterations in many genes. According to the multistage theory of cancer, the clonal tumor emerges as a result of a number of mutations in a single cell (Armitage and Doll 1954, 1957; Hemminki and Mutanen 2001; Herrero-Jimenez et al. 1998, 2000; Loeb 2001; Moolgavkar and Knudson Jr 1981; Moolgavkar and Luebeck 1992). The first mutation(s) occur in normal cells creating a slowly growing preneoplastic colony. Additional changes in a cell of the preneoplastic colony are believed to be necessary to create a neoplastic cell capable of growing as a tumor without further rate limiting genetic changes. The number of required mutations may vary and probably depends on the genes and tissues affected. An initial mutant clone may arise and thus increase the target size for subsequent promotional mutations. The adoption of known mutation rates, number of stem cells, and normal human life-span can accommodate a carcinogenic process with three or more mutations, such as two in the initiation stage and one or more in the promotional stage (Herrero-Jimenez et al. 1998, 2000).

When two or more genes are involved, it is difficult to observe mendelian inheritance in pedigrees (Hemminki and Mutanen 2001). With an increasing number of multifactorial genes, the likelihood decreases that an offspring will inherit the parental set of disease genes. In such pedigrees it is difficult to distinguish multifactorial inheritance from low penetrance single-gene or environmental effects, which is a major challenge to current segregation analyses (AITKEN et al. 1998; SHAM 1998). In the twin model, polygenic inheritance would be expressed as a much higher risk among monozygotic than dizygotic twins (RISCH 2001; VOGEL and MOTULSKY 1996). Another model where polygenic inheritance could be distinguished is in multiple primary cancers in the same individual (DONG and HEMMINKI 2001b; HEMMINKI 2001a). Both of these models will be discussed later.

C. Familial Cancer

Heritable effects would lead to a clustering of cancer in families, i.e., offspring and parents, or siblings, would present with the same cancer. However, familial clustering can also be caused by shared environment, life-style or even by chance, and an increased familial risk does not tell whether the reason is heritable or environmental. Shared environmental effects can be found in lung, stomach, and genital cancers and in melanoma (HEMMINKI et al. 2001a). However, in cancers where strong environmental effects do not exist, most of familial clustering appears to be due to inheritance (HEMMINKI et al. 2001a).

Numerous studies on familial cancer have been carried out (EASTON 1994; HOULSTON and PETO 1996; LINDOR et al. 1998). A large majority of them are case-control studies, in which cases and controls are asked about cancers in their first- or second-degree relatives. A general problem in this design is that people are not well informed about cancers in their family members. There is ample literature indicating over- and underreporting, and false reporting of cancers in family members (for discussion see DHILLON et al. 2001; HEMMINKI 2001b; LAGERGREN et al. 2000). These errors may partially neutralize each other, and for cancer sites on which many studies have been carried out, the results approach values that have also been observed in cohort studies (PHAROAH et al. 1997; STRATTON et al. 1998). A limited number of cohort studies on familial cancer have been carried out outside Sweden (CARSTENSEN et al. 1996; EASTON et al. 1996; FUCHS et al. 1994; GOLDGAR et al. 1994; PETO et al. 1996). Because of its unique datasets, Sweden has been the main source of cohort studies of familial cancer (HEMMINKI 2001a).

Statistics Sweden created a family database, "Second Generation Register," in 1995. Initially it included offspring born in Sweden in 1941 with their biological parents as families, a total of 6 million individuals. It was expanded in the beginning of 2001 to 10.2 million individuals. It covers offspring (second generation) born after 1931 with their parents, and has been renamed to "Multigeneration Register." We have linked this Register to the Swedish Cancer Registry (started in 1958) to make the Family-Cancer Database in four expanded versions in 1996 1997 1999, and 2001 (HEMMINKI et al. 2001c). The number of cancers in the second generation increased from 20,000 in 1996 to

158,000 in 1999; in the parental generation the increase was from 500,000 to over 600,000 invasive cancers. The Family-Cancer Database has been the largest population-based dataset ever used for studies on familial cancer. For comparison, The Utah Population Database, successfully used in many cancer studies, has a different structure in containing more than two generations, and 42,000 cancers in 1994 (Goldgar et al. 1994). Regarding the Family-Cancer Database, it is worth pointing out that the parents have been registered at the time of birth of the child. Thus it is possible to track biological parents in spite of divorce and remarriage. The national personal identification code has been deleted from the Database. The Database is population-based and is not sensitive to selection or reporting biases because both the family relations and cancers in family members have been obtained from recorded sources. The Database has been used in over 100 studies so far, including familial studies at most common sites.

We have carried out a systematic comparison of cancer risks between parents and offspring for putative dominant effects (Dong and Hemminki 2001a). Standardized incidence ratios (SIRs) were calculated for offspring who had an affected parent and they were compared to all offspring. The results are summarized in Table 1. Among the 18 cancer sites, all the risks were significantly increased, and they ranged from 6.9 for thyroid cancer to 1.5 for kidney and bladder cancer. For the population burden of familial cancer, the

Table 1. Standardized incidence ratios (SIRs), familial proportions (% of all affected offspring with an affected parent) and population attributable fractions (PAFs) for parent–offspring familial relationships among 0–61-year-old offspring, based on the Swedish Family-Cancer Database (modified from Dong and Hemminki 2001c; Hemminki 2001a)

Site	SIR	Proportion (%)	Familial PAF (%)
Stomach	1.7	4.5	1.9
Colorectum	2.0	9.8	4.9
Lung	1.6	5.6	2.1
Breast, female	1.9	8.1	3.8
Cervix	1.9	4.0	1.9
Endometrium	2.9	3.1	2.0
Ovary	2.8	3.1	2.0
Prostate	2.7	17.2	10.8
Testis	4.3	0.4	3.1
Kidney	1.5	2.9	1.4
Bladder	1.5	3.4	1.7
Melanoma	2.4	2.3	1.3
Skin, squamous	2.2	3.4	1.9
Nervous system	1.7	2.5	1.0
Thyroid	6.9	2.5	2.1
Other endocrine	2.5	2.1	1.4
Lymphoma	1.6	1.0	0.4
Leukemia	1.8	2.4	1.1

prevalence of familial cases is important. This is shown in column "Proportion," giving the percentage of offspring who have an affected parent. Population attributable fraction (PAF) is a measure used to quantify the effect at the population level, or in other words, the reduction in the particular cancers if the familial effect would not exist. PAFs for familial cancer range from 10.8% for prostate cancer to 0.4% for lymphoma. The population analyzed was 0–61 years old. Because heritable cancers usually show the highest risks at young age, the PAFs of Table 1 are likely to be higher than those that would be found in a fully aged population. In other words, prostate cancer is an old age disease, and the cases occurring by age 62 years would be likely to be enriched in heritable cases. Thus the PAF of 10.8% is likely to be much higher than that found among all men. The PAF values cites in Table 1 are much lower than the figures sometimes cited in the literature (RISCH 2001). As was discussed under Cancer Models, the analysis of familial risks between parents and offspring may be inefficient in detecting polygenic effects and it would miss recessive effects. Analysis of cancer between siblings without affected parents is informative of recessive effects and such results have also been presented from the Family-Cancer Database (DONG and HEMMINKI 2001a; HEMMINKI et al. 2001d).

D. Cancer in Twins

The Nordic countries have twin and cancer registries that cover a long period of time. A cancer study was carried out by pooling data from the Swedish, Finnish, and Danish twin registries for a joint analysis (LICHTENSTEIN et al. 2000). The aim of this study was to provide reliable estimates of genetic and environmental effects for the most common cancer sites and to assess the modification of such estimates by age at diagnosis. Data from 90,000 twins were combined to assess the cancer risks at 28 sites for co-twins of twins with cancer. At least one malignancy was observed among 10,803 individuals among 9,512 twin pairs. Risk increases for co-twins of affected twins were detected for several sites including stomach, colorectum, lung, breast, and prostate cancer. Structural equation modeling was used to determine the relative importance of heritable and environmental effects on cancers at 11 sites.

The results from model-fitting are presented in Table 2. For stomach cancer heritability was estimated to account for 28%, shared environmental effects for 10%, and nonshared environmental effects for the remaining 62% of the variation in liability. Statistically significant heritability estimates, where the 95% confidence interval did not include zero, were detected for cancers of the colorectum (35%), breast (27%), and prostate (42%). The estimates for the shared environmental effects ranged from 0% to 20% but none were statistically significant. There were no significant differences between sexes at any of the sites.

Table 2. Heritable and environmental effects for cancers among Swedish, Danish, and Finnish twins (modified from LICHTENSTEIN et al. 2000)

Cancer site	Proportion of variance attributed to		
	Heritable effects	Shared environment effects	Nonshared environment effects
Stomach	0.28	0.10	0.62*
Colorectum	0.35*	0.05	0.60*
Pancreas	0.36	0	0.64*
Lung	0.26	0.12	0.62*
Breast	0.27*	0.06	0.67*
Cervix uteri	0	0.20	0.80*
Corpus uteri	0	0.17	0.82*
Ovary	0.22	0	0.78*
Prostate	0.42*	0	0.58*
Bladder	0.31	0	0.69*
Leukemia	0.21	0.12	0.66*

*95% CI does not include 0.0, i.e., the estimate is statistically significant.

The results quantified the effect of nonshared environment to range from 58% to 82% for different cancers. Nonshared environment encompasses anything that is not hereditary and not shared between the twins: sporadic causes of cancer. It is of interest to note that this effect was large, 80% or more for uterine and cervical cancer. Shared environment, summing up common family experiences and habits of the twins, accounted for 0%–24% of etiology but none of these proportions were significant statistically. The proportions were 20% or more for cervical cancer. The twin model can accommodate both dominant and recessive mendelian modes and polygenic modes of inheritance. Thus the results on heritability summarize the total genetic effects, which for colorectal, breast and prostate cancer were between 27% and 42%, clearly higher than the PAF values of Table 1. For all cancer, the heritable effect was 26%. Moreover, we found evidence for heritability of cancers at stomach, pancreas, lung, ovary, and bladder, and for leukemia, but these estimates, ranging from 21% to 36%, did not reach statistical significance. If the range of heritable effects for colorectal, breast, and prostate cancer of 27%–42% turns out to be true, there are major gaps in the understanding of the genetic basis of these diseases. The frequencies of mutations in the known high-risk susceptibility genes, *BRCA1* and *BRCA2* in breast cancer and DNA mismatch repair genes in hereditary nonpolyposis colorectal cancer (HNPCC), are so low that they explain at most 10% of the heritability noted (PETO et al. 1999; SALOVAARA et al. 2000). For prostate cancer, candidate genes have been mapped but not identified (GRÖNBERG et al. 1999; XU et al. 1998). These findings suggest that other genes are yet to be identified but because they are likely to be relatively common and of moderate risk only, the incrimination will be difficult.

E. Multiple Primary Cancers

Multiple primary cancers in the same individual are one of the hallmarks of hereditary cancers (LINDOR et al. 1998). Patients belonging to BRCA or HNPCC families are characterized by an increased risk of multiple primary cancers (THE BREAST CANCER LINKAGE CONSORTIUM 1999; LYNCH and SMYRK 1996). In studies from the Family-Cancer Database, patients with a family history are at a highly elevated risk of second primaries (DONG and HEMMINKI 2001b; HEMMINKI et al. 2001b; VAITTINEN and HEMMINKI 2000). An increased occurrence of second primary cancers can also result from intensive medical surveillance after first diagnosis, therapy-induced exposure to X-rays and carcinogens, and shared environmental causes between the first and second cancer. As 98% of new primary cancers are verified histopathologically or cytologically in the Swedish Cancer Registry, it is unlikely that intensive medical surveillance is causing diagnostic misclassification. However, the diagnosis of second cancer is arrived at earlier, causing an increase in incidence during the first year of follow-up and a deficit later. On the other hand, therapy-induced carcinogenic effects usually occur about a decade or more after treatment. Thus, second cancer offers an interesting possibility for study of risk factors of cancer, including heritable factors.

In Table 3 we show the risks for second primary cancer at two follow-up times from the Swedish Family-Cancer Database (DONG and HEMMINKI 2001d). The risks for second cancer were calculated for the total population

Table 3. Risk for subsequent primary cancer from the Family-Cancer Database (DONG and HEMMINKI 2001d)

Initial cancer site	Follow-up interval (years)	
	0–9	10–38
	SIR	SIR
Oral etc.	8.2	6.0
Colon	3.4	2.6
Nose	31.8	39.0
Breast	2x 3.8	2x 2.2
Female genitals	6.7	8.8
Testis	5.3	6.8
Kidney	1.5	2.0
Urinary bladder	2.2	3.1
Melanoma	8.7	6.1
Skin	15.9	9.2
Connective tissue	20.3	7.9
Lymphoma	3.8	4.4
Leukemia	6.9	12.2

All SIRs are significant statistically. Follow-up time is the interval between the first and second cancer diagnoses.

(offspring and parents). The risks (SIRs) are very much higher than the offspring risks cited in Table 1. Remarkably high SIRs for second cancer were noted for nose, skin (squamous cell carcinoma), connective tissue and leukemia. The SIRs for breast cancer were multiplied by 2 because only one, contralateral breast, is at risk. We have analyzed the effect of family history on some cancers, such as breast cancer, and it is an important factor but affects a relatively small proportion of patients with second breast cancer (VAITTINEN and HEMMINKI 2000). The data suggest that patients with second cancer include a subgroup with a strong genetic predisposition to cancer, which cannot often be predicted by a family history. The findings are consistent with a recessive or polygenic effect.

F. Cancer in Migrants

The classical migrant studies on Japanese immigrants to the USA and on European immigrants to Australia have been strong arguments for the predominant environmental etiology in cancer (HAENSZEL and KURIHARA 1968; McMICHAEL et al. 1980). Subsequently, numerous other migrant studies have appeared from these geographic areas, from Israel, South America and some European countries (BALZI et al. 1993; McCREDIE et al. 1999a,b; PARKIN et al. 1990; STEINITZ et al. 1989). Common to these studies has been, with a few exceptions, that the incidence of cancer has moved to the level of the new host population in one or two generations (DOLL and PETO 1981; IARC 1990; PARKIN and KHLAT 1996). While these studies on practically all main cancers, and decreasing and increasing rates, leave little doubt about the overall importance of changing environmental factors in cancer, there are some features in migrant studies that have deserved limited attention, including movement of people between approximately the same socio-economic backgrounds and between small geographic distances. Such movements, typical of inter-European migration, may entail relatively fast cultural mixing with the recipient population and uninterrupted contacts to the native population. A set of studies has recently been completed based on the Swedish Family-Cancer Database, covering the large European migration to Sweden (HEMMINKI and LI 2002a,b; HEMMINKI et al. 2002). The findings of these studies are very much in line with the earlier studies, reinforcing the argument for environmental cancer etiology.

The main challenge to the current and future immigrant studies is whether it is possible to pinpoint the environmental factors that cause the change, either increasing or decreasing, in the incidence of cancer upon migration. Another challenge is to identify cancer rates that would truly differ between ethnic groups and thus suggest genetic factors predisposing to cancer. Although humans are thought be genetically identical to more than 99.9% (THE INTERNATIONAL SNP MAP WORKING GROUP 2001; VENTER et al. 2001), there are ethnic differences in genotypes that may or may not have an impact on the risk of cancer (CAVALLI-SFORZA 1998; IARC 1999). Such effects may be small and their demonstration would require unbiased epidemiological studies of high statistical power (MCCREDIE 1998; PARKIN and KHLAT 1996). Thus, immigrant studies may eventually serve in showing the effects of inherited genotypes on the risk of cancer.

G. Conclusions

There are no available data on the etiology of cancer that would refute the predominant role of environment as a causative factor. However, since the epochal review by DOLL and PETO in 1981 (DOLL and PETO 1981), disappointingly little progress has taken place in the search for new causes of environmental carcinogenesis. One likely reason is that environmental carcinogenesis is due to the interaction of external and host factors that cannot be unraveled by epidemiological or molecular biological means alone. There is hope that merging of these approaches into molecular epidemiology, or even better, into molecular genetic epidemiology, will tool the exogenous/endogenous interphase of human carcinogenesis.

All the main neoplasms appear to have a familial component that ranges, as measured in PAFs, from 10% down to below 1% of all cancer at a particular site. When strong environmental risk factors do not exist, the familial risk primarily constitutes inherited risk factors. A larger proportion of cancer may be due to inherited effects, but the mode of inheritance has remained uncharacterized. At a cellular level, cancer is attributed to an accumulation of genetic alterations in cells (HANAHAN and WEINBERG 2000). Familial risks observed among twins and among patients with multiple primary cancers provide support for the multistage carcinogenesis in human cancers at a population level. There are at least two practical implications from such findings. One is that in the search for new susceptibility factors in cancer, association studies with a case-control design may turn out to be the tools of choice, but large sample sizes are needed because of the expected small risks (EASTON 1999; HEMMINKI and MUTANEN 2001; REICH et al. 2001; REICH and LANDER 2001; RISCH and MERIKANGAS 1996). The second implication is that in clinical counseling polygenic and recessive conditions imply uncertainty. The disease strikes apparently randomly even though there is an inherited background.

References

Aarnio M, Sankila R, Pukkala E, Salovaara R, Aaltonen L, De La Chapelle A, Peltomäki P, Mecklin J-P, Järvinen H (1999) Cancer risk in mutation carriers of DNA-mismatch-repair genes. Int J Cancer 81:214–218

Aitken J, Bailey-Wilson J, Green A, MacLennen R, Martin N (1998) Segregation analysis of cutaneous melanoma in Queensland. Genet Epidemiol 15:391–401

Armitage P, Doll R (1954) The age distribution of cancer and a multi-stage theory of carcinogenesis. Br J Cancer 8:1–12

Armitage P, Doll R (1957) A two-stage theory of carcinogenesis in relation to the age distribution of human cancer. Br J Cancer 9:161–169

Balzi D, Buiatti E, Geddes M, Khlat M, Masuyer E, Parkin DM (1993) Cancer in Italian migrant populations. Summary of the results by site. IARC Sci Publ 123:193–292

Carstensen B, Soll-Johanning H, Villadsen E, Söndergaard J, Lynge E (1996) Familial aggregation of colorectal cancer in the general population. Int J Cancer 68:428–435

Cavalli-Sforza L (1998) The DNA revolution in population genetics. Trends Genet 14:60–65

Connor M, Ferguson-Smith M (1997) Essential Medical Genetics. Oxford: Blackwell Science

The Breast Cancer Linkage Consortium (1999) Cancer risks in BRCA2 mutation carriers. J Natl Cancer Inst 91:1310–1306

Dhillon PK, Farrow DC, Vaughan TL, Chow WH, Risch HA, Gammon MD, Mayne ST, Stanford JL, Schoenberg JB, Ahsan H, Dubrow R, West AB, Rotterdam H, Blot WJ, Fraumeni JF Jr (2001) Family history of cancer and risk of esophageal and gastric cancers in the United States. Int J Cancer 93:148–152

Doll R (1998) Epidemiological evidence of the effects of behaviour and the environment on the risk of human cancer. Recent Results Cancer Res 154:3–21

Doll R, Peto R (1981) The causes of cancer. J Natl Cancer Inst 66:1191–1309

Dong C, Hemminki K (2001a) Modification of cancer risks in offspring by sibling and parental cancers from 2,112,616 nuclear families. Int J Cancer 91:144–150

Dong C, Hemminki K (2001b) Multiple primary cancers at colon, breast and skin (melanoma) as models for polygenic cancers. Int J Cancer 92:883–887

Dong C, Hemminki K (2001c) Second primary breast cancer in men. Breast Cancer Res Treat 66:171–172

Dong C, Hemminki K (2001d) Second primary neoplasms in 633964 cancer patients in Sweden 1958–1996. Int J Cancer 93:155–161

Easton D (1994) The inherited component of cancer. Br Med Bull 50:527–535

Easton D (1999) How many more breast cancer predisposition genes are there? Breast Cancer Res 1:14–17

Easton D, Matthews F, Ford D, Swerdlow A, Peto J (1996) Cancer mortality in relatives of women with ovarian cancer: the OPCS study. Int J Cancer 65:284–294

Fearon ER (1997) Human cancer syndromes: clues to the origin and nature of cancer. Science 278:1043–1050

Fuchs C, Giovannucci E, Colditz G, Hunter D, Speizer F, Willett W (1994) A prospective study of family history and the risk of colorectal cancer. N Engl J Med 331:1669–1674

Goldgar DE, Easton DF, Cannon-Albright LA, Skolnick MH (1994) Systematic population-based assessment of cancer risk in first-degree relatives of cancer probands. J Natl Cancer Inst 86:1600–1607

The International SNP Map Working Group (2001) A map of human genome sequence variation containing 1.42 million single nucleotide polymorphisms. Nature 409:928–933

Grönberg H, Smith J, Emanuelsson M, Jonsson BA, Bergh A, Carpten J, Isaacs W, Xu J, Meyers D, Trent J, Dambert JE (1999) In Swedish families with hereditary prostate cancer, linkage to the HPC1 locus on chromossome 1q24–25 is restricted to families with early-onset prostate cancer. Am J Hum Genet 65:134–40

Haenszel W, Kurihara M (1968) Studies of Japanese migrants. I. Mortality from cancer and other diseases in Japanese in the United States. J Natl Cancer Inst 40:43–68

Hanahan D, Weinberg R (2000) The hallmarks of cancer. Cell 100:57–70

Hemminki K (2001a) Genetic epidemiology: science and ethics on familial cancers. Acta Oncol 40:439–444

Hemminki K (2001b) Re: Characterization of hereditary nonpolyposis colorectal cancer families from a population-based series of cases. J Natl Cancer Inst 93:651

Hemminki K, Dong C, Vaittinen P (2001a) Cancer risks to spouses and offspring in the Family-Cancer Database. Genet Epidemiol 20:247–257

Hemminki K, Li X (2002a) Cancer risks in childhood and adolescence among second generation immigrants to Sweden. Br J Cancer 86:1414–1418

Hemminki K, Li X (2002b) Cancer risks in second-generation immigrants to Sweden. Int J Cancer 99:229–237

Hemminki K, Li X, Czene K (2002) Cancer risks in first generation immigrants to Sweden. Int J Cancer 99:218–228

Hemminki K, Li X, Dong C (2001b) Second primary cancers after sporadic and familial colorectal cancer. Cancer Epidemiol Biomarkers Prev 10:793–798

Hemminki K, Li X, Plna K, Granström C, Vaittinen P (2001c) The nation-wide Swedish Family-Cancer Database: updated structure and familial rates. Acta Oncol 40:772–777.

Hemminki K, Mutanen P (2001) Genetic epidemiology of multistage carcinogenesis. Mut Res 473:11–21

Hemminki K, Vaittinen P, Dong C, Easton D (2001d) Sibling risks in cancer: clues to recessive or X-linked genes? Br J Cancer 84:388–391

Herrero-Jimenez P, Thilly G, Southam P, Tomita-Mitchell A, Morgenthaler S, Furth E, Thilly W (1998) Mutation, cell kinetics, and subpopulations at risk for colon cancer in the United States. Mut Res 400:553–578

Herrero-Jimenez P, Tomita-Mitchell A, Furth E, Morgenthaler S, Thilly W (2000) Population risk and physiological rate parameters for colon cancer. The union of an explicit model for carcinogenesis with the public health records of the United States. Mut Res 447:73–116

Higginson J (1968) Present trends in cancer epidemiology. Canadian cancer conference 8:40–75

Houlston R, Peto J (1996) Genetics and the common cancers. In Genetic Predisposition to cancer, ed. R Eeles, B Ponder, D Easton A. Horwich. London: Chapman & Hall 1996, pp 208–226

IARC (1990) Cancer: Causes, Occurrence and Control. Lyon: IARC

IARC (1999) Metabolic polymorphisms and susceptibility to cancer. IARC Sci Publ 148:1–510

Lagergren J, Ye W, Lindgren A, Nyren O (2000) Heredity and risk of cancer of the esophagus and gastric cardia. Cancer Epidemiol Biomarkers Prev 9:757–760

Lichtenstein P, Holm N, Verkasalo P, Illiado A, Kaprio J, Koskenvuo M, Pukkala E, Skytthe A, Hemminki K (2000) Environmental and heritable factors in the causation of cancer. N Engl J Med 343:78–85

Lindor N, Greene M (1998) A concise handbook of family cancer syndromes. J Natl Cancer Inst 90:1039–1071

Loeb L (2001) A mutator phenotype in cancer. Cancer Res 61:3230–3239

Lynch H, Smyrk T (1996) Hereditary nonpolyposis colorectal cancer (Lynch syndrome). Cancer 78:1149–1167

McCredie M (1998) Cancer epidemiology in migrant studies. Recent Results Cancer Res 154:298–305

McCredie M, Williams S, Coates M (1999a) Cancer mortality in East and Southeast Asian migrants to New South Wales, Australia 1975–1995. Br J Cancer 79:1277–1282

McCredie M, Williams S, Coates M (1999b) Cancer mortality in migrants from the British Isles and continental Europe to New South Wales, Australia 1975–1995. Int J Cancer 83:179–185

McMichael AJ, McCall MG, Hartshorne JM, Woodings TL (1980) Patterns of gastrointestinal cancer in European migrants to Australia: the role of dietary change. Int J Cancer 25:431–437

Moolgavkar S, Knudson Jr A (1981) Mutation and cancer: a model for human carcinogenesis. J Natl Cancer Inst 66:1037–1052

Moolgavkar S, Luebeck E (1992) Multistage carcinogenesis: population-basedmodel for colon cancer. J Natl Cancer Inst 84:610–618

Parkin DM, Khlat M (1996) Studies of cancer in migrants: rationale and methodology. Eur J Cancer 32A:761–771

Parkin DM, Steinitz R, Khlat M, Kaldor J, Katz L, Young J (1990) Cancer in Jewish migrants to Israel. Int J Cancer 45:614–621

Peto J, Collins N, Barfoot R, Seal S, Warren W, Rahman N, Easton D, Evans C, Deacon J, Stratton M (1999) Prevalence of BRCA1 and BRCA2 gene mutations in patients with early-onset breast cancer. J Natl Cancer Inst 91:943–949

Peto J, Easton D, Matthews F, Ford D, Swerdlow A (1996) Cancer mortality in relatives of women with breast cancer: the OPCS study. Int J Cancer 65:275–283

Pharoah P, Day N, Duffy S, Easton D, Ponder B (1997) Family history and the risk of breast cancer: a systematic review and meta-analysis. Int J Cancer 71:800–809

Reich DE, Cargill M, Bolk S, Ireland J, Sabeti PC, Richter DJ, Lavery T, Kouyoumjian R, Farhadian SF, Ward R, Lander ES (2001) Linkage disequilibrium in the human genome. Nature 411:199–204

Reich DE, Lander ES (2001) On the allelic spectrum of human disease. Trends Genet 17:502–510

Risch N (2001) The genetic epidemiology of cancer: interpreting family and twin studies and their implications for molecular genetic approaches. Cancer Epidemiol Biomarkers Prev 10:733–741

Risch N, Merikangas K (1996) The future of genetic studies of complex diseases. Science 273:1516–1517

Rothman K, Greenland S (1998) Modern Epidemiology. Philadelphia: Lippincott-Raven

Salovaara R, Loukola A, Kristo P, Kaariainen H, Ahtola H, Eskelinen M, Harkonen N, Julkunen R, Kangas E, Ojala S, Tulikoura J, Valkamo E, Jarvinen H, Mecklin J, Aaltonen L, de la Chapelle A (2000) Population-based molecular detection of hereditary nonpolyposis colorectal cancer. J Clin Oncol 18:2193–2200

Sham P (1998) Statistics in Human Genetics. New York: John Wiley & Sons

Steinitz R, Parkin DM, Young JL, Bieber CA, Katz L (1989) Cancer incidence in Jewish migrants to Israel 1961–1981. IARC Sci Publ 98:1–311

Stratton J, Pharoah P, Smith S, Easton D, Ponder B (1998) A systematic review and meta-analysis of family history and risk of ovarian cancer. Br J Obstet Gynaecol 105:493–499

Syrjäkoski K, Vahteristo P, Eerola H, Tamminen A, Kivinummi K, Sarantaus L, Holli K, Blomqvist C, Kallioniemi OP, Kainu T, Nevanlinna H (2000) Population-based study of BRCA1 and BRCA2 mutations in 1035 unselected Finnish breast cancer patients. J Natl Cancer Inst 92:1529–1531

Vaittinen P, Hemminki K (2000) Risk factors and age-incidence relationships for contralateral breast cancer. Int J Cancer 88:998–1002

Venter J, Adams M, Myers E, Li P, Mural R, Sutton G, Smith H, Yandell M et al. (2001) The sequence of the human genome. Science 291:1304–1351

Vogel F, Motulsky A (1996) Human Genetics: problems and approaches. Heidelberg: Springer

Vogelstein B, Kinzler KW, Editors (1998) The genetic basis of human cancer. New York: McGraw-Hill

Xu J, Meyers D, Freije D, Isaacs S, Wiley K, Nusskern D, Ewing C et al. (1998) Evidence for a prostate cancer susceptibility locus on the X chromosome. Nat Genet 20:175–179

CHAPTER 3

Genetic Pathways to Human Cancer

H. OHGAKI, W. YASUI, and J. YOKOTA

Carcinogenesis is a multi-step process and it is generally accepted that morphological changes that occur in malignant progression reflect the sequential acquisition of genetic alterations. Sequences of genetic alterations appear to be tissue- and cell type-specific. In this chapter, we summarize and discuss genetic pathways leading to brain tumors, stomach cancer, and lung cancer.

A. Genetic Pathways to Brain Tumors

I. Astrocytic Brain Tumors

Diffusely infiltrating astrocytomas are the most frequent intracranial neoplasms and account for more than 60% of all primary brain tumors. Low-grade diffuse astrocytomas (WHO grade II) are well-differentiated tumors that typically develop in young adults. They grow slowly, but diffusely infiltrate the surrounding brain tissues. Therefore they tend to recur, and recurrence is often associated with progression to more malignant histologic types, i.e., anaplastic astrocytoma (WHO grade III) and glioblastoma (secondary glioblastoma WHO grade IV) (KLEIHUES et al. 2000). The mean time till progression from low-grade diffuse astrocytoma to glioblastoma is 4–5 years. Secondary glioblastomas are considered to account for less than 20% of all glioblastomas and occur in young patients (mean age, 40 years). In contrast, the majority of glioblastomas develop very rapidly without clinical, radiological, or morphologic evidence of a less malignant precursor lesion. These glioblastomas develop typically in older patients (mean age, 55 years), and are termed primary or de novo glioblastoma.

Primary and secondary glioblastomas share similar morphological features, but recent genetic analyses have shown that they are genetically quite different (Fig. 1) (BIERNAT et al. 1997a,b; FUJISAWA et al. 2000; KLEIHUES and OHGAKI 2000; NAKAMURA et al. 2000, 2001a,b; TOHMA et al. 1998; WATANABE et al. 1996). Primary glioblastomas are characterized by frequent *EGFR* amplification/overexpression, *MDM2* amplification/overexpression, *PTEN* mutations, and loss of heterozygosity (LOH) on the entire chromosome 10 (BIERNAT et al. 1997a; FUJISAWA et al. 2000; TOHMA et al. 1998; WATANABE et al. 1996). Secondary glioblastomas frequently contain *p53* mutations, of which more than 90% are already present in low-grade astrocytomas (WATANABE et

Glioblastoma

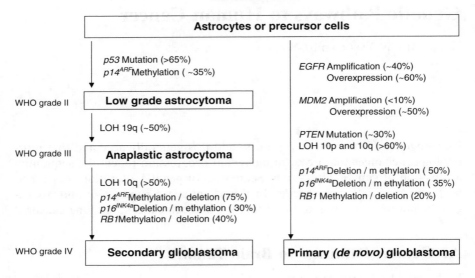

Fig. 1. Glioblastoma

al. 1997). Promoter methylation of the *p14^ARF* gene has also been found in one third of low-grade astrocytomas (NAKAMURA et al. 2001a). The pathway to secondary glioblastomas is further characterized by LOH on chromosome 19q, *RB1* methylation, and LOH on chromosome 10q (FUJISAWA et al. 1999, 2000; NAKAMURA et al. 2000, 2001b).

Since primary and secondary glioblastomas are usually histologically indistinguishable, at least one genetic alteration should be common if the phenotype of these lesions is a reflection of genetic alterations. Neuropathologists occasionally observe an abrupt transition from low-grade or anaplastic astrocytoma to glioblastoma, suggesting the emergence of a new tumor clone. Such glioblastoma foci have been microdissected and the chromosome 10 status was compared with that of the respective low-grade or anaplastic astrocytoma areas from the same tumor. In glioblastoma foci, deletions were typically detected distal from *PTEN* at 10q25-qter, covering the *DMBT1* and *FGFR2* loci (FUJISAWA et al. 1999), suggesting that the acquisition of a highly malignant glioblastoma phenotype is associated with loss of a putative tumor-suppressor gene on 10q25-qter.

More subtypes of glioblastoma may exist with intermediate clinical and genetic profiles. Giant cell glioblastoma, a rare glioblastoma variant characterized by predominance of multinucleated giant cells, occupies a hybrid position, sharing with primary glioblastomas a short clinical history, the absence of a less malignant precursor lesion and a 30% frequency of *PTEN* mutations. With secondary glioblastomas, it has in common a younger patient age at manifestation and a high frequency (>70%) of *p53* mutations (OHGAKI et al. 2000b). Another rare glioblastoma variant, gliosarcoma, has a genetic profile similar to that of primary glioblastomas but appears to lack their most typical genetic change, i.e., *EGFR* amplification (OHGAKI et al. 2000a).

II. Oligodendrogliomas

Oligodendrogliomas account for approximately 4% of all primary brain tumors and represent 5%–18% of all gliomas. Oligodendroglioma (WHO grade II) is genetically characterized by concurrent LOH on chromosomes 1p and 19q (up to 80%–90%) (REIFENBERGER et al. 2000b), which is associated with longer survival (SMITH et al. 2000a). Promoter methylation of the *p14^ARF* gene has been found in 20% of oligodendrogliomas (WATANABE et al. 2001a,b; Fig. 2). About half of oligodendrogliomas show strong expression of *EGFR* mRNA and protein in the absence of *EGFR* amplification (REIFENBERGER et al. 1996). Platelet-derived growth factors A and B, as well as the corresponding receptors, are coexpressed in most oligodendrogliomas (DI ROCCO et al. 1998).

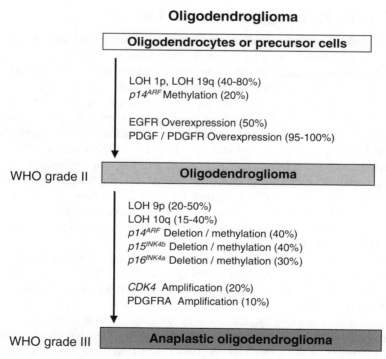

Fig. 2. Oligodendroglioma

Anaplastic oligodendrogliomas (WHO grade III) share LOH on 1p and 19q with grade II oligodendrogliomas, and this is associated with sensitivity to chemotherapy and longer survival of patients (Cairncross et al. 1998). In addition, anaplastic oligodendrogliomas carry several genetic alterations, including LOH on 9p and 10, and gain of chromosome 7 (10%–40%; Fig. 2) (Reifenberger et al. 2000a). In anaplastic oligodendrogliomas, the RB1/CDK4/p16^{INK4a}/p15^{INK4b} pathway was altered in 13/20 (65%) cases, by either *RB1* alteration, *CDK4* amplification or *p16^{INK4a}/p15^{INK4b}* homozygous deletion or promoter hypermethylation. Among anaplastic oligodendrogliomas, 50% showed alterations in the p53 pathway through promoter hypermethylation or homozygous deletion of the *p14^{ARF}* gene and, less frequently, through *p53* mutation or *MDM2* amplification (Watanabe et al. 2001b). It is notable that simultaneous disruption of the RB1/CDK4/p16^{INK4a}/p15^{INK4b} and the p53/p14^{ARF}/MDM2 pathways occurs in 45% of anaplastic oligodendrogliomas (Watanabe et al. 2001b), whereas no oligodendroglioma WHO grade II showed simultaneous disruption of these pathways. Amplifications of the *CDK4* and *PDGFRA* genes were found in 20% and 10% of anaplastic oligodendrogliomas, respectively (Smith et al. 2000b; Watanabe et al. 2001b).

B. Genetic Pathways to Stomach Cancer

In the course of multi-step stomach carcinogenesis, various genetic and epigenetic alterations of oncogenes, tumor-suppressor genes, DNA repair genes, cell cycle regulators and cell adhesion molecules are involved (Tahara 1993; Yasui et al. 2000; Yokozaki et al. 2001). Stomach cancer is histologically divided into two types, namely the intestinal and diffuse types. Genetic alterations typical of the intestinal type of gastric cancer include K-*ras* mutations, *APC* mutations, *pS2* methylation, *hMLH1* methylation, *p16^{INK4a}* methylation, *p73* deletion and c-*erbB*-2 amplification, while those typical of the diffuse type of gastric cancer are *CDH1* gene alterations and K-*sam* amplification (Figs. 3, 4). Other genetic alterations, including telomere reduction, hTERT expression, telomerase activation, genetic instability, overexpression of the cyclin E, CDC25B, and E2F1 genes, *p53* mutations, reduced expression of p27, CD44 aberrant transcripts, and amplification of the c-*met* and *cyclin E* genes, are common in both pathways (Figs. 3, 4).

Telomerase activation and genetic instability are involved in the initial step of carcinogenesis in the pathways of both diffuse and intestinal types (Yasui et al. 2000; Yokozaki et al. 2001). Maintenance of telomeres by telomerase activation induces cellular immortalization (Kim et al. 1994). Most stomach cancers possess strong telomerase activity with overexpression of the catalytic subunit of telomerase (hTERT), regardless of the histological type and tumor stage (Yasui et al. 1998). Approximately 30% of primary stomach cancers, including early cancers, show a low frequency of micro-

Intestinal type gastric cancer

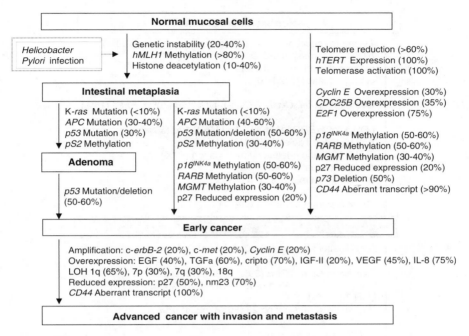

Fig. 3. Intestinal type gastric cancer

satellite instability (MSI-L) (YOKOZAKI et al. 2001). Approximately 50% of adenomas and 25% of intestinal metaplasias also show MSI-L (HAMAMOTO et al. 1997).

I. Histone Deacetylation

Acetylation of histones disrupts nucleosome structure, which leads to DNA relaxation and thus increased accessibility for transcription factors to enhance expression of various genes, including p21$^{WAF1/cip1}$, CBP, Bak and cyclin E (GRUNSTEIN 1997; SUZUKI et al. 2000). More than 70% of stomach cancers show reduced levels of histone acetylation. Reduced telomerase activity and histone acetylation have also been detected in adenomas and less frequently in intestinal metaplasias (YASUI et al. 1999a).

II. Cell Cycle Regulatory Genes

Abnormalities in cell cycle regulators are involved in the development and progression of stomach cancer (YASUI et al. 2000; YOKOZAKI et al. 2001). Cyclin

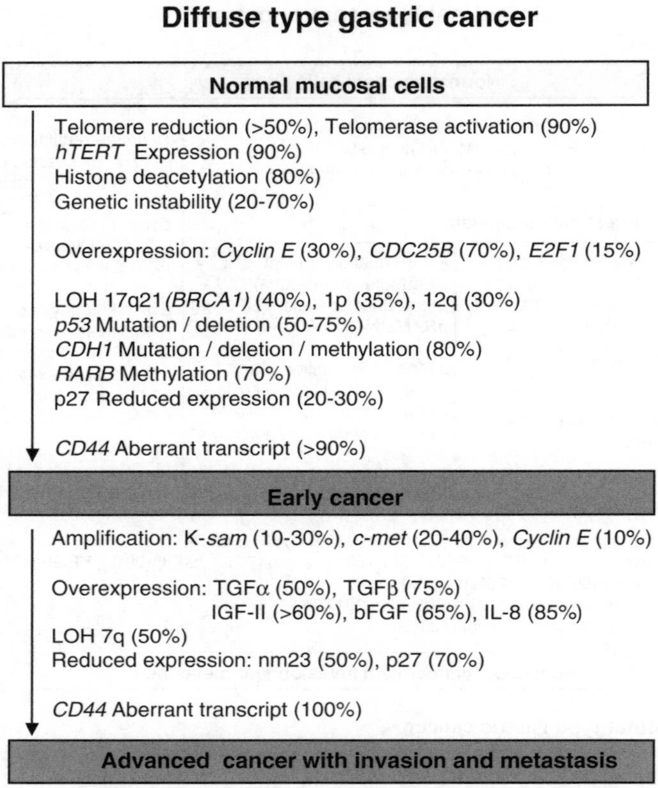

Diffuse type gastric cancer

Normal mucosal cells

Telomere reduction (>50%), Telomerase activation (90%)
hTERT Expression (90%)
Histone deacetylation (80%)
Genetic instability (20-70%)

Overexpression: *Cyclin E* (30%), *CDC25B* (70%), *E2F1* (15%)

LOH 17q21 *(BRCA1)* (40%), 1p (35%), 12q (30%)
p53 Mutation / deletion (50-75%)
CDH1 Mutation / deletion / methylation (80%)
RARB Methylation (70%)
p27 Reduced expression (20-30%)

CD44 Aberrant transcript (>90%)

Early cancer

Amplification: K-*sam* (10-30%), *c-met* (20-40%), *Cyclin E* (10%)

Overexpression: TGFα (50%), TGFβ (75%)
            IGF-II (>60%), bFGF (65%), IL-8 (85%)
LOH 7q (50%)
Reduced expression: nm23 (50%), p27 (70%)

CD44 Aberrant transcript (100%)

Advanced cancer with invasion and metastasis

Fig. 4. Diffuse type gastric cancer

E overexpression occurs in both diffuse and intestinal types of gastric cancer and tends to correlate with their aggressiveness (Yasui et al. 1999b). Cyclin E amplification was detected in 15%–20% of advanced gastric carcinomas (Yokozaki et al. 2001). Reduced $p27^{Kip1}$ expression without genetic alterations is preferentially found in adenomas that progress to carcinomas, and also significantly correlates with depth of tumor invasion and the presence of lymph-node metastasis (Yasui et al. 1999b). E2F-1, a target of cyclins/CDKs at G1/S transition, is overexpressed in approximately 75% of intestinal type of stomach cancer (Suzuki et al. 1999).

III. Oncogenes and Growth Factors

K-*ras* mutation and c-*erb*B2 amplification preferentially occurs in the intestinal type, while amplification of the K-*sam* and c-*met* genes is frequently found in diffuse-type stomach cancer (Yokozaki et al. 2001). In particular, amplification of c-*erb*B2, K-*sam* and c-*met* is significantly associated with advanced stomach cancers, suggesting that it contributes to invasion and metastasis. Overexpression of growth factors or cytokines such as EGF, TGFα, bFGF and VEGF promotes progression through multiple autocrine and paracrine loops modulating cell growth and microenvironment including neovascularization.

IV. Tumor-Suppressor Genes

Mutations of the *p53* gene are important in the initial stage of carcinogenesis of both the intestinal and diffuse types, while mutations and LOH on the *APC* gene locus occur at an early stage of carcinogenesis of the intestinal type of stomach cancer (YOKOZAKI et al. 2001). LOH on the *p73* locus occurs exclusively in the intestinal type with a foveolar epithelial phenotype (YOKOZAKI et al. 1999). Since LOH on 1q, 7p, and 18q has been found in advanced carcinomas of the intestinal type, certain genes located at these loci may have a suppressor function for malignant progression (SANO et al. 1991). The diffuse type frequently shows LOH on 17q21 (BRCA1 locus), 1p and 12q.

One of the epigenetic mechanisms of loss of expression of tumor-suppressor genes is methylation of CpG islands in their regulatory (e.g., promoter) sequences. Methylation of *hMLH1*, O^6-methylguanine DNA methyltransferase *(MGMT)*, *p16^{INK4a}* and *pS2* associated with loss of expression is detected in 20%–30% of stomach cancers, especially of the intestinal type (FUJIMOTO et al. 2000; OUE et al. 2001, 2002; TOYOTA et al. 1999). Since *hMLH1* methylation already occurs in intestinal metaplasias, reduced hMLH1 expression due to methylation may be an initial event which leads to accumulation of genetic abnormalities in stomach carcinogenesis. In contrast, *CDH-1* (E-cadherin) promoter methylation and consistent reduced E-cadherin expression participate exclusively in diffuse-type stomach cancer (OUE et al. 2002). Promoter methylation and reduced expression of retinoic acid receptor β (RARB) has been detected in both the intestinal and diffuse types (OUE et al. 2002).

C. Genetic Pathways to Lung Cancer

Lung cancer is histologically classified into three major types: adenocarcinoma (AdC), squamous cell carcinoma (SqC) and small cell lung cancer (SCLC). The term non-small cell lung cancer (NSCLC) is often used for AdC and SqC together, since these have similar clinical behavior, being mostly chemoresistant and therefore being treated primarily by surgery. In contrast, SCLCs are chemosensitive and are treated primarily by chemotherapy and radiotherapy.

The origins of AdC are considered to be alveolar epithelial cells (in particular, type II alveolar epithelial cells and Clara cells) and those of SqC are

Non-small cell lung cancer

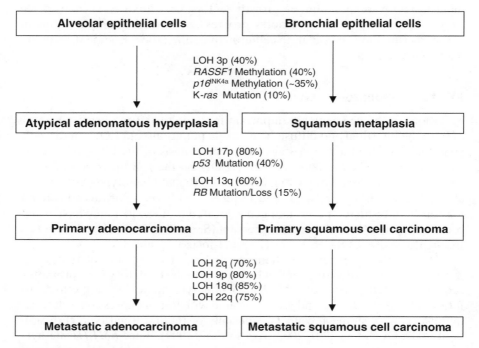

Fig. 5. Non-small cell lung cancer

bronchial epithelial cells. Atypical adenomatous hyperplasia (AAH) and squamous metaplasia (SM) are considered to be precancerous lesions for SqC and AdC, respectively. SCLC is considered to originate from neuroendocrine epithelial cells. It is not clear if there are precancerous lesions for SCLC, since the majority of SCLC is already in an advanced stage at the time of diagnosis.

Several genes have been identified as being genetically and/or epigenetically altered in lung cancer cells, and the timing of the occurrence of these alterations has been assessed by molecular analyses of cancer cells at various stages of progression. Several genetic alterations are common between NSCLCs and SCLCs and others are unique to a certain type only (Figs. 5, 6) (Kohno and Yokota 1999; Wistuba et al. 2001). The most frequent alterations are *p53* mutations, which have been reported in more than 90% of SCLCs and in more than 50% of NSCLCs. The *RB1* gene is also inactivated in over 90% of SCLCs but in only 15% of NSCLCs. In contrast, the $p16^{INK4a}$ gene is inactivated in more than 50% of NSCLCs but rarely in SCLCs. Since RB1 and p16^{INK4a} are components of the same signaling pathway

Small cell lung cancer

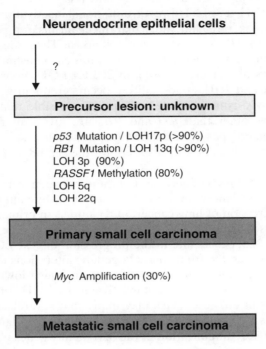

Fig. 6. Small cell lung cancer

regulating the G_1/S transition in the cell cycle, the biological significance of abnormalities in the RB1 pathway appears to be similar in SCLCs and NSCLCs.

What genes are involved in the early stages of lung carcinogenesis? Relevant information has been obtained from analysis of atypical adenomatous hyperplasia for AdC and squamous metaplasia for SqC, but is not available for SCLC for the reasons described in Sect. C (BOYLE et al. 2001; NIKLINSKI et al. 2001; WISTUBA et al. 1999, 2000). The results indicate that chromosome 3p and p16^{INK4a} abnormalities occur before *p53* alterations in NSCLCs. The K-*ras* gene is mutated in a small subset of NSCLCs, preferentially in AdC, and this occurs earlier than *p53* alterations, as in the case of colorectal cancer. There are several candidate tumor-suppressor genes inactivated by LOH on chromosome 3p. The strongest candidate at present is the *RASSF1* gene at chromosome 3p21.3, since the promoter region of this gene is hypermethylated and its expression is downregulated in a considerable fraction of both SCLCs and NSCLCs (DAMMANN et al. 2000). Another candidate is the *FHIT* gene, which was isolated from a common fragile site, FRA3B, at chromosome 3p14.3 (Croce et al. 1999). Expression of Fhit protein is greatly reduced in the majority of lung cancers and this is preferentially observed in tumors with LOH at 3p14. However, mutational inactivation of the *RASSF1* and *FHIT* genes is rare and molecular mechanisms for promoter hyper-methylation of the *RASSF1* gene are unknown. Thus, the possibility that another tumor-suppressor gene is present on this chromosome arm cannot be excluded (Baylin and Herman 2001). In SCLCs, LOH on 3p, 5q and 22q, in addition to p53 and RB1 abnormalities, occurs frequently in any stage of progression (Kawanishi et al. 1997). Thus, it is possible that several tumor-suppressor genes other than *p53* and *RB1* are involved in the formation of aggressive phenotypes typical of SCLC, although target genes on these chromosomes are still unidentified, except for the candidate *RASSF1* gene on chromosome 3p.

Comparative analyses of genetic alterations between primary lung cancers and metastatic lung cancers indicate that further genetic alterations accumulate during progression of lung cancer. LOH studies in primary NSCLCs and brain metastases indicate that LOH on several chromosome arms, including 2q, 9p, 18q, and 22q, occurs late in the progression of NSCLC (Shiseki et al. 1994, 1996). However, the frequencies of genetic alterations in known tumor-suppressor genes on these chromosome arms are much lower than those of LOH in NSCLC. Thus, target genes inactivated by LOH for these chromosome arms are still unknown. This may imply that several unknown tumor-suppressor genes are involved in the formation of more malignant phenotypes in NSCLC. In SCLC, amplification of the *Myc* family genes occurs frequently in tumors with more aggressive phenotypes. Since the presence or absence of metastasis is a critical factor for the prognosis of patients with lung cancer, it is very important to identify genes whose alterations are associated with metastatic potential of lung cancer cells.

Deletion mapping studies have already defined more than 30 regions dispersed on 21 different chromosome arms as candidate tumor-suppressor loci (Kohno and Yokota 1999). Moreover, a recent genome-wide allelotyping study using approximately 400 polymorphic markers distributed at around 10 cM resolution across the human genome has indicated that, on average, approximately 20 chromosomal loci show LOH in individual tumors in both SCLC and NSCLC (Girard et al. 2000). Some "hot spots" for LOH are common for both SCLC and NSCLC, and others are unique for each type. These results indicate that there are still several unidentified tumor-suppressor genes in the human genome, which are involved in the pathogenesis and/or progression of lung cancer. The results also suggest that a set of tumor-suppressor genes for SCLC is partly the same as, but significantly different from, that for NSCLC. Therefore, it is indispensable to identify several additional tumor-suppressor genes in order to fully understand the molecular pathways for lung carcinogenesis (Kuramochi et al. 2001; Xu et al. 2001).

The etiology of lung cancer is strongly tied to cigarette smoking. Thus, several possible genetic targets of tobacco carcinogens have been identified, such as p53, FHIT and p16^{INK4a} (CROCE et al. 1999; SANCHEZ-CESPEDES et al. 2001b; YOON et al. 2001). The frequencies of genetic alterations in these genes are considerably lower in lung cancers in nonsmokers (SANCHEZ-CESPEDES et al. 2001a). These findings indicate that lung cancers in nonsmokers arise through genetic alterations distinct from those in smokers. Since the incidence of AdC in nonsmokers has increased in recent years, and AdC has replaced SqC as the most frequent histological type of lung cancer (CHARLOUX et al. 1997; THUN et al. 1997), it is important to elucidate the molecular pathways to AdC in nonsmokers.

D. Summary

In this review, we show that progression to a more malignant phenotype is a reflection of sequential acquisition of genetic alterations in human neoplasms. Accordingly, malignant neoplasms tend to contain a larger number of genetic alterations than benign lesions. Some neoplasms develop de novo without evidence of less malignant precursor lesions (e.g., primary glioblastomas, small cell lung cancer). However, this refers to the lack of an identifiable precursor lesion but should not be taken to imply that the lesion results from a single-step malignant transformation. There is also increasing evidence that not only genetic changes but also epigenetic changes are important. Promoter methylation is frequently associated with loss of expression of tumor-suppressor genes.

The sequence of genetic alterations appears to be highly cell- and tissue-specific. For example, p53 mutations are gatekeeper lesions in the pathway leading to secondary glioblastomas, gastric cancer and lung cancer, as summarized in this chapter, while they occur at a late stage in colon carcinogenesis (AUGENLICHT 1998; CHO and VOGELSTEIN 1992).

Similar histologic phenotypes may arise through different genetic pathways, as observed in primary and secondary glioblastomas. In such cases, at least one genetic alteration may be responsible for the common histologic phenotype. LOH on 10q25-qter is a common alteration in primary and secondary glioblastomas (FUJISAWA et al. 2000), and has been demonstrated to be associated with acquisition of the glioblastoma phenotype (FUJISAWA et al. 1999).

In contrast, different histologic subtypes may share similar genetic pathways, as is observed in adenocarcinomas and squamous cell carcinomas of the lung. However, more extensive genetic analyses and identification of novel tumor-suppressor genes on chromosomes where LOH is frequent, may lead to the finding of different genetic alterations in these histologic types of lung cancer.

References

Augenlicht LH (1998) The molecular genetics of colonic cancer. Cancer Treat Res 98:351–382

Baylin SB, Herman JG (2001) Promoter hypermethylation–can this change alone ever designate true tumor suppressor gene function? J Natl Cancer Inst 93:664–665

Biernat W, Kleihues P, Yonekawa Y, Ohgaki H (1997a) Amplification and overexpression of MDM2 in primary (de novo) glioblastomas. J Neuropathol Exp Neurol 56:180–185

Biernat W, Tohma Y, Yonekawa Y, Kleihues P, Ohgaki H (1997b) Alterations of cell cycle regulatory genes in primary (de novo) and secondary glioblastomas . Acta Neuropathol 94:303–309

Boyle JO, Lonardo F, Chang JH, Klimstra D, Rusch V, Dmitrovsky E (2001) Multiple high-grade bronchial dysplasia and squamous cell carcinoma: concordant and discordant mutations. Clin Cancer Res 7:259–266

Cairncross JG, Ueki K, Zlatescu MC, Lisle DK, Finkelstein DM, Hammond RR, Silver JS, Stark PC, Macdonald DR, Ino Y, Ramsay DA, Louis DN (1998) Specific genetic predictors of chemotherapeutic response and survival in patients with anaplastic oligodendrogliomas. J Natl Cancer Inst 90:1473–1479

Charloux A, Quoix E, Wolkove N, Small D, Pauli G, Kreisman H (1997) The increasing incidence of lung adenocarcinoma: reality or artifact? A review of the epidemiology of lung adenocarcinoma. Int J Epidemiol 26:14–23

Cho KR, Vogelstein B (1992) Suppressor gene alterations in the colorectal adenoma-carcinoma sequence. J Cell Biochem Suppl 16G: 137–141

Croce CM, Sozzi G, Huebner K (1999) Role of FHIT in human cancer. J Clin Oncol 17:1618–1624

Dammann R, Li C, Yoon JH, Chin PL, Bates S, Pfeifer GP (2000) Epigenetic inactivation of a RAS association domain family protein from the lung tumor suppressor locus 3p21.3. Nat Genet 25:315–319

Di Rocco F, Carroll RS, Zhang J, Black PM (1998) Platelet-derived growth factor and its receptor expression in human oligodendrogliomas. Neurosurgery 42:341–346

Fujimoto J, Yasui W, Tahara H, Tahara E, Kudo Y, Yokozaki H, Tahara E (2000) DNA hypermethylation at the pS2 promoter region is associated with early stage of stomach carcinogenesis. Cancer Lett 149:125–134

Fujisawa H, Kurrer M, Reis RM, Yonekawa Y, Kleihues P, Ohgaki H (1999) Acquisition of the glioblastoma phenotype during astrocytoma progression is associated with LOH on chromosome 10q25-qter. Am J Pathol 155:387–394

Fujisawa H, Reis RM, Nakamura M, Colella S, Yonekawa Y, Kleihues P, Ohgaki H (2000) Loss of heterozygosity on chromosome 10 is more extensive in primary (de novo) than in secondary glioblastomas. Lab Invest 80:65–72

Girard L, Zochbauer-Muller S, Virmani AK, Gazdar AF, Minna JD (2000) Genome-wide allelotyping of lung cancer identifies new regions of allelic loss, differences between small cell lung cancer and non-small cell lung cancer, and loci clustering. Cancer Res 60:4894 –4906

Grunstein M (1997) Histone acetylation in chromatin structure and transcription. Nature 389:349–352

Hamamoto T, Yokozaki H, Semba S, Yasui W, Yunotani S, Miyazaki K, Tahara E (1997) Altered microsatellites in incomplete-type intestinal metaplasia adjacent to primary gastric cancers. J Clin Pathol 50:841–846

Kawanishi M, Kohno T, Otsuka T, Adachi J, Sone S, Noguchi M, Hirohashi S, Yokota J (1997) Allelotype and replication error phenotype of small cell lung carcinoma. Carcinogenesis 18:2057 –2062

Kim NW, Piatyszek MA, Prowse KR, Harley CB, West MD, Ho PL, Coviello GM, Wright WE, Weinrich SL, Shay JW (1994) Specific association of human telomerase activity with immortal cells and cancer. Science 266:2011–2015

Kleihues P, Burger PC, Collins VP, Newcomb EW, Ohgaki H, Cavenee WK (2000) Glioblastoma (2000) In: Pathology and Genetics of Tumours of the Nervous System. Eds. P. Kleihues and K. Cavenee, IARCPress, Lyon, pp 29–39

Kleihues P, Ohgaki H (2000) Phenotype vs genotype in the evolution of astrocytic brain tumors. Toxicol Pathol 28:164–170

Kohno T, Yokota J (1999) How many tumor suppressor genes are involved in human lung carcinogenesis? Carcinogenesis 20:1403–1410

Kuramochi M, Fukuhara H, Nobukuni T, Kanbe T, Maruyama T, Ghosh HP, Pletcher M, Isomura M, Onizuka M, Kitamura T, Sekiya T, Reeves RH, Murakami Y (2001) *TSLC1* is a tumor-suppressor gene in human non-small-cell lung cancer. Nat Genet 27:427–430

Nakamura M, Watanabe T, Klangby U, Asker CE, Wiman KG, Yonekawa Y, Kleihues P, Ohgaki H (2001a) *P14^{Arf}* deletion and methylation in genetic pathways to glioblastomas. Brain Pathol 11:159–168

Nakamura M, Yang F, Fujisawa H, Yonekawa Y, Kleihues P, Ohgaki H (2000) Loss of heterozygosity on chromosome 19 in secondary glioblastomas. J Neuropathol Exp Neurol 59:539–543

Nakamura M, Yonekawa Y, Kleihues P, Ohgaki H (2001b) Promoter hypermethylation of the *RB1* gene in glioblastomas. Lab Invest 81:77–82

Niklinski J, Niklinska W, Chyczewski L, Becker HD, Pluygers E (2001) Molecular genetic abnormalities in premalignant lung lesions: biological and clinical implications. Eur J Cancer Prev 10:213–226

Ohgaki H, Biernat W, Reis R, Hegi M, Kleihues P (2000a) Gliosarcoma. In: Pathology and Genetics of Tumours of the Nervous System. Eds. P. Kleihues and K. Cavenee, IARCPress, Lyon, pp 42–44

Ohgaki H, Peraud A, Nakazato Y, Watanabe K, von Deimling A (2000b) Giant cell glioblastoma. In: Pathology and Genetics of Tumours of the Nervous System. Eds. P. Kleihues and K. Cavenee, IARCPress, Lyon, pp 40–41

Oue N, Motoshita J, Yokozaki H, Hayashi K, Tahara E, Taniyama K, Matsusaki K, Yasui W (2002) Distinct promoter hypermethylation of *p16^{INK4a}*, *CDH1*, and *RAR-beta* in intestinal, diffuse-adherent, and diffuse-scattered-type gastric carcinomas. J Pathol, 198:55–59

Oue N, Shigeishi H, Kuniyasu H, Yokozaki H, Kuraoka K, Ito R, Yasui W (2001) Promoter hypermethylation of *MGMT* is associated with protein loss in gastric carcinoma. Int J Cancer, 93:805–809

Reifenberger G, Kros JM, Burger PC, Louis DN, Collins VP (2000a) Anaplastic oligodendroglioma. In: Pathology and Genetics of Tumours of the Nervous System. Eds. P. Kleihues and K. Cavenee, IARCPress, Lyon, pp 62–64

Reifenberger G, Kros JM, Burger PC, Louis DN, Collins VP (2000b) Oligodendroglioma. In: Pathology and Genetics of Tumours of the Nervous System. Eds. P. Kleihues and K. Cavenee, IARCPress, Lyon, pp 56–61.

Reifenberger J, Reifenberger G, Ichimura K, Schmidt EE, Wechsler W, Collins VP (1996) Epidermal growth factor receptor expression in oligodendroglial tumors. Am J Pathol 149:29–35

Sanchez-Cespedes M, Ahrendt SA, Piantadosi S, Rosell R, Monzo M, Wu L, Westra WH, Yang SC, Jen J, Sidransky D (2001a) Chromosomal alterations in lung adenocarcinoma from smokers and nonsmokers. Cancer Res 61:1309–1313

Sanchez-Cespedes M, Decker PA, Doffek KM, Esteller M, Westra WH, Alawi EA, Herman JG, Demeure MJ, Sidransky D, Ahrendt SA (2001b) Increased loss of chromosome 9p21 but not *p16* inactivation in primary non-small cell lung cancer from smokers. Cancer Res 61:2092–2096

Sano T, Tsujino T, Yoshida K, Nakayama H, Haruma K, Ito H, Nakamura Y, Kajiyama G, Tahara E (1991) Frequent loss of heterozygosity on chromosomes 1q, 5q, and 17p in human gastric carcinomas. Cancer Res 51:2926–2931

Shiseki M, Kohno T, Adachi J, Okazaki T, Otsuka T, Mizoguchi H, Noguchi M, Hirohashi S, Yokota J (1996) Comparative allelotype of early and advanced stage non-small cell lung carcinomas. Genes Chromosomes Cancer 17:71–77

Shiseki M, Kohno T, Nishikawa R, Sameshima Y, Mizoguchi H, Yokota J (1994) Frequent allelic losses on chromosomes 2q, 18q, and 22q in advanced non-small cell lung carcinoma. Cancer Res 54:5643–5648

Smith JS, Perry A, Borell TJ, Lee HK, O'Fallon J, Hosek SM, Kimmel D, Yates A, Burger PC, Scheithauer BW, Jenkins RB (2000a) Alterations of chromosome arms 1p and 19q as predictors of survival in oligodendrogliomas, astrocytomas, and mixed oligoastrocytomas. J Clin Oncol 18:636–645

Smith JS, Wang XY, Qian J, Hosek SM, Scheithauer BW, Jenkins RB, James CD (2000b) Amplification of the platelet-derived growth factor receptor-A (PDGFRA) gene occurs in oligodendrogliomas with grade IV anaplastic features. J Neuropathol Exp Neurol 59:495–503

Suzuki T, Yasui W, Yokozaki H, Naka K, Ishikawa T, Tahara E (1999) Expression of the E2F family in human gastrointestinal carcinomas. Int J Cancer 81:535–538

Suzuki T, Yokozaki H, Kuniyasu H, Hayashi K, Naka K, Ono S, Ishikawa T, Tahara E, Yasui W (2000) Effect of trichostatin A on cell growth and expression of cell cycle- and apoptosis-related molecules in human gastric and oral carcinoma cell lines. Int J Cancer 88:992–997

Tahara E (1993) Molecular mechanism of stomach carcinogenesis. J Cancer Res Clin Oncol 119:265–272

Thun MJ, Lally CA, Flannery JT, Calle EE, Flanders WD, Heath CW, Jr. (1997) Cigarette smoking and changes in the histopathology of lung cancer. J Natl Cancer Inst 89:1580–1586

Tohma Y, Gratas C, Biernat W, Peraud A, Fukuda M, Yonekawa Y, Kleihues P, Ohgaki H (1998) PTEN (MMAC1) mutations are frequent in primary glioblastomas (de novo) but not in secondary glioblastomas. J Neuropathol Exp Neurol 57:684–689

Toyota M, Ahuja N, Suzuki H, Itoh F, Ohe-Toyota M, Imai K, Baylin SB, Issa JP (1999) Aberrant methylation in gastric cancer associated with the CpG island methylator phenotype. Cancer Res 59:5438–5442

Watanabe K, Sato K, Biernat W, Tachibana O, von Ammon K, Ogata N, Yonekawa Y, Kleihues P, Ohgaki H (1997) Incidence and timing of p53 mutations during astrocytoma progression in patients with multiple biopsies. Clin Cancer Res 3:523–530

Watanabe K, Tachibana O, Sato K, Yonekawa Y, Kleihues P, Ohgaki H (1996) Overexpression of the EGF receptor and p53 mutations are mutually exclusive in the evolution of primary and secondary glioblastomas. Brain Pathol 6:217–224

Watanabe T, Nakamura M, Yonekawa Y, Kleihues P, Ohgaki H (2001a) Promoter hypermethylation and homozygous deletion of the $p14^{ARF}$ and $p16^{INK4a}$ genes in oligodendrogliomas. Acta Neuropathol 101:185–189

Watanabe T, Yokoo H, Yokoo M, Yonekawa Y, Kleihues P, Ohgaki H (2001b) Concurrent inactivation of RB1 and TP53 pathways in anaplastic oligodendrogliomas. J Neuropathol Exp Neurol 60:1181–1189

Wistuba II, Behrens C, Milchgrub S, Bryant D, Hung J, Minna JD, Gazdar AF (1999) Sequential molecular abnormalities are involved in the multistage development of squamous cell lung carcinoma. Oncogene 18:643–650

Wistuba II, Berry J, Behrens C, Maitra A, Shivapurkar N, Milchgrub S, Mackay B, Minna JD, Gazdar AF (2000) Molecular changes in the bronchial epithelium of patients with small cell lung cancer. Clin Cancer Res 6:2604–2610

Wistuba II, Gazdar AF, Minna JD (2001) Molecular genetics of small cell lung carcinoma. Semin Oncol 28:3–13

Xu XL, Wu LC, Du F, Davis A, Peyton M, Tomizawa Y, Maitra A, Tomlinson G, Gazdar AF, Weissman BE, Bowcock AM, Baer R, Minna JD (2001) Inactivation of Human SRBC, Located within the 11p15.5-p15.4 Tumor Suppressor Region, in Breast and Lung Cancers. Cancer Res 61:7943–7949

Yasui W, Tahara E, Tahara H, Fujimoto J, Naka K, Nakayama J, Ishikawa F, Ide T, Tahara
    E (1999a) Immunohistochemical detection of human telomerase reverse tran-
    scriptase in normal mucosa and precancerous lesions of the stomach. Jpn J Cancer
    Res 90:589–595
Yasui W, Tahara H, Tahara E, Fujimoto J, Nakayama J, Ishikawa F, Ide T, Tahara E
    (1998) Expression of telomerase catalytic component, telomerase reverse tran-
    scriptase, in human gastric carcinomas. Jpn J Cancer Res 89:1099–1103
Yasui W, Yokozaki H, Fujimoto J, Naka K, Kuniyasu H, Tahara E (2000) Genetic and
    epigenetic alterations in multistep carcinogenesis of the stomach. J Gastroenterol
    35 Suppl 12:111–115
Yasui W, Yokozaki H, Shimamoto F, Tahara H, Tahara E (1999b) Molecular-patholog-
    ical diagnosis of gastrointestinal tissues and its contribution to cancer histopathol-
    ogy. Pathol Int 49:763–774
Yokozaki H, Shitara Y, Fujimoto J, Hiyama T, Yasui W, Tahara E (1999) Alterations of
    p73 preferentially occur in gastric adenocarcinomas with foveolar epithelial phe-
    notype. Int J Cancer 83:192–196
Yokozaki H, Yasui W, Tahara E (2001) Genetic and epigenetic changes in stomach
    cancer. Int Rev Cytol 204:49–95
Yoon JH, Smith LE, Feng Z, Tang M, Lee CS, Pfeifer GP (2001) Methylated CpG din-
    ucleotides are the preferential targets for G-to-T transversion mutations induced
    by benzo[a]pyrene diol epoxide in mammalian cells: similarities with the p53 muta-
    tion spectrum in smoking-associated lung cancers. Cancer Res 61:7110–7117

CHAPTER 4

Signalling Pathways as Targets in Cancer Prevention

M.M. Manson, L.M. Howells, and E.A. Hudson

A. Introduction

Normal cells constantly receive signals from their external and internal environments which determine whether they proliferate, differentiate, arrest cell growth, or undergo apoptosis. Transformed cells either fail to respond or receive inappropriate signals which favor proliferation and avoidance of apoptosis. Thus, it is no coincidence that many oncogenes and tumor suppressor genes are components of signalling pathways. Despite the great variety of cancer cell genotypes, it has been suggested that transformation is a result of a few essential changes in cell physiology which collectively dictate malignant phenotype. These acquired characteristics are self-sufficiency in growth signals, insensitivity to growth inhibitory signals, evasion of apoptosis, limitless replicative potential, sustained angiogenesis, and tissue invasion and metastasis (HANAHAN and WEINBERG 2000). There are now examples, at least from in vitro studies, of chemopreventive agents which influence each of these acquired characteristics, suggesting the possibility of intervention at many stages of the carcinogenic process. As our understanding of the cell circuitry involved increases (HANAHAN and WEINBERG 2000), exciting new opportunities to target deregulated signalling pathways present themselves. Already enormous research effort is being expended on the discovery and design of molecules such as hormone or growth factor antagonists (DERYNCK et al. 2001), inhibitors of growth factor receptor autophosphorylation (LEVITT and KOTY 1999; KIRSCHBAUM and YARDEN 2000; BUNDRED et al. 2001), inhibitors of cyclin dependent kinases (FISCHER and LANE 2000), angiogenesis (BERGERS et al. 1999; DORMOND et al. 2001), and cyclooxygenase 2 (COX2) (LIU et al. 1998; HSU et al. 2000; WILLIAMS et al. 2000;) and modulators of the tumor suppressor p53 (HUPP and LANE 2000; HIETANEN et al. 2000; KOMOROVA and GUDKOV 2001).

Here, several of the major pathways involved in cell proliferation and apoptosis are briefly described, along with examples of chemopreventive agents which have been shown to target them. Further examples of signalling pathways modulated by natural products are summarized in several reviews (AGARWAL 2000; MANSON et al. 2000a,b; PRIMIANO et al. 2001). However, it should be emphasized that, while there are now many examples of agents affecting signal transduction, in most instances the precise targets, particularly for naturally occurring chemopreventive agents, have not yet been identified.

B. MAPK Cascades and Proliferation

The extensively studied and ubiquitous mitogen activated protein kinase (MAPK) cascades are important in regulation of cell proliferation, differentiation, movement, and death (Ichijo 1999; Davis 2000; Schlessinger 2000). Typically they consist of a hierarchy of three kinases (Fig. 1). The family of MAPKs, extracellular signal regulated kinases (ERK1 and 2), c-jun N-terminal kinases (JNKs), and p38, are phosphorylated by MAPK kinases (MEKs or MKKs), which are phosphorylated by MAPK kinase kinases (MAP3Ks). The MAP3Ks are activated by interaction with a family of small GTPases, such as ras or other protein kinases, linking the pathways to cell surface receptors and/or extracellular growth factors or other stimuli. A major consequence of signalling through these pathways is an increase in transcriptional activity, for example via the activator protein 1 (AP-1) complex. Oncogenic ras (one of the most commonly mutated oncogenes in human cancer) will stimulate this pathway continuously without need for external signalling through the receptor. In addition, many tumors exhibit enhanced production

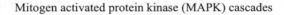

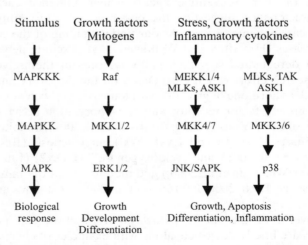

Fig. 1. MAPK cascades. The mitogen activated protein kinases (MAPK) are widely conserved among eukaryotes. They phosphorylate their substrates on serine/threonine and are thereby involved in a wide range of cellular processes. They are phosphorylated by upstream MAPK kinases, which are phosphorylated by MAPKK kinases. These MAP3Ks are activated by interactions with small GTPases and/or other protein kinases, linking the cascade to the cell surface receptor or external stimuli

of growth factors, therefore, clearly, inhibitors of this pathway could have significant chemopreventive action.

C. Cell Cycle Checkpoints

The cell cycle is divided into distinct phases G_0, G_1, S, G_2, and M. Many signalling molecules are involved at each stage and there are checkpoints which help to determine whether the cell is ready to progress to the next phase. The crucial G_1/S checkpoint ensures that the cell is ready to undergo the DNA synthesis (S) phase (Fig. 2). Two kinase complexes cdk4/6-cyclin D and cdk2-cyclin E and a transcription complex containing Rb and E2F are pivotal in this control. During the G_1 phase, Rb binding to the E2F complex inhibits transcription of genes which allow progression through S phase. Phosphorylation of Rb by the two kinase complexes allows dissociation of the Rb repressor

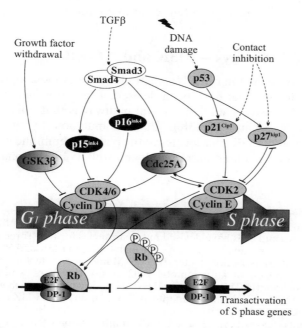

Fig. 2. Signalling components involved in G_1 to S phase transition during the cell cycle. The G_1/S checkpoint controls the passage of cells towards DNA replication. Two complexes, containing cdk4/6-cyclin D and cdk2-cyclin E, along with a transcription complex containing the retinoblastoma tumor suppressor (*Rb*) and the transcription factor E2F, are involved. Many different stimuli exert control over this checkpoint, causing cells to arrest in G_1, including DNA damage, growth factor withdrawal, contact inhibition, senescence, and transforming growth factor β (*TGFβ*). In many instances cell cycle inhibitors, p15, p16, p21, and p27, which prevent the phosphorylation of Rb by cdks, are upregulated. Chemopreventive agents have been shown to modulate the levels or activity of cdk2, cdk4/6, p21, p27, Rb, p53 and cyclins D and E

complex to facilitate transcription of S phase genes which activate the G_1 to S phase switch. However, under many conditions such as damage to DNA, withdrawal of growth factors, contact inhibition, replicative senescence or presence of inhibitory factors such as TGFβ, progression to S phase is inappropriate. Under these conditions induction of members of the INK4 or Kip/Cip families of cell cycle kinase inhibitors helps to retain cells in G_1. TGFβ, while inducing expression of cell cycle inhibitory proteins p15 and p16, also inhibits transcription of cdc25A, a phosphatase which activates the cell cycle kinases. Growth factor withdrawal activates GSK3β which in turn phosphorylates cyclin D leading to its ubiquitination and degradation. Damage to the cell DNA can lead to an increase in the tumor suppressor p53, which in turn leads to an increase in cell cycle inhibitory proteins.

In tumor cells, however, signals which would retain cells in G_0 or G_1 are absent or ignored (MALUMBRES and BARBACID 2001). In cells where inappropriate proliferation is occurring, compounds which can reinstate cell cycle arrest, either in G_1 or during later stages of the cycle, will slow down the growth of tumors, and such arrest will often result in apoptosis.

D. Survival Pathways – PI3K and NF-κB

A key feature of many tumor cells is their ability to evade apoptosis. Numerous strategies for survival have been devised, a few of which are illustrated in Fig. 3. One intensively studied survival pathway is that signalling through phosphoinositide 3-kinase (PI3K). Upon stimulation by growth factors, cytokines or insulin, PI3K translocates to the plasma membrane where it phosphorylates the phospholipid phosphotidylinositol 4,5 bisphosphate (PIP2) to

---

Fig. 3. Signalling pathways involved in cell survival. Survival requires the active inhibition of apoptosis and cells have devised many strategies for this. Three key pathways signal through GFRs, ras and the MAPKs, through GFRs to PI3K and PKB or through the TNFR to the transcription factor NF-κB. Many growth factors and cytokines increase the expression of antiapoptotic Bcl2 family members, which protect the integrity of mitochondria. This prevents release of cytochrome c, which would activate caspase 9, one of the executioners of apoptosis. Stimulation of the PI3K pathway results in activated PKB, which inhibits proapoptotic Bad (another Bcl2 family member), again preventing release of cyt c. It also directly inhibits caspase 9 and additional apoptotic pathways linked to GSK3 and forkhead (*FKHR*) transcription factors. The latter activate the Fas ligand, a death-inducing molecule which binds to cell surface death receptors. TNF induces apoptosis by activating caspases 8 and 9, but can effectively inhibit the process by activating the NF-κB pathway. This transcription factor activates a number of survival genes, including inhibitors of apoptosis (*IAPs*), cyclin D1, COX2 and Bcl-X$_L$. Inhibition of NF-κB can result in an increase in proapoptotic Bax, which is also regulated by p53 following DNA damage. Chemopreventive agents have been shown to inhibit phosphorylation of ERKs and PKB, to inhibit translocation, activation, and DNA-binding of NF-κB, and to upregulate proapoptotic and downregulate antiapoptotic Bcl2 family members

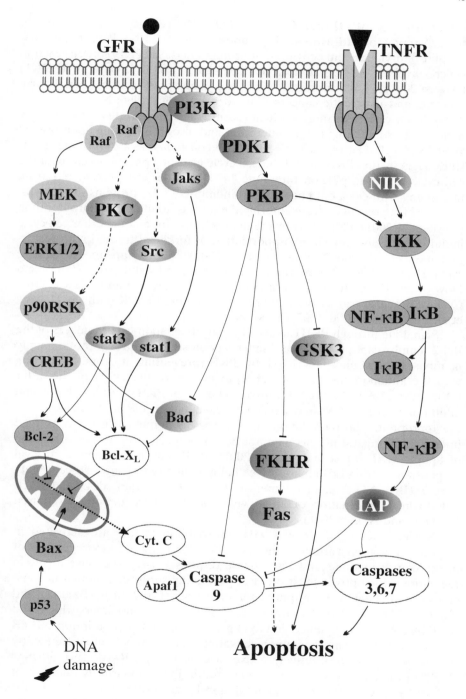

form PtdIns(3,4,5)P3 (PIP3) (Cantrell 2001). This reaction is reversed by the tumor suppressor PtdIns (3,4,5)P3 3-phosphatase (PTEN). PIP3 is essential for phosphorylation and activation of protein kinase B (PKB/Akt), a reaction which involves 3-phosphoinositide-dependent protein kinase 1 (PDK1) (Alessi 2001). PKB, isoforms of which are overexpressed in ovarian, breast, prostate, and pancreatic cancers (Cheng et al. 1992, 1996; Nakatani et al. 1999), has a variety of targets. Much recent research indicates it to be a key molecule in stimulating cell proliferation and also in inhibiting apoptosis by virtually all cell-death-inducing agents (Lawlor and Alessi 2001). One recent study suggests that PKB can inhibit cell cycle arrest by phosphorylation of the cell cycle inhibitor, p21, on threonine 145. This does not prevent p21 from interacting with cdks, but encourages binding to 14-3-3 proteins in the cytoplasm, which prevents it from entering the nucleus to inhibit cell proliferation (Zhou et al. 2001). PKB also downregulates transcription of another cell cycle inhibitor, p27, possibly via phosphorylation of forkhead transcription factors (Medema et al. 2000; Nakamura et al. 2000). It also appears to regulate cyclin D, at the level of transcription, translation, and stabilization (Gille and Downward 1999; Muise-Helmericks et al. 1998; Lawlor and Alessi 2001). Cyclin D1 is also transcriptionally regulated by the MAPK pathway (Lavoie et al. 1996; Weber et al. 1997; Cheng et al. 1998).

Signalling through PKB can also directly affect apoptosis. Members of the Bcl-2 family can promote or hinder apoptosis. The proapoptotic family member Bad is phosphorylated by PKB, preventing it from interacting with the antiapoptotic protein Bcl-X$_L$ to neutralize the effect of the latter (Downward 1999). Another downstream target for PKB phosphorylation and inhibition is caspase 9, caspases being the executioners of apoptosis. However, the appropriate phosphorylation site in caspase 9 in humans is not conserved in evolution, suggesting this may not be a key mechanism in the regulation of apoptosis (Lawlor and Alessi 2001). PKB may also promote survival by phosphorylating IκB kinase α (see below), the breast cancer susceptibility gene 1 (BRCA1), human telomerase, the GTPases Rac1/cdc42 and Raf1, but further confirmation of an in vivo role for these targets is required (Lawlor and Alessi 2001).

Nuclear factor κB (Rel/NF-κB) transcription factors are activated in response to a great variety of signals (Pahl 1999) and are key regulators of inflammatory, immune, and acute phase responses. They also have a role in regulation of apoptosis, most often in promoting survival, although in some cases they appear to be required for induction of apoptosis (Barkett and Gilmore 1999). Rel/NF-κB proteins form hetero- or homodimers which bind to DNA consensus sequences in target genes to regulate transcription. NF-κB usually refers to the most common activating dimer, p50/p65, and is frequently overexpressed or constitutively active in cancer cells (Rayet and Gelinas 1999). In the inactive state it is sequestered in the cytoplasm by inhibitor of κB (IκB α, β or ε). Upon phosphorylation by an upstream complex, IκB is degraded allowing NF-κB to become active and translocate to the nucleus.

The complex which phosphorylates IκB contains two IκB kinases (IKKα and β) and a structural component IKKγ, otherwise known as NF-κB essential modulator (NEMO) (ISRAEL 2000). IKKγ is required for activation of the complex by upstream components including the MAP3Ks – NF-κB inducing kinase (NIK), MEKK1 or TGFβ activated kinase 1 (TAK1). PKB/Akt has also been reported to activate NF-κB, although whether this occurs through interaction with the IKK complex (OZES et al. 1999; ROMASHKOVA and MAKAROV 1999), or through direct phosphorylation of the p65 subunit of NF-κB, without degradation of IκB (SIZEMORE et al. 1999) is still unclear. It may also be possible that IKKs have the potential to autophosphorylate in stimulated cells. Thus, compounds which compromise the ability of NF-κB to prevent apoptosis have the potential to be clinically useful (WADDICK and UCKUN 1999).

E. Cross-Reactivity of Signalling Pathways

Because of the degree of overlap and interdependence of signalling pathways, therapeutic intervention aimed at a single key target could have profound effects on the growth and survival of tumor cells (McCormick 2000). The complex nature of signalling was explored by FAMBROUGH et al. (1999) in a study which examined the relationship between receptor tyrosine kinase (RTK) activated signalling pathways and the transcriptional induction of immediate early genes (IEGs). By screening an array of 6,000 genes this group identified 66 IEGs (including *c-fos, junB, c-jun, IκB, NF-κB*, and *Cox2*) which were induced in fibroblasts via platelet-derived growth factor receptor β (PDGFRβ) signalling. Following ligand binding, RTKs dimerise and autophosphorylation of key tyrosines initiates signalling through diverse pathways, including the Ras GTPase-activating protein, SHP2 phosphatase, phospholipase Cγ, and PI3K pathways. By constructing a mutant receptor lacking five of the critical tyrosine binding sites required to activate these various pathways, FAMBROUGH and co-workers found that 64 of the genes were still inducible, albeit to a lesser extent. Comparison of IEG induction via PDGFRβ with that via fibroblast growth factor receptor 1 showed similar levels of induction of essentially the same set of genes. However, signalling through the much less abundant epidermal growth factor receptor (EGFR) induced only a subset of the genes to lower levels. These results suggested that while the five key tyrosine residues were not absolutely essential for induction of most of the IEGs, nonetheless, together they determined the level of induction. Thus, RTKs appeared to transduce signals to the nucleus by employing multiple signalling pathways that interact to modulate the quantitative level of transcription of a common group of IEGs. This type of strategy is likely to apply to other effector genes.

Many chemopreventive agents, particularly those of dietary origin, appear to have multiple modes of action. *N*-acetyl cysteine, for example, as well as being an antioxidant, is reported to modulate metabolism, DNA repair, effects in mitochondria, gene expression, signal transduction, and cell survival, to have antiangiogenic and anti-inflammatory activity, and to influence immunological effects, cell cycle, invasion, and metastasis (DE FLORA et al. 2001). Given the complex, interactive nature of signal transduction and the fact that oncogenes and tumor suppressors depend on one another for their selective advantage, affecting multiple pathways that intersect and overlap (MCCORMICK 2000), it is perhaps not surprising that a single agent should affect so many aspects of cellular biochemistry. However, responses differ from one cell type to another and may also be significantly more specific in vivo compared to culture conditions, so that listing all the possible mechanisms of action of a particular compound may give an unrealistic picture of its true physiological effects. Equally, assuming that a mechanism identified in one cell type is generic may also be misleading. A further complication is the fact that for many chemopreventive agents mechanism of action is dose-dependent, even to the extent that opposite effects may be achieved at high and low dose.

From the cell's point of view, another factor to bear in mind is that oncogenic signalling may differ significantly from normal signalling. For instance, ras plays a minor role in normal signalling to PI3K from growth factor receptors, but oncogenic ras is a potent activator of PI3K. Thus, a molecule such as ras could contribute to tumor development through multiple pathways that change as tumors develop (MCCORMICK 2000). This allows for the possibility that a chemopreventive agent may behave differently in tumor versus normal cells, inducing apoptosis in one but not the other for example.

F. Chemoprevention by Growth Arrest or Apoptosis

Tumor development requires abnormal cells to proliferate and resist apoptosis. Signal transduction pathways that mediate the activation of transcription factors, caspases, or cell cycle control proteins are all likely targets for prevention (KONG et al.1999). A number of signalling pathways, including those outlined above, involving growth factor receptors and MAPKs, PI3K, or NF-κB, are involved in these processes, offering many possible targets for chemopreventive activity.

While tamoxifen and its analogues have proved useful in the treatment and prevention of estrogen receptor (ER) positive breast cancer (WISEMAN 1994; JORDAN 2001), PARDEE and his colleagues have turned their attention to ER negative tumors. They proposed that a major pathway of cell cycle progression and resistance to apoptosis in ER negative breast cancer is the activation of NF-κB by epidermal growth factor stimulation (BISWAS et al. 2000). In breast cell lines, signalling from the EGFR appeared to be dependent on PI3K and protein kinase C (PKC), as demonstrated by the inhibitors LY294002 and the indolocarbazole Go6796 respectively. NF-κB was shown to transactivate cyclin D1, leading to increased phosphorylation of Rb and enhanced proliferation. In a subsequent in vivo study by the same group in which an ER-ve mouse mammary epithelial tumor line was implanted into syngeneic mice, local administration of Go9796 (an inhibitor of PKCα and β) led to extensive regression of tumors. In addition, the tumorigenic potential of the implanted cell line was lost upon expression of dominant negative mutants of IKK β, which also blocked overexpression of cyclin D1 (Biswas et al. 2001). They concluded that NF-κB is a potential target for therapy of ER-negative breast cancers overexpressing EGFR family receptors.

Sulforaphane, derived from cruciferous vegetables, is an effective chemo-preventive agent in a number of animal models, including dimethyl benzanthracene-induced preneoplastic lesions in mouse mammary glands (Gerhauser et al. 1997), rat mammary tumorigenesis (Zhang et al. 1994), and azoxymethane-induced aberrant crypt foci in rat colon (Chung et al. 2000). A recent study by Heiss et al. (2001) suggests that anti-inflammatory mechanisms involving inhibition of NF-κB transactivation may account in part for sul-foraphane's anticancer activity. While it did not inhibit degradation of IκB or translocation of NF-κB to the nucleus, it did inhibit DNA binding by the transcription factor, resulting in a downregulation of lipopolysaccharide-stimulated nitric oxide synthase (iNOS), Cox2, and tumor necrosis factor α expression in RAW macrophages. The suggested mechanism by which sulforaphane targeted NF-κB in this study was by modulation of intracellular redox conditions via dithiocarbamoylation of essential thiol groups involved in activation of the transcription factor.

Another chemopreventive agent, also derived from green vegetables and already in clinical trial for breast cancer because of its effect on estrogen metabolism, is indole-3-carbinol (I3C) (Bradlow et al. 1994). This compound inhibits growth of a number of different cell types including the nontumori-genic HBL100 and tumorigenic MDA-MB-468 breast cell lines, but the latter is much more sensitive. Because the MDA line lacks the tumor suppressor PTEN, it contains higher basal levels of phosphorylated PKB. Inhibition of this phosphorylation by I3C only in the tumor cells correlated with an inhibition of DNA binding by NF-κB without affecting the translocation of p65 to the nucleus or the ability of IKK to phosphorylate IκB. This in turn correlated with induction of apoptosis in the MDA-MB-468 cell line (Howells et al. 2001).

In a study by Cover et al. (1998), in MCF7 and MDA-MB 231 breast tumor cell lines, I3C was found to cause arrest in the G_1 phase of the cell cycle. This was attributed to inhibition of cdk6 expression, which resulted in a lack of phosphorylation of Rb. An increase in the cell cycle inhibitors p21 and p27 was also observed. Inhibition of cdk6 was subsequently shown to result from disruption of Sp1 transcription factor interactions in the promoter region of the gene (Cram et al. 2001). A number of other potential chemopreventive mechanisms have been described in breast cells for I3C. These include nega-tive regulation of estrogen receptor α signalling by downregulating estrogen responsive genes and upregulating the tumor suppressor BRCA1 (Meng et al. 2000a); inhibition of adhesion, invasion, and spreading with concomitant increase in expression of PTEN and E-cadherin, a regulator of adhesion

(Meng et al. 2000b,c); and facilitation of apoptosis in ErbB2-expressing cells by inducing expression and translocation of the proapoptotic Bcl-2 family member Bax to the mitochondria, while also downregulating antiapoptotic Bcl-2 (Rahman et al. 2000).

Epigallocatechin-3-gallate, a major component of green tea, has been shown to inhibit proliferation of a range of cell types. In breast tumor cells it caused G_1 arrest and was shown to inhibit phosphorylation of Rb, inhibit activity of cdk2 and cdk4, decrease expression of cyclins D and E, and increase levels of p21, p27, and p53 (Liang et al. 1999).

Nonsteroidal anti-inflammatory agents, which inhibit the activity of cyclooxygenases, have been found to lower mortality from colorectal cancer. Celecoxib, which was designed as a specific inhibitor of COX2, was found to inhibit the growth of colon cancer cell lines and to induce apoptosis, independently of COX2 (Williams et al. 2000). However, the same group found, encouragingly, that attenuation of HCA-7 xenografts in nude mice occurred at much lower concentrations of celecoxib in plasma than had been used in cell culture, with no in vivo effect on normal gut cells. Celecoxib also induced apoptosis in prostate cells, an effect which was selective for tumor lines and correlated with COX2 levels (Hsu et al. 2000). In this study, the ability of celecoxib to block phosphorylation of PKB was considered to contribute to apoptosis, since overexpression of constitutively active PKB protected cells from apoptosis. However, the exact mechanism of action was unclear since in vivo celecoxib did not adversely affect PI3K, nor could okadaic acid, a phosphatase 2A inhibitor, rescue the inhibition of PKB phosphorylation.

There is extensive evidence that another chemopreventive agent, curcumin, a major component of turmeric, may be effective against colon cancer. Amongst its mechanisms of action, curcumin inhibited transcriptional activation by NF-κB by inhibiting phosphorylation and degradation of IκB and translocation of the p65 subunit to the nucleus (Singh and Aggarwal 1995; Bierhaus et al. 1997; Chan et al. 1998; Kumar et al. 1998). It appeared to inhibit the ability of the IKK complex to phosphorylate IκB (Jobin et al. 1999; Plummer et al.1999). Curcumin also inhibits signalling through the EGFR family (Korutla et al. 1995; Hong et al. 1999; Manson et al. 2000a), MAPK pathway involving JNK (Chen and Tan 1998; Manson et al. 2000a) and transcription via AP-1 (Huang et al. 1991; Bierhaus et al. 1997).

G. Conclusions

The last few years have seen an explosion of data relating to potential mechanisms of action of chemopreventive agents, particularly with respect to ways in which they might suppress tumor growth where initiation has already taken place. The examples cited here, both of signalling molecules and of putative agents, merely give a hint of what is possible. Perhaps one of the most striking properties of dietary agents in particular is just how potent and wide-ranging is their ability to alter cell biochemistry. However, in light of experiments such as that described in Sect. E by FAMBROUGH et al.(1999), it appears that what at first sight seems to be a rather specific ligand-receptor interaction can result in multiple downstream consequences. Because of the complexity of cross-talk and the high degree of redundancy in signalling networks, the higher up a signalling pathway an agent can exert its influence, the more wide-ranging should be its effects. On the other hand, a compound which interacts very specifically with the active site or binding site of a component close to the transcriptional end of the pathway might be expected to have a much more selective or even invisible effect on the fate of the cell. It seems from available evidence that many dietary chemopreventive agents belong to the former category, although as already noted, they may demonstrate more promiscuous effects in culture than in vivo.

Abbreviations

AP-1	activator protein 1
Apaf1	apoptotic protease activating factor 1
ASK1	apoptosis signal regulating kinase 1
Bad	Bcl2-antagonist of cell death
Bax	Bcl2-associated X protein
Bcl2	B-cell CLL/lymphoma 2
BRCA1	breast cancer susceptibility gene 1
cdc25A	cell division cycle 25A
cdk	cyclin dependent kinase
cip1	cyclin dependent kinase inhibitor, p21
COX2	cyclooxygenase 2
CREB	cAMP responsive element binding protein
DP-1	transcription factor dimerization partner-1
ErbB2	v-erb-b2 avian erythroblastic leukemia viral oncogene homolog 2, (EGFR family member)
EGFR	epidermal growth factor receptor
ER	estrogen receptor
ERK	extracellular signal regulated kinase
FKHR	forkhead transcription factor
GFR	growth factor receptor
GSK3	glycogen synthase kinase 3
IAP	inhibitor of apoptosis
I3C	indole-3-carbinol
IEG	immediate early gene
IκB	inhibitor of kappa B
IKK	IκB kinase
INK4	inhibitor of cdk4
JAK	Janus kinase

JNK	c-jun N terminal kinase
Kip1	cyclin-dependent kinase inhibitor, p27
MAPK	mitogen-activated protein kinase
MEKK (MKKK, MAP3K)	MAP kinase kinase kinase
MKK (MEK)	MAP kinase kinase
MLK	mixed lineage kinase
NEMO	NF-κB essential modulator
NF-κB	nuclear factor κB
NIK	NF-κB inducing kinase
iNOS	inducible nitric oxide synthase
PDK1	3-phosphoinositide-dependent protein kinase 1
PI3K	phosphoinositide 3-kinase
PIP2/ PIP3	phosphotidylinositol 4,5 bisphosphate/3,4,5 triphosphate
PDGFR	platelet-derived growth factor receptor
PKB	protein kinase B
PKC	protein kinase C
PTEN	phosphatase and tensin homolog deleted on chromosome ten
Rb	retinoblastoma tumor suppressor
p90RSK	ribosomal s6 kinase
RTK	receptor tyrosine kinase
SAPK	stress-activated protein kinase
Smad	homolog of mothers against decapentaplegic, (*Drosophila*)
STAT	signal transducer and activator of transcription
TAK	TGFβ-activated kinase
TGFβ	transforming growth factor β
TNFR	tumor necrosis factor receptor

References

Agarwal R (2000) Cell signalling and regulators of cell cycle as molecular targets for prostate cancer prevention by dietary agents. Biochem Pharmacol 6:1051–1059

Alessi DR (2001) Discovery of PDK1, one of the missing links in insulin signal transduction. Biochem Soc Trans 29:1–14

Barkett M, Gilmore TD (1999) Control of apoptosis by Rel/NF-κB transcription factors. Oncogene 18:6910–6924

Bergers G, Javaherian K, Lo K-M, Folkman J, Hanahan D (1999) Effects of angiogenesis in multistage carcinogenesis in mice. Science 284:808–812

Bierhaus A, Zhang Y, Quehenberger P, Luther T, Haase M, Muller M, Mackman N, Ziegler R, Nawroth PP (1997) The dietary pigment curcumin reduces endothelial tissue factor gene by inhibiting binding of AP-1 to the DNA and activation of NF-κB. Thrombosis Haemostasis 77:772–782

Biswas DK, Cruz AP, Gansberger E, Pardee AB (2000) Epidermal growth factor-induced nuclear factor κB activation: a major pathway of cell cycle progression in estrogen-receptor negative breast cancer cells. Proc Natl Acad Sci USA 97: 8542–8547

Biswas DK, Dai SC, Cruz A, Weiser B, Graner E, Pardee AB (2001) The nuclear factor kappa B (NF-κB): a potential therapeutic target for estrogen receptor negative breast cancers. Proc Natl Acad Sci USA 98:10386–10391

Bradlow HL, Michnovicz JJ, Halsper M, Miller DG, Wong GY, Osborne MP (1994) Long term responses of women to I3C or a high fibre diet. Cancer Epidemiol Biomarkers Prev 3:591–595

Bundred NJ, Chan K, Anderson NG (2001) Studies of epidermal growth factor inhibition in breast cancer. Endocr Relat Cancer 8:183–189

Cantrell D (2001) Phosphoinositide 3-kinase signalling pathways. J Cell Sci 114: 1439–1445

Chan MM-Y, Huang HI, Fenton MR, Fong D (1998) In vivo inhibition of nitric oxide synthase gene expression by curcumin, a cancer preventive natural product with antiinflammatory properties. Biochem Pharmacol 55:1955–1962

Chen Y-R, Tan T-H (1998) Inhibition of c-jun N-terminal kinase (JNK) signalling pathway by curcumin. Oncogene 17:173–178

Cheng JQ, Godwin AK, Bellacosa A, Taguchi T, Franke TF, Hamilton YC, Tsichlis PN Testa JR (1992) Akt2, a putative oncogene encoding a member of a sub family of protein-serine/threonine kinases, is amplified in ovarian cancer. Proc Natl Acad Sci USA 89:9267–9271

Cheng JQ, Ruggeri B, Klein WM, Sonoda G, Altomare DA, Watson DK, Testa JR (1996) Amplification of Akt2 in human pancreatic cells and inhibition of Akt2 expression and tumorigenicity by antisense RNA. Proc Natl Acad Sci USA 93:3636–3641

Cheng M, Sexl V, Sherr CJ, Roussel MF (1998) Assembly of cyclin D-dependent kinase and titration of p27^{kip1} regulated by mitogen-activated protein kinase kinase (MEK1) Proc Natl Acad Sci USA 95:1091–1096

Cover CM, Hsieh SJ, Tran SH, Hallden G, Kim GS, Bjeldanes LF, Firestone GL (1998) Indole-3-carbinol inhibits the expression of cyclin-dependent kinase-6 and induces a G_1 cell cycle arrest of human breast cancer cells independent of estrogen receptor signalling. J Biol Chem 273:3838–3847

Cram EJ, Liu BD, Bjeldanes LF and Firestone GL (2001) Indole-3-carbinol inhibits CDK6 expression in human MCF-7 breast cancer cells by disrupting Sp1 transcription factor interactions with a composite element in the CDK6 gene promoter. J Biol Chem 276:22332–22340

Chung FL, Conaway CC, Rao CV, Reddy BS (2000) Chemoprevention of colonic aberrant crypt foci in Fischer rats by sulforaphane and phenethyl isothiocyanate. Carcinogenesis 21:2287–2291

Davis RJ (2000) Signal transduction by the JNK group of MAP kinases. Cell 103: 239–252

De Flora S, Izzotti A, D'Agostini F, Balansky RM (2001) Mechanisms of N-acetylcysteine in the prevention of DNA damage and cancer, with special reference to smoking related end-points. Carcinogenesis 22:999–1013

Derynck R, Akhurst R, Balmain A (2001) TGFβ signalling in tumor suppression and cancer progression. Nature Genetics 29:117–129

Dormond O, Foletti A, Paroz C, Ruegg C, (2001) NSAIDs inhibit αVb3 integrin-mediated and Cdc42/Rac-dependent endothelial-cell spreading, migration and angiogenesis. Nature Med 7:1041–1047

Downward J (1999) How Bad phosphorylation is good for survival. Nature Cell Biol 1:E33–E35

Fambrough D, McClure K, Kaslauskas A, Lander E (1999) Diverse signalling pathways activated by growth factor receptors induce broadly overlapping, rather than independent sets of genes. Cell 97:727–741

Fischer PM, Lane DP (2000) Inhibitors of cyclin-dependent kinases as anticancer therapeutics. Curr Med Chem 7:1213–1245

Gerhauser C, You M, Lui J, Moriaty RM, Hawthorne M, Mehta RG, Moon RC, Pezzuto JM (1997) Cancer chemopreventive potential of sulforamate, a novel analogue of sulforaphane that induces phase 2 drug-metabolizing enzymes. Cancer Res 57: 272–278

Gille H, Downward J (1999) Multiple ras effector pathways contribute to G_1 cell cycle progression. J Biol Chem 274:22033–22040

Hanahan D, Weinberg RA (2000) The hallmarks of cancer. Cell 100:57–70

Heiss E, Herhaus C, Klimo K, Bartsch H, Gerhauser C (2001) Nuclear factor κB is a molecular target for sulforaphane-mediated antiinflammatory mechanisms. J Biol Chem 276:32008–32015

Hietanen S, Lain S, Krausz E, Blattner C, Lane DP (2000) Activation of p53 in cervical carcinoma cells by small molecules. Proc Natl Acad Sci USA 97:8501–8506

Hong R-L, Spohn WH, Hung M-C (1999) Curcumin inhibits tyrosine kinase activity of $p185^{neu}$ and also depletes $p185^{neu1}$. Clin Cancer Res 5:1884–1891

Howells L, Gallacher-Horley B, Hudson EA, Manson MM (2001) Indole-3-carbinol inhibits PKB/Akt phosphorylation in a human breast tumor cell line. Proc Am Assoc Cancer Res 42:312

Hsu A-L, Ching T-T, Wang D-S, Song X, Rangnekar VM, Chen C-S (2000) The cyclooxygenase-2 inhibitor celecoxib induces apoptosis by blocking Akt activation in human prostate cancer cells independently of Bcl-2. J Biol Chem 275: 11397–11403

Huang T-S, Lee S-C, Lin J-K (1991) Suppression of c-Jun/AP-1 activation by an inhibitor of tumor promotion in mouse fibroblast cells. Proc Natl Acad Sci 88: 5292–5296

Hupp TR, Lane DP, Ball KL (2000) Strategies for manipulating the p53 pathway in the treatment of human cancer. Biochem J 352:1–17

Ichijo H (1999) From receptors to stress-activated MAP kinases. Oncogene 18: 6087–6093

Israel A (2000) The IKK complex: an integrator of all signals that activate NF-κB? Trends Cell Biol 10:129–133

Jobin C, Bradham CA, Russo MP, Juma B, Narula AS, Brenner DA, Sartor RB (1999) Curcumin blocks cytokine-mediated NF-κB activation and proinflammatory gene expression by inhibiting inhibitory factor I-κB kinase activity. J Immunol 163: 3474–3483

Jordan VC (2001) Selective estrogen receptor modulation: a personal perspective. Cancer Res 61:5683–5687

Kirschbaum MH, Yarden Y (2000) The ErbB/HER family of receptor tyrosine kinases: a potential target for chemoprevention of epithelial neoplasms. J Cell Biochem 34:52–60

Komarova EA, Gudkov AV (2001) Chemoprotection from p53-dependent apoptosis: potential clinical applications of p53 inhibitors. Biochem Pharmacol 62:657–667

Kong AN, Mandlekar S, Yu R, Lei W, Fasanmande A (1999) Pharmacodynamics and toxicodynamics of drug action: signalling in cell survival and cell death. Pharm Res 16:790–798

Korutla L, Cheung JY, Mendelsohn J, Kumar R (1995) Inhibition of ligand-induced activation of epidermal growth factor receptor tyrosine phosphorylation by curcumin. Carcinogenesis 16:1741–1745

Kumar A, Dhawan S, Hardegen NJ, Aggarwal BB (1998) Curcumin (diferuloylmethane) inhibition of tumor necrosis factor (TNF)-mediated adhesion of monocytes to endothelial cells by suppression of cell surface expression of adhesion molecules and of nuclear factor-κB activation. Biochem Pharmacol 55:775–783

Liang Y-C, Lin-Shiau S-Y, Chen C-F, Lin J-K (1999) Inhibition of cyclin-dependent kinases 2 and 4 activities as well as induction of Cdk inhibitors p21 and p27 during growth arrest of human breast carcinoma cells by (-)-epigallocatechin-3-gallate. J Cell Biochem 75:1–12

Lawlor MA, Alessi, DR (2001) PKB/Akt: a key mediator of cell proliferation, survival and insulin response? J Cell Science 114:2903–2910

Lavoie JN, L'Allemain G, Brunet A, Mueller R, Pouyssegur J (1996) Cyclin D1 expression is regulated positively by the p42/p44 ^{MAPK} and negatively by the p38/HOG^{MAPK} pathway. J Biol Chem 271:20608–20616

Levitt ML, Koty PP (1999) Tyrosine kinase inhibitors in preclinical development. Invest New Drugs 17:213–226

Liu K-H, Yao S, Kirschenbaum A, Levine AC (1998) NS398, a selective cyclooxygenase-2 inhibitor, induces apoptosis and down regulates Bcl-2 expression in LNCaP cells. Cancer Res 58; 4245–4249

McCormick F (2000) Signalling networks that cause cancer. Trends Cell Biol 9:M53–M56

Malumbres M, Barbacid M (2001) To cycle or not to cycle: a critical decision in cancer. Nature Rev Cancer 1:222–231

Manson MM, Holloway KA, Howells LM, Hudson EA, Plummer SM, Squires MS, Prigent SA (2000) Modulation of signal-transduction pathways by chemopreventive agents. Biochem Soc Trans 28:7–12

Manson MM, Gescher A, Hudson EA, Plummer SM, Squires MS, Prigent SA (2000) Blocking and suppressing mechanisms of chemoprevention by dietary constituents. Toxicol Letters 112–113:499–505

Medema RH, Kops GJ, Bos JL, Burgering BM (2000) AFX-like Forkhead transcription factors mediate cell cycle regulation by Ras and PKB through p27^{kip1}. Nature 404:782–787

Meng Q, Yuan F, Goldberg ID, Rosen EM, Auborn K, Fan S (2000a) Indole-3-carbinol is a negative regulator of estrogen receptor α signalling in human tumor cells, J Nutr 130:2927–2931

Meng Q, Goldberg ID, Rosen EM, Fan S (2000b) Inhibitory effect of indole-3-carbinol on invasion and migration in human breast cancer cells. Breast Cancer Res Treat 63:147–152

Meng Q, Qi M, Chen D-Z, Yuan R, Goldberg ID, Rosen EM, Auborn K, Fan S (2000c) Suppression of breast cancer invasion and migration by indole-3-carbinol:associated with upregulation of BRCA1 and E-cadherin/catenin complexes, J Mol Med 78:155–165

Muise-Helmericks RC, Grimes HL, Bellacosa A, Malstrom SE, Tsichlis PN, Rosen N (1998) Cyclin D expression is controlled post-transcriptionally via a phosphatidylinositol 3-kinase/Akt-dependent pathway. J Biol Chem 273:29864–29872

Nakamura N, Ramaswamy S, Vazquez F, Signoretti S, Loda M, Sellers WR (2000) Forkhead transcription factors are critical effectors of cell death and cell cycle arrest downstream of PTEN. Mol Cell Biol 20:8969–8982

Nakatani K, Thompson DA, Barthel A, Sakaue H, Liu W, Weigel RJ, Roth RA (1999) Up-regulation of Akt3 in estrogen receptor-deficient breast cancers and androgen-independent prostate cancer cell lines. J Biol Chem 274:21528–21532

Ozes ON, Mayo LD, Gustin JA, Pfeffer SR, Pfeffer LM, Donner DB (1999) NF-κB activation by tumor necrosis factor requires the Akt serine-threonine kinase. Nature 401:82–85

Pahl HL (1999) Activators and target genes of Rel/NF-κB transcription factors. Oncogene 18:6853–6866

Plummer SM, Holloway KA, Manson MM, Munks RJL, Kaptein A, Farrow S, Howells L (1999) Inhibition of cyclo-oxygenase 2 expression in colon cells by the chemopreventive agent curcumin involves inhibition of NF-κB activation via the NIK/IKK signalling complex. Oncogene 18:6013–6020

Primiano T, Yu R, Kong A-N T (2001) Signal transduction events elicited by natural products that function as cancer chemopreventive agents. Pharm Biol 39:83–107

Rahman KMW, Aranha O, Glazyrin A, Chinni SR, Sarkar FH (2000) Translocation of Bax to mitochondria induces apoptoic cell death in indole-3-carbinol (I3C) treated breast cancer cells. Oncogene 19:5764–5771

Rayet B, Gelinas C (1999) Aberrant rel/nf-κb genes and activity in human cancer. Oncogene 18:6938–6947

Romashkova JA, Makarov SS (1999) NF-κB is a target of Akt in antiapoptotic PDGF signalling. Nature 401:86–90

Singh S, Aggarwal BB, (1995) Activation of transcription factor NF-κB is suppressed by curcumin (diferulolylmethane). J Biol Chem 270:24995–25000

Sizemore N, Leung S, Stark GR (1999) Activation of phosphotidylinositol-3-kinase in response to interleukin-1 leads to phosphorylation and activation of the NF-κB p65/Rel A subunit. Mol Cell Biol 19:4798–4805

Schlessinger J (2000) Cell signalling by receptor tyrosine kinases. Cell 103:211–225

Waddick KG, Uckun FM (1999) Innovative treatment programs against cancer. II Nuclear factor κB (NF-κB) as a molecular target. Biochem Pharmacol 57:9–17

Weber JD, Hu W, Jefcoat SC, Raben DM, Baldassare JJ (1997) Ras-stimulated extracellular signal-related kinase 1 and RhoA activities coordinate platelet-derived growth factor-induced G1 progression through the independent regulation of cyclin D1 and p27kip1. J Biol Chem 272:32966–32971

Williams CS, Watson AJM, Sheng H, Helou R, Shao J, DuBois RN (2000) Celecoxib prevents tumor growth in vivo without toxicity to normal gut: lack of correlation between in vitro and in vivo models. Cancer Res 60:6045–6051

Wiseman H (1994) Tamoxifen: molecular basis of use in cancer treatment and prevention. John Wiley and Sons, Chichester, UK

Zhang Y, Kensler TW, Cho CG, Posner GH, Talalay P (1994) Anticarcinogenic activities of sulforaphane and structurally related synthetic norbornyl isothiocyanates. Proc Natl Acad Sci USA 91:3147–3150

Zhou BP, LiaoY, Xia W, Spohn B, Lee MH, Hung MC (2001) Cytoplasmic localization of p21Cip1/WAF1 by Akt-induced phosphorylation in HER-2/neu-overexpressing cells. Nature Cell Biol 3:245–252

CHAPTER 5
TP53 in Carcinogenesis and Cancer Prevention

E. GORMALLY and P. HAINAUT

A. Introduction

Since its discovery in 1979, the tumor suppressor gene TP53 has been one of the main focuses of cancer research. This gene is altered at high frequency in most types of human cancers and studies on TP53-deficient mice have shown that lack of p53 protein function predisposes to early cancers (DONEHOWER et al. 1992). In humans, inheritance of a TP53 mutation is the molecular basis of Li-Fraumeni syndrome (LFS), a rare syndrome predisposing to multiple early cancers (MALKIN et al. 1990; SRIVASTAVA et al. 1990). Extensive experimental evidences support that p53 is essential in the control of genetic stability of cells exposed to genotoxic stress. These observations have led to identify TP53 as "the ultimate tumor suppressor gene" (OREN 1992), or "the only thing that stands between us and early death by cancer" (LANE 1992).

The p53 protein lies at the crossroad of many signaling pathways controlling DNA repair and cell proliferation, survival and differentiation. This functional diversity is considered as the main reason why TP53 is mutated in many types of cancers. The functional consequences of TP53 mutation may differ according to the nature and position of the mutation, the cell type and the timing of occurrence in cancer progression. In several instances tumor specific mutation patterns have been identified. In cancers of the skin, liver and lung, it has been shown that mutation patterns could be read as the "signatures" of particular environmental insults.

During the past 10 years studies on TP53 mutations have concentrated on carcinogen fingerprint patterns (molecular epidemiology) or on diagnosis and prognosis of cancer (molecular pathology). These aspects are discussed in several recent reviews (HAINAUT and HOLLSTEIN 2000; HUSSAIN et al. 2001b). However, the TP53 gene and its product may also represent interesting endpoints in cancer prevention. First, the analysis of TP53 mutation patterns provides clues on significant mutagens (or mutagenic mechanisms). This knowledge may help to design preventive strategies to limit the impact of these mutagens. Second, it is possible to detect the presence of TP53 mutations in the tissues of individuals at high cancer risk (AGUILAR et al. 1993; BARRETT et al. 1999; HUSSAIN et al. 2001a; MANDARD et al. 2000). Monitoring of mutations may thus be useful for evaluating preventive strategies. Third, the p53 protein may be a target for pharmacological preventive intervention.

Indeed, p53 is an important regulator of homeostasis under genotoxic stress. "Boosting" its function using chemicals may be an effective way to increase the protection of cells against such stresses.

In this chapter, we summarize characteristics of TP53 relevant for its potential in cancer prevention. We also discuss current hypotheses on the significance of TP53 mutations, as well as on the pharmacological modulation of p53 protein functions.

B. TP53: Structure and Functions

I. TP53 Is a Member of a Multi-Gene Family

The TP53 gene (OMIM 191170) is located on chromosome 17p13 and contains 11 exons in a 20-kilobase locus. The coding sequence is well-conserved in vertebrates but sequences found in invertebrates show only a distant resemblance with mammalian TP53 (SOUSSI and MAY 1996). Two related genes have been recently identified on chromosome 1p36 (TP73, OMIM 601990) and on chromosome 3p28 (TP63, OMIM 603273). They both encode proteins with high structural homology to p53. All three family members oligomerize and are sequence-specific transcription factors (Fig. 1; LEVRERO et al. 2000). The three proteins bind as tetramer to DNA sequences containing repeats of the consensus $RRRC^A/_T{}^A/_TGYYY$ (where R is a purine and Y a pyrimidine) (EL DEIRY et al. 1993). Thus, they share the capacity to regulate the transcription of a common set of genes, suggesting functional redundancies. However, the three genes differ by their pattern of expression. Whereas TP53 is ubiquitously expressed as a single mRNA, the expression of TP73 and TP63 is tissue-specific and is regulated by alternative splicing, resulting in multiple isoforms with different N- or C-terminal regions. Furthermore, inactivation of these genes in mouse results in very distinct phenotypes. TP53-deficient mice develop almost normally but are prone to multiple, early cancers (DONEHOWER et al. 1992). TP73-deficient mice do not show increased tumorigenesis but have a complex pattern of neurosensorial and inflammatory defects (YANG et al. 2000). TP63-deficient mice show limb malformations and impaired development of squamous epithelia (YANG et al. 1999).

In human cancers, only TP53 is mutated at a significant frequency. Most of the mutations are scattered in the central domain, with "hotspots" at codons 175, 245, 248, 282, and 273. Recent evidence indicates that TP63 is amplified in some squamous carcinomas. But the mechanism by which amplification contributes to cancer is poorly understood. TP73 is located in a chromosomal region often deleted in neuroblastomas, but absence of mutations in the remaining allele indicates that TP73 is not a neuroblastoma gene (KAGHAD et al. 1997).

II. The p53 Protein Is Responsive to Many Stress Signals

Most of p53 regulation in normal cells occurs at the posttranslational level. The protein is permanently produced in most tissues, but does not accumulate

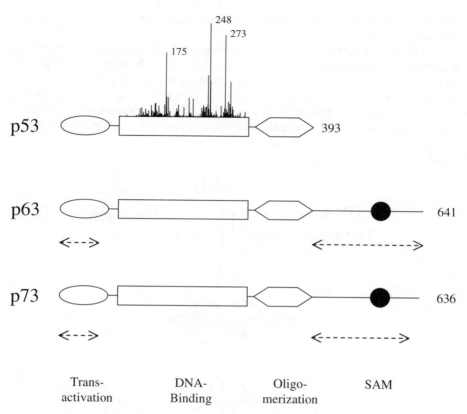

Fig. 1. Protein structure of p53, p63 and p73. The three proteins have a transactivation domain (*oval*), a DNA binding domain (*rectangle*) and an oligomerization domain (*diamond*). P63 and p73 have a sterile alpha motif (*SAM; black circle*), a protein–protein interaction domain usually found in proteins involved in development (LEVRERO 2000). Only the longest isoforms of p63 and p73 are shown. *Dashed arrows* indicate regions affected by alternative splicing. The number of amino acids contained in each protein is shown on the *right*. The TP53 mutation spectrum mostly spanning the DNA binding domain is depicted on top of p53. The length of bars is proportional to the number of mutations. Major "Hotspot" codons are indicated

due to its rapid degradation (within minutes) by the proteasome. The key regulator of p53 protein stability is mdm2. The MDM2 gene ("Mouse double minutes") is the human homologue of a gene amplified in aberrant mouse chromosomes (MOMAND et al. 1992). Mdm2 binds p53 in the N-terminus, mediates its export from the nucleus into the cytoplasm, where it triggers degradation by the proteasome (BOTTGER et al. 1997; HAUPT et al. 1997; KUBBUTAT et al. 1997), with a turnover of only a few minutes in most normal cells. Interestingly, MDM2 is a transcriptional target of p53 (JUVEN 1992). After p53 activation, levels of mdm2 protein increase within the cell, helping to bring p53 back to basal levels. These two proteins are thus interconnected by a feedback loop which determines the extent of p53 accumulation in the nucleus (Lane and Hall 1997).

Activation of p53 requires the temporary interruption of this feedback loop for p53 to escape mdm2-mediated degradation. Three main mechanisms can activate p53 through different signaling pathways (Fig. 2; Pluquet and Hainaut 2001). The extent and duration of p53 activation differ, depending on the exact nature of the inducing agent. The best known mechanism is DNA-damage signaling. Many physical and chemical genotoxic agents (UV, irradia-

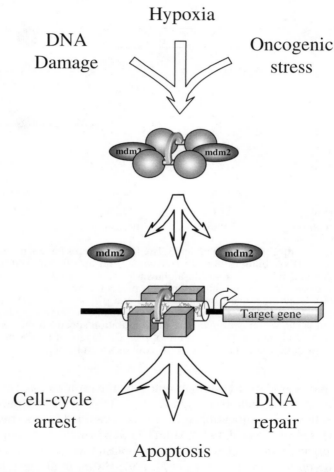

Fig. 2. Activation of p53. Inactive p53 (*sphere*) is shown as a tetramer bound to two molecules of mdm2. After activation by various stress mechanisms (*upper part*), the p53 tetramer undergoes conformational changes (*cubes*) and escapes mdm2 mediated degradation. After binding to DNA, p53 regulates several biological processes (*lower part*)

tion, carcinogens, chemotherapeutic drugs, and oxidative stress) can turn p53 from a "latent" to an "active" state. This process requires the phosphorylation of p53 by several kinases, including the cell-cycle regulatory kinase chk2, and atm, the product of the *Ataxia-Telangiectasia* gene, a complex syndrome characterized by radiosensitivity. Both kinases phosphorylate p53 in the mdm2-binding domain, inducing the dissociation of the p53-mdm2 complex (APPELLA and ANDERSON 2000). The second mechanism is oncogenic stress signaling (KAMIJO et al. 1997; POMERANTZ et al. 1998). Oncogenic stresses arise when hyperproliferative signals are constitutively activated within the cell, for example after mutations of genes involved in the RAS/MAPKinase cascade, or of the β Catenin/MYC pathway. The central effector in this pathway is p14^{arf}, the alternative product of a locus (9p31) that also encodes the cell-cycle inhibitory protein p16 (STONE et al. 1995). When activated, p14^{arf} binds and neutralizes mdm2 allowing p53 to accumulate (KAMIJO et al. 1998; TAO and LEVINE 1999; ZHANG et al. 1998). A less well-described, third mechanism involves nongenotoxic stresses such as hypoxia (GRAEBER et al. 1994, 1996). Solid tumors with limited oxygen supply may undergo growth suppression when p53 is activated by low oxygen pressure. Thus the p53 response to hypoxia might represent an important limiting factor for tumor growth.

III. P53 Controls Several Antiproliferative Responses

After activation, p53 coordinates antiproliferative responses, including effects on cell-cycle progression, apoptosis, and DNA repair (Fig. 2). In turn, these cellular responses have an impact on senescence, differentiation, angiogenesis, and, possibly, on development (OREN 1999; OREN and ROTTER 1999; PRIVES and HALL 1999). Two biochemical properties are essential for p53 activity: sequence-specific DNA binding (and transcriptional regulation) and protein–protein complex formation. Within the wide range of biological responses, only a selected subset of targets are affected, depending on the activating agent, the dose, and the cell type (Table 1). P53 is involved at multiple levels in each of these processes. In cell-cycle, p53 exerts negative effects at all phases. In apoptosis, although p53 is not part of the apoptotic machinery, it regulates several of the initiating pathways. The role of p53 in DNA repair is less understood and results, at least in part, in the elimination of unrepaired cells by cell cycle arrest or apoptosis. Nevertheless, p53 also plays direct roles in DNA repair (LIU and KULESZ-MARTIN 2001).

What are the biological consequences of p53 activation? In cultured cell lines, p53 induces either cell death, or transient cell cycle arrest that facilitates proper DNA repair. The p53 protein thus appears to act as a referee for the decision between life and death. In primary cells and in normal tissues, however, these responses may both contribute to the permanent elimination of damaged cells from the pool of cells with replicative potential. Indeed, arrested primary cells do not appear to reenter cell cycle after p53 activation (LINKE et al. 1997). In vivo, such arrested cells may undergo senescence or

Table 1. p53 transcriptional and protein targets. Examples of genes transcriptionally regulated by p53 (left hand side) and proteins interacting with p53 (right hand side)

	Transcriptional regulation	References	Protein–protein interaction	References
Cell Cycle	p21[waf-1]	EL DEIRY et al. 1993	RPA	DUTTA et al. 1993
	14–3–3σ	HERMEKING et al. 1997		
	GADD45	KASTAN et al. 1992		
Apoptosis	BAX–1	MIYASHITA et al. 1994		
	APO1/Fas	OWEN-SCHAUB et al. 1995		
	Killer/DR5	SHEIKH et al. 1998		
	AIPI	ODA et al. 2000		
	PIG3	POLYAK et al. 1997		
DNA repair	MSH2	SCHERER et al. 2000	PCNA	SHIVAKUMAR et al. 1995
	0⁶MGMT	HARRIS et al. 1996	XRCC2/3	WANG et al. 1996
			p33[ING1]	CHEUNG et al. 2001

enter terminal differentiation (WILSON et al. 1998). Thus, both responses should be seen as complementary rather than antagonistic.

C. Alteration of TP53 in Carcinogenesis

TP53 is often affected by mutations in most types of human cancers (Fig. 3). The highest mutation prevalence is observed in esophageal cancers (50%). In contrast, cancers of the cervix rarely contain TP53 mutations (5%). This is due to the fact that the E6 antigen of human papillomavirus, an important etiological agent in cervical cancer, binds to wild-type p53 and induces its degradation, thus bypassing the need for mutation. Over 70% of mutations are missense and fall within the central portion of the gene, encoding the DNA-binding domain (Fig. 1; HAINAUT and HOLLSTEIN 2000). These mutations prevent correct binding of the protein to DNA sequences, thus abrogating transcriptional activation. It is not clear whether they also abrogate the capacity of p53 to bind to other proteins. Loss of heterozygosity at the TP53 locus is also common in human cancer, but the wild-type allele is not systematically lost in cancer cells that carry mutant TP53.

Cells with mutant TP53 are allowed to proliferate in conditions where normal cells undergo stress-induced growth suppression. The multi-functional

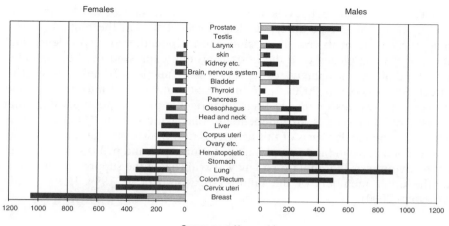

Fig. 3. Cancer cases and the estimated number of TP53 mutations worldwide. The worldwide estimates of cancer cases (in thousands) are shown as histograms (*dark gray areas*). Within each histogram bar cancers estimated to carry a TP53 mutation are shown as *light gray areas*. Data from Globocan 2000 (PARKIN 2000) (cancer estimates) and IARC TP53 mutation database (TP53 mutation estimates; http://www.iarc.fr/p53)

character of p53 may explain why mutations occur as early events in some cancers and as late events in others (GUIMARAES and HAINAUT, 2002). For example, TP53 mutation seems to occur as a very early event (sometimes detected in exposed, normal tissues) in cancers of the lung and of the head and neck. In these cancers, tumor cells generally emerge from portions of the epithelium exposed to exogenous damaging agents such as tobacco smoke. Early loss of p53 function may thus favor the escape of cells on the path to tumorigenesis. In other cancers, however, TP53 mutation is not detectable until late stages, for example in colon or breast cancers. This observation suggests that these tumors develop despite the presence of a wild-type TP53, but that loss of p53 function provides a selective advantage at a later stage of tumor development.

The paradigm for tumor suppressor genes (KNUDSON 1971) implies that mutation results in loss of function, which in due course is reflected by the disappearance of the protein from cancer cells. In the case of TP53, however, many missense mutations have a stabilizing effect and lead to the accumulation of mutant protein in the nucleus of cancer cells, allowing the detection of "mutant" p53 by immunohistochemistry in cancer tissues (BRAMBILLA and BRAMBILLA 1997). While there is a fairly good correlation between the two phenomena, many mutations do not result in protein accumulation (e.g., nonsense mutations, insertions, and deletions) and wild-type p53 accumulation may also occur as a consequence of exposure to stress. Thus, care should be exercised in the use of immunohistochemistry as a surrogate for mutation analysis.

The presence of high levels of mutant p53 in cancer cells, and the frequent retention of a wild-type allele, has led to speculate that the mutant protein may play a role of its own in carcinogenesis. Indeed, there is evidence that mutant p53 complexes with the normal protein expressed by the remaining wild-type allele and inactivates its suppressor functions (dominant-negative effect; BLAGOSKLONNY 2000). Introduction of mutant TP53 into p53-deficient cancer cells can also enhance their tumorigenic phenotype, suggesting that mutant p53 behaves as an independent, oncogenic protein (DITTMER et al. 1993). The molecular basis of this activity is not known, but the recent finding that mutant p53 can bind to and inactivate some p63 and p73 isoforms has led to the hypothesis that mutant p53 may also abrogate the suppressor functions of the other members of the family (BLANDINO et al. 1999; LOHRUM and VOUSDEN 2000).

D. TP53 and Cancer Prevention

A large body of literature deals with the significance of TP53 as a biomarker in clinical studies (HOLLSTEIN et al. 1991; SIDRANSKY and HOLLSTEIN 1996). Intensive investigations have been performed to evaluate whether TP53 mutation might be a predictor of bad prognosis in molecular pathology. Overall, these studies have shown that, if TP53 mutation often correlates with aggressive tumors, the presence of a mutation is generally not an independent predictor of malignancy. Many studies have also addressed the question of whether mutant TP53 may determine poor response of tumor cells to cytotoxic therapies (LOWE et al. 1993; LOWE 1995). Indeed, in vitro, p53 is a crucial effector of apoptosis in response to drugs used in cancer therapy. However, studies in patients do not confirm that wild-type TP53 predicts a better response to treatment.

In contrast with clinical studies, the significance of TP53 for cancer prevention has not been fully assessed. Four distinct aspects may be considered. First, TP53 polymorphisms may be associated with susceptibility to cancer. Second, TP53 mutations may be seen as molecular "signatures" of cancer-causing agents in the human population and designing strategies to counteract their effects is important. Third, TP53 mutations might be detectable in surrogate tissues such as sputum, urine, or plasma, sometimes ahead of the appearance of a detectable tumor. Fourth, the p53 protein may be an interesting endpoint for pharmacological intervention aimed at preventing cancer. These four aspects are developed in the paragraphs below.

I. TP53 Polymorphisms and Risk of Cancer

Table 2 provides a list of 14 known polymorphisms in the human TP53 gene. Four are in the coding sequence and only two, at positions 47 and 72, entail a change in amino acids (IARC TP53 database,

Table 2. List of TP53 polymorphism from the LARC TP53 database. The 14 polymorphisms found in the exons and introns of TP53 are described. Only two polymorphisms in exon 4 at codon 47 and 72 result in amino-acid substitutions. Data on allelic ratio are available only for a few polymorphisms. For details, see IARC TP53 mutation database

Polymorphisms	Codon/nucleotide	Nucleotide variants	Codon variants	Allelic ratio
Exon 4	47	CCG to TCG	Pro to Ser	<0.015
Exon 4	72	CGC to CCC	Arg to Pro	0.2–0.6
Exon 2	21	GAC to GAT	None	?
Exon 4	36	CCG to CCA	None	0.04
Exon 6	213	CGA to CGG	None	<0.11
Intron 1	8545	T to A	None	?
Intron 1	8703	$(AAAAT)_n$	None	?
Intron 1	?	HAEIII RFLP	None	?
Intron 2	11827	G to C	None	?
Intron 3	11951	+16 bp	None	?
Intron 6	13484	G to A	None	?
Intron 7	14201	T to G	None	?
Intron 7	14181	C to T	None	?
Intron 9	14766	T to C	None	?

http://www.iarc.fr/P53). The codon 47 polymorphism (proline to serine) is extremely rare (allele ratio: less than 0.015) and has only been reported so far in the African population (BECKMAN et al. 1994; WESTON et al. 1992; WESTON et al. 1994). Its association with disease is unknown. The codon 72 polymorphism (arginine, R to proline, P) is widespread and is detected in all populations with different allelic ratios. In Western populations, the most frequent allele is R72 (0.6–0.8). However, in East Asian and in African populations, P72 is the major allele. This polymorphism shows a north to south cline, with a high proportion of P72 near the equator, falling to less than 20% near the poles (BECKMAN et al. 1994). It is not known whether this geographic variation is associated with cancer susceptibility.

In 1998, STOREY et al. have shown that the R72 p53 protein variant showed greater in vitro sensitivity than the P72 variant to degradation by the E6 protein of human papilloma viruses (HPV; STOREY et al. 1998). They speculated that this increased sensitivity may predispose R72 homozygotes to cancer of the cervix. This observation launched a flurry of studies aimed at assessing the significance of the codon 72 polymorphisms for the risk of HPV-associated cancers. However, to date, most of the publications based on well-defined, epidemiological series have not confirmed the existence of an increased risk of HPV-associated cancer (KLUG et al. 2001). Several studies have suggested associations between codon 72 polymorphism and risk of other cancers, including cancer of the lung (FAN et al. 2000; JIN et al. 1995), and squamous cell carcinoma of the esophagus in a Taiwanese population (LEE et al. 2000).

Recent experiments provide a new basis for a functional difference between the R72 and P72 variants. In tumors with TP53 mutations, the mutant p53 often binds to other proteins, including the homologous protein p73. Mutant forms of the R72 variant bind better to p73 than mutant forms of the P72 variant. Moreover, the R72 allele is preferentially mutated and retained in squamous cell tumors arising in R72/P72 heterozygotes. Thus, a polymorphic residue may affect mutant p53 behavior by controlling inactivation of p53 family members (Marin et al. 2000).

II. TP53 Mutations as "Signatures" for Carcinogenic Exposures

In several cancers, particular mutation patterns may be seen as molecular "signatures" of environmental carcinogens. Clear examples of such signatures are observed in nonmelanoma skin cancers (CC to TT transitions, UV damage), in lung cancers (G to T transversions, damage by polycyclic aromatic hydrocarbons of tobacco smoke) and in liver cancers (G to T transversions, damage by aflatoxins). However, the majority of TP53 mutations detected in cancer are primarily the result of endogenous mutation mechanisms, such as the spontaneous deamination of 5'-methylcytosine to generate thymine (C to T mutations) within poly-pyrimidine repeats (CpG sites) (Wink et al. 1991; Yang et al. 1996).

1. Sunlight UVs and Nonmelanoma Skin Cancers

DNA damage by UV induces p53 stabilization and activation, with increased expression of the target protein p21^{waf-1}. In skin cancers, TP53 is often mutated and about 10% of these mutations are double CC to TT transitions. This type of mutation also represents 4.2% of all TP53 mutations in cancers of the lip, but are virtually absent in cancers of internal organs (IARC TP53 database). CC to TT transitions are consequences of inefficient DNA repair of a frequent photoproduct, the cyclobutane pyrimidine dimer. Over half of the CC to TT transitions in TP53 are within CpG sequences. This distribution may be explained by the fact that absorption of near-UV by 5-methylcytosine (which is often present at CpG sites) is 5- to 10-fold higher than by cytosine (Tommasi et al. 1997). Moreover, repair of UV-induced lesions in vitro is exceptionally slow at codons 177, 196, and 278 of TP53, corresponding to mutational "hotspots" in human skin cancers (Tornaletti and Pfeifer 1994). In skin tumors of individuals with *Xeroderma pigmentosum*, a complex DNA repair-deficiency syndrome with increased susceptibility to skin cancer, CC to TT transitions represent almost 50% of all mutations (Dumaz et al. 1993). Thus, CC to TT transitions may be seen as molecular "signatures" of DNA damage by UVB.

CC to TT transitions are also detectable in normal, UV exposed skin cells in both humans (Nakazawa et al. 1994) and mice (Ananthaswamy et al. 1997). In mice experimentally exposed to UV, CC to TT mutations are found in the skin up to 6 months before the appearance of skin tumors. Applying sunscreens before irradiation reduces both the occurrence of skin cancers and the early detection of TP53 mutations (ANANTHASWAMY et al. 1999). Thus, inhibition of TP53 mutations is a useful early endpoint for photoprotection in ultraviolet carcinogenesis.

2. Tobacco Smoke and Lung Cancer

TP53 mutations are frequent in cancers associated with tobacco smoking, and the mutation load increases with the extent of tobacco consumption in cancers of the lung, of the head and neck and of the esophagus (squamous cell carcinoma) (HAINAUT and PFEIFER 2001). Cigarette smoking is responsible for 90% of lung cancers worldwide. The pattern of mutations in TP53 shows a high prevalence of G to T transversions (30%) in lung cancers of smokers, but are less frequent in lung cancer of nonsmokers (11%) or in cancers not directly related to smoking such as brain, breast, or colon cancers (average of 10%). Moreover, in vitro, these G to T mutations cluster at 5 codons (157, 158, 248, 245, and 273) that are sites of DNA adducts formation by metabolites of polycyclic aromatic hydrocarbons such as benzo(a)pyrene (DENISSENKO et al. 1996; SMITH et al. 2000). Mutations at codon 157 and 158, in particular, are rare in cancers other than lung cancers of smokers, and may be seen as tobacco-specific mutations (HAINAUT and PFEIFER 2001). Recent studies have shown that exposure of primary bronchial cells to benzo(a)pyrene in vitro induces mutations at codon 157. The same mutation is detectable in the nontumoral lung tissue of smokers with lung cancers (HUSSAIN et al. 2001a), making them potentially useful as early biomarkers in prevention studies against tobacco-induced tumors. However, these mutations seem to be specific to lung cancers and are not as frequent in other smoking-related cancers such as oral, esophageal or bladder cancers.

3. Aflatoxin B1 and Liver Cancer (Hepatocellular Carcinoma)

About 80% of hepatocellular carcinomas (HCC) arise in developing countries, with high incidences of chronic infection by hepatitis viruses B or C. In these regions, staple diets often contain high levels of aflatoxin B1, a mycotoxin contaminant. In regions of sub-Saharan Africa and of Eastern Asia where both risk factors are present, HCC has often a characteristic TP53 mutation at codon 249 (AGG to AGT). This mutation is rarely observed in HCC in Western countries (JACKSON and GROOPMAN 1999; MONTESANO et al. 1997; SMELA et al. 2001).

Metabolites of AFB1 can bind to codon 249 in TP53 and induce this particular type of mutation. However, AFB1 can similarly damage other sites in TP53, and the reasons why only codon 249 mutation is observed in HCC are still not understood (DENISSENKO et al. 1998). It has been proposed that selection of codon 249 may result from cooperative effects between AFB1 and the

HBx protein of HBV, which may modulate cell survival and DNA repair (SOHN et al. 2000).

Given the role of AFB1 in liver carcinogenesis, chemopreventive approaches have been developed to limit hepatic DNA damage by this agent (WILD and HALL 2000). The drug oltipraz decreases the metabolization of AFB1 by CYP1A2 and increases its detoxification by GST in liver cells. This drug is currently used in chemoprevention trials in an area of high incidence of HCC in China.

4. C to T Transitions at CpG Sites and Cancers Linked to Inflammatory Diseases

C to T transition is the most frequent type of mutation in all human cancers. About 50% of these mutations fall at 6 codons corresponding to a CpG site, codons 175, 213, 245, 248, 273, and 282 (IARC TP53 database). This type of mutation may arise without the direct intervention of environmental carcinogens. In the human genome, 3%–5% of all cytosines at CpG sites are methylated in the 5′ position (HOLLIDAY and GRIGG 1993). Spontaneous deamination of 5′-methylcytosine (5mC) generates thymine, creating a mismatch that, if not taken over by repair mechanisms, gives rise to a C to T transition (ROBERTSON and JONES 2000; YANG et al. 1995). Spontaneous deamination of 5mC is enhanced by exposure to oxyradicals and, in particular, to nitric oxide (NO; MURATA et al. 1997; WINK et al. 1991). The prevalence of C to T transition is thus high in cancers that arise in the context of an inflammatory lesion, for example colorectal cancers (arising in the context of ulcerative colitis), esophageal adenocarcinomas (often arising in the context of Barrett's mucosa) and stomach cancers (often associated with chronic infection by *Helicobacter pylori*; AMBS et al. 1999). In patients with colorectal cancers, there is a correlation between levels of expression of the inducible form of nitric oxide synthase (NOS2), and CpG transitions in the tumor. Thus, this type of mutation might be efficiently prevented by agents inhibiting the production of NO (WATANABE et al. 2000).

III. Detection of TP53 Mutations in Surrogate Tissues

Low levels of mutant DNA may be found in surrogate tissues in subjects who do not show clinically detectable lesions. For example, mutant TP53 has been detected in DNA extracted from plasma, sputum, urine, bile, or feces (Tables 3, 4; SIDRANSKY 1997). Obtaining these surrogate tissues does not entail invasive and painful interventions for the subject. Surrogate material may represent a flexible alternative to tumor biopsy in large-scale, follow-up programs. Intensive research is currently aimed at identifying TP53 mutations (as well as other mutations in cancer genes) in surrogate material ahead of tumor development.

Table 3. Detection of TP53 mutations in different surrogate materials. The proportion of patients with a TP53 mutation in the tumor and in the corresponding surrogate material is shown. The concordance is the percentage of tumors and corresponding surrogate materials that had a TP53 mutation

Surrogate	Cancer	Surrogate	Percentage	References
Bladder wash	Bladder	6/13	46	VET et al. 1996
Bile	Cholangiosarcoma	4/12	33	ITOI et al. 1999
Sputum	Lung	30/54	55.5	WANG et al. 2001
Plasma	Lung	13/35	37	GONZALES et al. 2000
Plasma	Liver	19/53	36	KIRK et al. 2000

Table 4. Concordance between TP53 mutation in surrogate and in tumor tissues. The number of surrogate material carrying a TP53 mutation is indicated over the total number of tested samples

Cancer	Surrogate	Mutations in				References
		Tumor[a]	Surrogate[b]	n	Concordance (%)	
Bladder	Bladder wash	38	33	49	84	PRESCOTT et al. 2001
Bladder	Urine sediments	46	29	28	61	XU et al. 1996
Colon	Feces	44	28	25	64	EGUCHI et al. 1996
Colon	Feces	59	59	51	100	DONG et al. 2001
NSCLC	Sputum	13	7	15	50	MAO et al. 1994
Lung	Bronchoalveolar lavage fluid	56	22	50	39	ARHENDT et al. 1999
Breast	Plasma	36.5	24	126	65	SHAO et al. 2000
HCC	Plasma	55	30	20	55	JACKSON et al. 2001
Colon	Serum	30	21	33	70	HIBI et al. 1998

[a] Percentage of tumors with a TP53 mutation.
[b] Percentage of surrogate with a TP53 mutation.
n, Number of cases.

Bladder cancer provides a good example of the interest of surrogate material for detection of TP53 mutations. Most bladder cancers are superficial transitional cell carcinoma (TCC), which are treatable by local intervention, but reoccur and progress towards an invasive phenotype in 15%–20% of the patients (PRESCOTT et al. 2001). TP53 mutation occur in over 30% of bladder cancers and are often associated with invasiveness (Vet et al. 1996). Presence of a TP53 mutation has been observed in bladder washes of patients treated for superficial TCC on average 8 months before recurrence (Vet et al. 1996). Screening for TP53 mutations in bladder washes of patients treated for TCC may help in the management of relapse.

Studies by Sidransky and collaborators have shown that detection of oncogene mutations in sputum could precede diagnosis of lung cancers. TP53 mutations or KRAS were identified in 10 of 15 (66%) normal subjects who were later diagnosed with adenocarcinoma of the lung. In eight out of these ten patients, the mutation found in sputum was identical to the one later detected in cancer tissues (Mao et al. 1994).

Plasma has long been recognized as containing small amounts of free DNA fragments. In normal, healthy subjects, levels of plasma DNA average 13 ng/ml, but levels up to 1,000 times higher can be detected in some cancer patients. How this DNA is released in plasma is still a matter of conjecture (Anker and Stroun 2000). In the past 5 years, a number of studies have demonstrated the presence of tumor-specific mutant DNA in the plasma of patients with overt cancers (reviewed in Anker and Stroun 2000). The molecular alterations detected in plasma DNA encompasses point mutations (KRAS, TP53), promoter hypermethylation (CDKN2a, O^{6}MGMT, DAPkinase, GSTP1), microsatellite instability and loss of heterozygosity (Anker and Stroun 2000; Chen et al. 1999; Esteller et al. 1999; Mulcahy et al. 1998).

We have analyzed TP53 mutations in plasma DNA in subjects from a case-control study of HCC in The Gambia, a region of high incidence in West Africa (Kirk et al. 2000). We have found that codon 249 mutation (see Sect. II.3) was detectable in 36% of cancer patients, 15% of individuals with liver cirrhosis, and 6% of healthy controls (Kirk et al. 2000). In cancer patients, presence of codon 249 mutation in the plasma correlates with the presence of this mutant in the majority of cancer cells (Jackson et al. 2001). In individuals with liver cirrhosis, detection of codon 249 mutation in the plasma may be a marker for the presence of asymptomatic cancer (e.g., diffuse groups of liver cancer cells that escape detection by ultrasonography). In healthy controls, however, the presence of codon 249 mutant DNA in the plasma may reflect high exposure to dietary AFB1 and thus behaves as a marker for identification of individuals at high risk of developing HCC. Further studies are in progress to address these questions.

Overall, only a subgroup of cancer patients with TP53 mutations have detectable anti-p53 antibodies (20%–40%) and there is no clear correlation between the presence of antibodies, clinical status or prognosis (Soussi 2000). In one interesting case, antibodies have been detected in an individual with chronic bronchitis several months ahead of cancer development (Lubin et al. 1995). This example shows that, in some instances, presence of anti-p53 antibodies in noncancer subjects may be an early marker of cancer development.

IV. The p53 Protein as a Target for Pharmacological Intervention

In recent years, several approaches have been tested to modulate p53 function in normal or cancer cells. Their effects depend upon the target cell, the TP53 mutation status and the clinical context (Fig. 4). Several approaches aim at "refolding" mutant p53 into wild-type form for therapeutic effects (FOSTER et al. 1999). In addition, wild-type p53 is in itself a potential target for pharmacological intervention aimed at "boosting" the cell's capacity to resist genotoxic damage. In tumor cells with wild-type p53, this activation may enhance the response to therapy. In contrast, in normal cells, enhancing p53 function may activate a physiological, "guardian of the genome" effect contributing to protection against toxic effects of cancer treatment. The same rationale can be extended to chemoprevention: drugs that activate p53 may facilitate either the elimination or the repair of cells under attack by DNA-damaging agents. In this paragraph, we summarize the biochemical basis of two recent approaches to modulate wild-type p53 protein function.

1. Stabilization of p53 by Disruption of Interactions with mdm2

Disruption of p53-mdm2 interactions leads to the accumulation of active, p53 in the nucleus of normal cells. In 1997, LANE and collaborators have designed

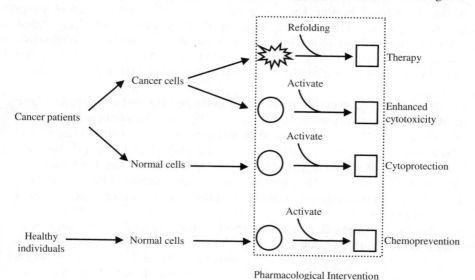

Pharmacological Intervention

Fig. 4. Rationale for the modulation of p53 function by pharmacological intervention. Different types of pharmacological interventions are proposed according to the status of the cells and p53 (dashed box). Mutant, inactive and active p53 are shown as *star*, *circle* and *square*, respectively. In cancer cells some mutant p53 forms could be refolded to their active form (*Therapy*) or normal p53 could be activated (*Enhanced Cytotoxicity*). In normal cells of cancer patients, inactive p53 could be activated (*Cytoprotection*). In normal cells of individuals at risk of developing cancer, p53 could be activated (*Chemoprevention*)

a synthetic mdm2-binding protein expressing a short segment of p53 within the active site of bacterial thioredoxin, which provides a stable scaffold for optimal peptide presentation (BOTTGER et al. 1997). When introduced into cells expressing wild-type p53, this synthetic protein neutralized mdm2 and caused a striking accumulation of endogenous p53. This accumulation was followed by activation of a p53-responsive reporter gene and by cell cycle arrest, mimicking the effects seen in these cells after exposure to UV or ionizing radiation. Microinjection of a monoclonal antibody to the p53-binding site of mdm2 achieved similar effects. Although the conditions for using this peptide for treatment or prevention remain to be established, these results demonstrate that it is possible to activate p53 and induce a protective, cell-cycle arrest response without causing DNA damage.

2. Pharmacological Control of p53 Protein Activity

The p53 protein shows an intrinsic sensitivity to oxidation-reduction conditions (MEPLAN et al. 2000b). This sensitivity is mediated by reactive cysteines located within the DNA-binding domain, three of them being involved in the binding of a zinc atom (HAINAUT and MILNER 1993). In vitro, the p53 protein requires reduction by thiol antioxidants for binding to specific DNA and activating gene transcription. There is good evidence that redox changes affect the folding of the DNA-binding domain of the protein. Many factors that alter the intracellular redox balance, such as strong oxidative or nitrosative stress, or exposure to heavy metals, inactivate wild-type p53 by turning the protein into a conformation similar to that of mutant p53 (HAINAUT and MANN 2001).

In vivo, several proteins are involved in the redox regulation of p53. These proteins include thioredoxin (UENO et al. 1999), metallothioneins (MEPLAN et al. 2000a) and Ref-1, a protein that interacts with the C-terminus of p53 (GAIDDON et al. 1999; JAYARAMAN and PRIVES 1995). Ref-1 is a dual-function enzyme with roles in redox regulation and DNA repair. Ref-1 may act as a functional link between DNA-damage recognition and modulation of p53 conformation. This pathway may represent a promising target for drugs aimed at modulating p53.

Another pathway that activates p53 involves polyamines (KRAMER et al. 1998). These short molecules are essential regulators of cell growth through multiple mechanisms, which are still poorly understood. Normal cell growth is accompanied by variations in polyamines biosynthesis, largely mediated by the rate-limiting enzyme ornithine decarboxylase (ODC). Difluoromethylornithine (DFMO), a suicide inhibitor of ODC, is an experimental cancer prevention agent that is evaluated in a number of current human cancer prevention trials (CARBONE et al. 2001; MEYSKENS JR. and GERNER 1999). Inhibition of polyamine metabolism has been proposed as an approach for the chemoprevention of colorectal cancer (WALLACE and CASLAKE 2001).

Synthetic polyamine analogues activate p53 function in cultured cell lines (KRAMER et al. 1999). Similar effects are observed after inhibition of ODC by DFMO (LI et al. 2001). The mechanisms by which polyamines activate p53 are still poorly understood. Recent evidence from our group indicates that polyamines may control p53 conformation and accumulation. We have studied the effects of a phosphoaminothiol, amifostine (WR2721), a drug currently used in the clinics as a radio/chemo protective drug (CAPIZZI 1999a,b). WR2721 is a prodrug that is converted to the active aminothiol compound WR1065 by alkaline phosphatase. A considerable amount of preclinical work suggests that this drug acts as an antimutagen in vitro and protects normal cells against the adverse effects of irradiation and of several anticancer drugs without inducing tumor protection (CAPIZZI 1999b; KURBACHER and MALLMANN 1998).

We have shown that amifostine activates p53, and induces a p53 dependent cell-cycle arrest in cultured cells (NORTH et al. 2000). This may be relevant for the protective activities of amifostine, since arrested cells appear to be more resistant than proliferating cells to DNA-damaging agents (NORTH et al. 2000). Treatment by the drug does not generate detectable DNA damage, does not perturb redox homeostasis, and does not induce p53 phosphorylation on serines located within the mdm2 binding site. Further studies have identified the c-Jun N-terminal Kinase (JNK) as a mediator of p53 activation in response to amifostine (Pluquet et al., submitted). The inactive form of JNK binds p53 in a domain distinct from mdm2 and induces p53 degradation in a pathway parallel to the one mediated by mdm2 (FUCHS et al. 1998). Activation of JNK disrupts the p53-JNK complex, resulting in the accumulation and activation of p53. Recent studies have shown that activation of JNK may be a common response to disruption of polyamine biosynthesis (RAY et al. 1999). Together, these results indicate the existence of a new, DNA damage independent pathway for p53 induction, involving disruption of endogenous polyamines as a key signal and JNK as the main effector. This pathway may be responsible for essential aspects of the chemopreventive effects of polyamines.

E. Conclusions and Perspectives

Within the 20 years following its discovery in 1979, TP53 has become the most studied cancer gene, with over 23,000 publications referenced in Medline. Despite the amount of information, the impact of TP53 in chemoprevention is still a matter of conjecture. The most promising area for immediate impact is in the field of molecular epidemiology. A better understanding of the mechanisms of formation of tumor-specific TP53 mutations will help to identify relevant carcinogens and hence to devise adequate preventive strategies. In the longer term, pharmacological approaches aimed at modulating p53 functions may prove beneficial in chemoprevention. However, the complexity of the biological processes regulated by p53 should not be underestimated and further studies are needed to determine whether chemopreventive, p53 activation is a realistic pharmacological target.

To exploit the promises of TP53 studies in chemoprevention, it will be necessary to improve our understanding of the mechanisms of TP53 mutagenesis in human tissues. It will also be very important to further explore the mechanisms by which a normal cell "chooses" between destructive (proapoptotic) or protective (cell-cycle arrest, DNA repair) responses when wild-type p53 is activated. The ultimate p53-dependent chemopreventive drug would need to activate p53 without inducing DNA-damage and to specifically enhance protective responses in normal cells. Thus, the main emphasis for further research should be on elucidating the molecular switches lying at the crossroads of the p53 pathway. It is very likely that these switches will involve many other proteins with important regulatory functions in growth control and in carcinogenesis.

Acknowledgments. E.G. is the recipient of an IARC Special Training Award funded by the EU contract number QLK4–1999–00927 (GENAIR). We are grateful to M. Olivier for providing the IARC TP53 database data from the R6 version for Fig. 3.

References

Aguilar F, Hussain SP, Cerutti P (1993) Aflatoxin B1 induces the transversion of G→T in codon 249 of the p53 tumor suppressor gene in human hepatocytes. Proc Natl Acad Sci U S A 90:8586–8590

Ahrendt SA, Chow JT, Xu LH, Yang SC, Eisenberger CF, Esteller M, Herman JG, Wu L, Decker PA, Jen J, Sidransky D (1999) Molecular detection of tumor cells in bronchoalveolar lavage fluid from patients with early stage lung cancer. J Natl Cancer Inst 91:332–339

Ambs S, Bennett WP, Merriam WG, Ogunfusika MO, Oser SM, Harrington AM, Shields PG, Felley-Bosco E, Hussain SP, Harris CC (1999) Relationship between p53 mutations and inducible nitric oxide synthase expression in human colorectal cancer. J Natl Cancer Inst 91:86–88

Ananthaswamy HN, Loughlin SM, Cox P, Evans RL, Ullrich SE, Kripke ML (1997) Sunlight and skin cancer: inhibition of p53 mutations in UV-irradiated mouse skin by sunscreens. Nat Med 3:510–514

Ananthaswamy HN, Ullrich SE, Mascotto RE, Fourtanier A, Loughlin SM, Khaskina P, Bucana CD, Kripke ML (1999) Inhibition of solar simulator-induced p53 mutations and protection against skin cancer development in mice by sunscreens. J Invest Dermatol 112:763–768

Anker P, Stroun M (2000) Circulating DNA in plasma or serum. Medicina (B Aires) 60:699–702

Appella E, Anderson CW (2000) Signaling to p53: breaking the posttranslational modification code. Pathol Biol (Paris) 48:227–245

Barrett MT, Sanchez CA, Prevo LJ, Wong DJ, Galipeau PC, Paulson TG, Rabinovitch PS, Reid BJ (1999) Evolution of neoplastic cell lineages in Barrett esophagus. Nat Genet 22:106–109

Beckman G, Birgander R, Sjalander A, Saha N, Holmberg PA, Kivela A, Beckman L (1994) Is p53 polymorphism maintained by natural selection? Hum Hered 44:266–270

Blagosklonny MV (2000) p53 from complexity to simplicity: mutant p53 stabilization, gain-of- function, and dominant-negative effect. FASEB J 14:1901–1907

Blandino G, Levine AJ, Oren M (1999) Mutant p53 gain of function: differential effects of different p53 mutants on resistance of cultured cells to chemotherapy. Oncogene 18:477–485

Bottger A, Bottger V, Garcia-Echeverria C, Chene P, Hochkeppel HK, Sampson W, Ang K, Howard SF, Picksley SM, Lane DP (1997) Molecular characterization of the hdm2-p53 interaction. J Mol Biol 269:744–756

Brambilla E, Brambilla C (1997) p53 and lung cancer. Pathol Biol (Paris) 45:852–863

Capizzi RL (1999a) Recent developments and emerging options: the role of amifostine as a broad-spectrum cytoprotective agent. Semin Oncol 26:1–2

Capizzi RL (1999b) The preclinical basis for broad-spectrum selective cytoprotection of normal tissues from cytotoxic therapies by amifostine. Semin Oncol 26:3–21

Carbone PP, Pirsch JD, Thomas JP, Douglas JA, Verma AK, Larson PO, Snow S, Tutsch KD, Pauk D (2001) Phase I chemoprevention study of difluoromethylornithine in subjects with organ transplants. Cancer Epidemiol Biomarkers Prev 10:657–661

Chen X, Bonnefoi H, Diebold-Berger S, Lyautey J, Lederrey C, Faltin-Traub E, Stroun M, Anker P (1999) Detecting tumor-related alterations in plasma or serum DNA of patients diagnosed with breast cancer. Clin Cancer Res 5:2297–2303

Cheung KJ, Jr., Mitchell D, Lin P, Li G (2001) The tumor suppressor candidate p33(ING1) mediates repair of UV-damaged DNA. Cancer Res 61:4974–4977

Denissenko MF, Koudriakova TB, Smith L, O'Connor TR, Riggs AD, Pfeifer GP (1998) The p53 codon 249 mutational hotspot in hepatocellular carcinoma is not related to selective formation or persistence of aflatoxin B1 adducts. Oncogene 17: 3007–3014

Denissenko MF, Pao A, Tang M, Pfeifer GP (1996) Preferential formation of benzo[a]pyrene adducts at lung cancer mutational hotspots in P53. Science 274: 430–432

Dittmer D, Pati S, Zambetti G, Chu S, Teresky AK, Moore M, Finlay C, Levine AJ (1993) Gain of function mutations in p53. Nat Genet 4:42–46

Donehower LA, Harvey M, Slagle BL, McArthur MJ, Montgomery CA, Jr., Butel JS, Bradley A (1992) Mice deficient for p53 are developmentally normal but susceptible to spontaneous tumors. Nature 356:215–221

Dong SM, Traverso G, Johnson C, Geng L, Favis R, Boynton K, Hibi K, Goodman SN, D'Allessio M, Paty P, Hamilton SR, Sidransky D, Barany F, Levin B, Shuber A, Kinzler KW, Vogelstein B, Jen J (2001) Detecting colorectal cancer in stool with the use of multiple genetic targets. J Natl Cancer Inst 93:858–865

Dumaz N, Brougard C, Sarasin A, Daya-Grosjean L (1993) Specific UV-induced mutation spectrum in the p53 gene of skin tumors from DNA-repair-deficient xeroderma pigmentosum patients. Proc Natl Acad Sci U S A 90:10529–10533

Dutta A, Ruppert JM, Aster JC, Winchester E (1993) Inhibition of DNA replication factor RPA by p53. Nature 365:79–82

Eguchi S, Kohara N, Komuta K, Kanematsu T (1996) Mutations of the p53 gene in the stool of patients with resectable colorectal cancer. Cancer 77:1707–1710

el Deiry WS, Tokino T, Velculescu VE, Levy DB, Parsons R, Trent JM, Lin D, Mercer WE, Kinzler KW, Vogelstein B (1993) WAF1, a potential mediator of p53 tumor suppression. Cell 75:817–825

Esteller M, Sanchez-Cespedes M, Rosell R, Sidransky D, Baylin SB, Herman JG (1999) Detection of aberrant promoter hypermethylation of tumor suppressor genes in serum DNA from non-small cell lung cancer patients. Cancer Res 59:67–70

Fan R, Wu MT, Miller D, Wain JC, Kelsey KT, Wiencke JK, Christiani DC (2000) The p53 codon 72 polymorphism and lung cancer risk. Cancer Epidemiol Biomarkers Prev 9:1037–1042

Foster BA, Coffey HA, Morin MJ, Rastinejad F (1999) Pharmacological rescue of mutant p53 conformation and function. Science 286:2507–2510

Fuchs SY, Adler V, Buschmann T, Yin Z, Wu X, Jones SN, Ronai Z (1998) JNK targets p53 ubiquitination and degradation in nonstressed cells. Genes Dev 12:2658–2663

Gaiddon C, Moorthy NC, Prives C (1999) Ref-1 regulates the transactivation and pro-apoptotic functions of p53 in vivo. EMBO J 18:5609–5621

Gonzalez R, Silva JM, Sanchez A, Dominguez G, Garcia JM, Chen XQ, Stroun M, Provencio M, Espana P, Anker P, Bonilla F (2000) Microsatellite alterations and TP53 mutations in plasma DNA of small- cell lung cancer patients: follow-up study and prognostic significance. Ann Oncol 11:1097–1104

Graeber TG, Osmanian C, Jacks T, Housman DE, Koch CJ, Lowe SW, Giaccia AJ (1996) Hypoxia-mediated selection of cells with diminished apoptotic potential in solid tumors. Nature 379:88–91

Graeber TG, Peterson JF, Tsai M, Monica K, Fornace AJ, Jr., Giaccia AJ (1994) Hypoxia induces accumulation of p53 protein, but activation of a G1-phase checkpoint by low-oxygen conditions is independent of p53 status. Mol Cell Biol 14:6264–6277

Guimaraes DP, Hainaut P (2002) TP53: a key gene in human cancer. Biochimie 84: 83–93

Hainaut P, Hollstein M (2000) p53 and human cancer: the first ten thousand mutations. Adv Cancer Res 77:81–137

Hainaut P, Mann K (2001) Zinc binding and redox control of p53 structure and function. Antioxid Redox Signal 3:611–623

Hainaut P, Milner J (1993) A structural role for metal ions in the "wild-type" conformation of the tumor suppressor protein p53. Cancer Res 53:1739–1742

Hainaut P, Pfeifer GP (2001) Patterns of p53 G→T transversions in lung cancers reflect the primary mutagenic signature of DNA-damage by tobacco smoke. Carcinogenesis 22:367–374

Harris LC, Remack JS, Houghton PJ, Brent TP (1996) Wild-type p53 suppresses transcription of the human O6-methylguanine- DNA methyltransferase gene. Cancer Res 56:2029–2032

Haupt Y, Maya R, Kazaz A, Oren M (1997) Mdm2 promotes the rapid degradation of p53. Nature 387:296–299

Hermeking H, Lengauer C, Polyak K, He TC, Zhang L, Thiagalingam S, Kinzler KW, Vogelstein B (1997) 14-3-3 sigma is a p53-regulated inhibitor of G2/M progression. Mol Cell 1:3–11

Hibi K, Robinson CR, Booker S, Wu L, Hamilton SR, Sidransky D, Jen J (1998) Molecular detection of genetic alterations in the serum of colorectal cancer patients. Cancer Res 58:1405–1407

Holliday R, Grigg GW (1993) DNA methylation and mutation. Mutat Res 285:61–67

Hollstein M, Sidransky D, Vogelstein B, Harris CC (1991) p53 mutations in human cancers. Science 253:49–53

Hussain SP, Amstad P, Raja K, Sawyer M, Hofseth L, Shields PG, Hewer A, Phillips DH, Ryberg D, Haugen A, Harris CC (2001a) Mutability of p53 hotspot codons to benzo(a)pyrene diol epoxide (BPDE) and the frequency of p53 mutations in nontumorous human lung. Cancer Res 61:6350–6355

Hussain SP, Hofseth LJ, Harris CC (2001b) Tumor suppressor genes: at the crossroads of molecular carcinogenesis, molecular epidemiology and human risk assessment. Lung Cancer 34 Suppl 2:S7–S15

Itoi T, Takei K, Shinohara Y, Takeda K, Nakamura K, Horibe T, Sanada A, Ohno H, Matsubayashi H, Saito T, Watanabe H (1999) K-ras codon 12 and p53 mutations in biopsy specimens and bile from biliary tract cancers. Pathol Int 49:30–37

Jackson PE, Groopman JD (1999) Aflatoxin and liver cancer. Baillieres Best Pract Res Clin Gastroenterol 13:545–555

Jackson PE, Qian GS, Friesen MD, Zhu YR, Lu P, Wang JB, Wu Y, Kensler TW, Vogelstein B, Groopman JD (2001) Specific p53 mutations detected in plasma and tumors of hepatocellular carcinoma patients by electrospray ionization mass spectrometry. Cancer Res 61:33–35

Jayaraman J, Prives C (1995) Activation of p53 sequence-specific DNA binding by short single strands of DNA requires the p53 C-terminus. Cell 81:1021–1029

Jin X, Wu X, Roth JA, Amos CI, King TM, Branch C, Honn SE, Spitz MR (1995) Higher lung cancer risk for younger African-Americans with the Pro/Pro p53 genotype. Carcinogenesis 16:2205–2208

Kaghad M, Bonnet H, Yang A, Creancier L, Biscan JC, Valent A, Minty A, Chalon P, Lelias JM, Dumont X, Ferrara P, McKeon F, Caput D (1997) Monoallelically expressed gene related to p53 at 1p36, a region frequently deleted in neuroblastoma and other human cancers. Cell 90:809–819

Kamijo T, Weber JD, Zambetti G, Zindy F, Roussel MF, Sherr CJ (1998) Functional and physical interactions of the ARF tumor suppressor with p53 and Mdm2. Proc Natl Acad Sci U S A 95:8292–8297

Kamijo T, Zindy F, Roussel MF, Quelle DE, Downing JR, Ashmun RA, Grosveld G, Sherr CJ (1997) Tumor suppression at the mouse INK4a locus mediated by the alternative reading frame product p19ARF. Cell 91:649–659

Kastan MB, Zhan Q, el Deiry WS, Carrier F, Jacks T, Walsh WV, Plunkett BS, Vogelstein B, Fornace AJ, Jr. (1992) A mammalian cell cycle checkpoint path way utilizing p53 and GADD45 is defective in ataxia-telangiectasia. Cell 71: 587–597

Kirk GD, Camus-Randon AM, Mendy M, Goedert JJ, Merle P, Trepo C, Brechot C, Hainaut P, Montesano R (2000) Ser-249 p53 mutations in plasma DNA of patients with hepatocellular carcinoma from The Gambia. J Natl Cancer Inst 92:148–153

Klug SJ, Wilmotte R, Santos C, Almonte M, Herrero R, Guerrero I, Caceres E, Peixoto-Guimaraes D, Lenoir G, Hainaut P, Walboomers JM, Munoz N (2001) TP53 polymorphism, HPV infection, and risk of cervical cancer. Cancer Epidemiol Biomarkers Prev 10:1009–1012

Knudson AGJ (1971) Mutation and cancer: statistical study of retinoblastoma. Proc Natl Acad Sci U S A 68:820–823

Kramer DL, Vujcic S, Diegelman P, Alderfer J, Miller JT, Black JD, Bergeron RJ, Porter CW (1999) Polyamine analogue induction of the p53-p21WAF1/CIP1-Rb pathway and G1 arrest in human melanoma cells. Cancer Res 59:1278–1286

Kramer DL, Vujcic S, Diegelman P, White C, Black JD, Porter CW (1998) Polyamine analogue-mediated cell cycle responses in human melanoma cells involves the p53, p21, Rb regulatory pathway. Biochem Soc Trans 26:609–614

Kubbutat MH, Jones SN, Vousden KH (1997) Regulation of p53 stability by Mdm2. Nature 387:299–303

Kurbacher CM, Mallmann PK (1998) Chemoprotection in anticancer therapy: the emerging role of amifostine (WR-2721). Anticancer Res 18:2203–2210

Lane DP (1992) Worrying about p53. Curr Biol 2:581–583

Lane DP, Hall PA (1997) MDM 2–arbiter of p53's destruction. Trends Biochem Sci 22: 372–374

Lee JM, Lee YC, Yang SY, Shi WL, Lee CJ, Luh SP, Chen CJ, Hsieh CY, Wu MT (2000) Genetic polymorphisms of p53 and GSTP1,but not NAT2,are associated with susceptibility to squamous-cell carcinoma of the esophagus. Int J Cancer 89: 458–464

Levrero M, De L, V, Costanzo A, Gong J, Wang JY, Melino G (2000) The p53/p63/p73 family of transcription factors: overlapping and distinct functions. J Cell Sci 113 (Pt 10): 1661–1670

Li L, Rao JN, Guo X, Liu L, Santora R, Bass BL, Wang JY (2001) Polyamine depletion stabilizes p53 resulting in inhibition of normal intestinal epithelial cell proliferation. Am J Physiol Cell Physiol 281:C941-C953

Linke SP, Clarkin KC, Wahl GM (1997) p53 mediates permanent arrest over multiple cell cycles in response to gamma-irradiation. Cancer Res 57:1171–1179

Liu Y, Kulesz-Martin M (2001) p53 protein at the hub of cellular DNA damage response pathways through sequence-specific and non-sequence-specific DNA binding. Carcinogenesis 22:851–860

Lohrum MA, Vousden KH (2000) Regulation and function of the p53-related proteins: same family, different rules. Trends Cell Biol 10:197–202

Lowe SW (1995) Cancer therapy and p53. Curr Opin Oncol 7:547–553

Lowe SW, Schmitt EM, Smith SW, Osborne BA, Jacks T (1993) p53 is required for radiation-induced apoptosis in mouse thymocytes. Nature 362:847–849

Lubin R, Zalcman G, Bouchet L, Tredanel J, Legros Y, Cazals D, Hirsch A, Soussi T (1995) Serum p53 antibodies as early markers of lung cancer. Nat Med 1:701–702

Malkin D, Li FP, Strong LC, Fraumeni JF, Jr., Nelson CE, Kim DH, Kassel J, Gryka MA, Bischoff FZ, Tainsky MA, . (1990) Germ line p53 mutations in a familial syndrome of breast cancer, sarcomas, and other neoplasms. Science 250:1233–1238

Mandard AM, Hainaut P, Hollstein M (2000) Genetic steps in the development of squamous cell carcinoma of the esophagus. Mutat Res 462:335–342

Mao L, Hruban RH, Boyle JO, Tockman M, Sidransky D (1994) Detection of oncogene mutations in sputum precedes diagnosis of lung cancer. Cancer Res 54: 1634–1637

Marin MC, Jost CA, Brooks LA, Irwin MS, O'Nions J, Tidy JA, James N, McGregor JM, Harwood CA, Yulug IG, Vousden KH, Allday MJ, Gusterson B, Ikawa S, Hinds PW, Crook T, Kaelin WG, Jr. (2000) A common polymorphism acts as an intragenic modifier of mutant p53 behaviour. Nat Genet 25:47–54

Meplan C, Richard MJ, Hainaut P (2000a) Metalloregulation of the tumor suppressor protein p53:zinc mediates the renaturation of p53 after exposure to metal chelators in vitro and in intact cells. Oncogene

Meplan C, Richard MJ, Hainaut P (2000b) Redox signaling and transition metals in the control of the p53 pathway. Biochem Pharmacol 59:25–33

Meyskens FL, Jr., Gerner EW (1999) Development of difluoromethylornithine (DFMO) as a chemoprevention agent. Clin Cancer Res 5:945–951

Miyashita T, Krajewski S, Krajewska M, Wang HG, Lin HK, Liebermann DA, Hoffman B, Reed JC (1994) Tumor suppressor p53 is a regulator of bcl-2 and bax gene expression in vitro and in vivo. Oncogene 9:1799–1805

Momand J, Zambetti GP, Olson DC, George D, Levine AJ (1992) The mdm-2 oncogene product forms a complex with the p53 protein and inhibits p53-mediated transactivation. Cell 69:1237–1245

Montesano R, Hainaut P, Wild CP (1997) Hepatocellular carcinoma: from gene to public health. J Natl Cancer Inst 89:1844–1851

Mulcahy HE, Lyautey J, Lederrey C, Qi C, X, Anker P, Alstead EM, Ballinger A, Farthing MJ, Stroun M (1998) A prospective study of K-ras mutations in the plasma of pancreatic cancer patients. Clin Cancer Res 4:271–275

Murata J, Tada M, Iggo RD, Sawamura Y, Shinohe Y, Abe H (1997) Nitric oxide as a carcinogen: analysis by yeast functional assay of inactivating p53 mutations induced by nitric oxide. Mutat Res 379:211–218

Nakazawa H, English D, Randell PL, Nakazawa K, Martel N, Armstrong BK, Yamasaki H (1994) UV and skin cancer: specific p53 gene mutation in normal skin as a biologically relevant exposure measurement. Proc Natl Acad Sci U S A 91:360–364

North S, El Ghissassi F, Pluquet O, Verhaegh G, Hainaut P (2000) The cytoprotective aminothiol WR1065 activates p21waf-1 and down regulates cell cycle progression through a p53-dependent pathway. Oncogene 19:1206–1214

Oda K, Arakawa H, Tanaka T, Matsuda K, Tanikawa C, Mori T, Nishimori H, Tamai K, Tokino T, Nakamura Y, Taya Y (2000) p53AIP1, a potential mediator of p53-dependent apoptosis, and its regulation by Ser-46-phosphorylated p53. Cell 102: 849–862

Oren M (1992) p53: the ultimate tumor suppressor gene? FASEB J 6:3169–3176

Oren M (1999) Regulation of the p53 tumor suppressor protein. J Biol Chem 274: 36031–36034

Oren M, Rotter V (1999) Introduction: p53–the first twenty years. Cell Mol Life Sci 55:9–11

Owen-Schaub LB, Zhang W, Cusack JC, Angelo LS, Santee SM, Fujiwara T, Roth JA, Deisseroth AB, Zhang WW, Kruzel E, . (1995) Wild-type human p53 and a temperature-sensitive mutant induce Fas/APO-1 expression. Mol Cell Biol 15:3032–3040

Parkin DM, Bray F, Ferlay J, Pisani P (2001) Estimating the world cancer burden: Globocan 2000. Int J Cancer 94:153–156

Pluquet O, Hainaut P (2001) Genotoxic and non-genotoxic pathways of p53 induction. Cancer Lett 174:1–15

Polyak K, Xia Y, Zweier JL, Kinzler KW, Vogelstein B (1997) A model for p53-induced apoptosis. Nature 389:300–305

Pomerantz J, Schreiber-Agus N, Liegeois NJ, Silverman A, Alland L, Chin L, Potes J, Chen K, Orlow I, Lee HW, Cordon-Cardo C, DePinho RA (1998) The Ink4a tumor suppressor gene product, p19Arf, interacts with MDM 2 and neutralizes MDM 2's inhibition of p53. Cell 92:713–723

Prescott JL, Montie J, Pugh TW, McHugh T, Veltri RW (2001) Clinical sensitivity of p53 mutation detection in matched bladder tumor, bladder wash, and voided urine specimens. Cancer 91:2127–2135

Prives C, Hall PA (1999) The p53 pathway. J Pathol 187:112–126

Ray RM, Zimmerman BJ, McCormack SA, Patel TB, Johnson LR (1999) Polyamine depletion arrests cell cycle and induces inhibitors p21(Waf1/Cip1), p27(Kip1), and p53 in IEC-6 cells. Am J Physiol 276:C684-C691

Robertson KD, Jones PA (2000) DNA methylation: past, present and future directions. Carcinogenesis 21:461–467

Scherer SJ, Maier SM, Seifert M, Hanselmann RG, Zang KD, Muller-Hermelink HK, Angel P, Welter C, Schartl M (2000) p53 and c-Jun functionally synergize in the regulation of the DNA repair gene hMSH2 in response to UV. J Biol Chem 275: 37469–37473

Shao ZM, Wu J, Shen ZZ, Nguyen M (2001) p53 mutation in plasma DNA and its prognostic value in breast cancer patients. Clin Cancer Res 7:2222–2227

Sheikh MS, Burns TF, Huang Y, Wu GS, Amundson S, Brooks KS, Fornace AJ, Jr., el Deiry WS (1998) p53-dependent and -independent regulation of the death receptor KILLER/DR5 gene expression in response to genotoxic stress and tumor necrosis factor alpha. Cancer Res 58:1593–1598

Shivakumar CV, Brown DR, Deb S, Deb SP (1995) Wild-type human p53 transactivates the human proliferating cell nuclear antigen promoter. Mol Cell Biol 15:6785–6793

Sidransky D (1997) Nucleic acid-based methods for the detection of cancer. Science 278:1054–1059

Sidransky D, Hollstein M (1996) Clinical implications of the p53 gene. Annu Rev Med 47:285–301

Smela ME, Currier SS, Bailey EA, Essigmann JM (2001) The chemistry and biology of aflatoxin B(1): from mutational spectrometry to carcinogenesis. Carcinogenesis 22:535–545

Smith LE, Denissenko MF, Bennett WP, Li H, Amin S, Tang M, Pfeifer GP (2000) Targeting of lung cancer mutational hotspots by polycyclic aromatic hydrocarbons. J Natl Cancer Inst 92:803–811

Sohn S, Jaitovitch-Groisman I, Benlimame N, Galipeau J, Batist G, Alaoui-Jamali MA (2000) Retroviral expression of the hepatitis B virus x gene promotes liver cell susceptibility to carcinogen-induced site specific mutagenesis. Mutat Res 460: 17–28

Soussi T (2000) p53 Antibodies in the sera of patients with various types of cancer: a review. Cancer Res 60:1777–1788

Soussi T, May P (1996) Structural aspects of the p53 protein in relation to gene evolution: a second look. J Mol Biol 260:623–637

Srivastava S, Zou ZQ, Pirollo K, Blattner W, Chang EH (1990) Germ-line transmission of a mutated p53 gene in a cancer-prone family with Li-Fraumeni syndrome. Nature 348:747–749

Stone S, Jiang P, Dayananth P, Tavtigian SV, Katcher H, Parry D, Peters G, Kamb A (1995) Complex structure and regulation of the P16 (MTS1) locus. Cancer Res 55:2988–2994

Storey A, Thomas M, Kalita A, Harwood C, Gardiol D, Mantovani F, Breuer J, Leigh IM, Matlashewski G, Banks L (1998) Role of a p53 polymorphism in the development of human papillomavirus- associated cancer [see comments]. Nature 393:229–234

Tao W, Levine AJ (1999) P19(ARF) stabilizes p53 by blocking nucleo-cytoplasmic shuttling of Mdm2. Proc Natl Acad Sci U S A 96:6937–6941

Tommasi S, Denissenko MF, Pfeifer GP (1997) Sunlight induces pyrimidine dimers preferentially at 5-methylcytosine bases. Cancer Res 57:4727–4730

Tornaletti S, Pfeifer GP (1994) Slow repair of pyrimidine dimers at p53 mutation hotspots in skin cancer. Science 263:1436–1438

Ueno M, Masutani H, Arai RJ, Yamauchi A, Hirota K, Sakai T, Inamoto T, Yamaoka Y, Yodoi J, Nikaido T (1999) Thioredoxin-dependent redox regulation of p53-mediated p21 activation. J Biol Chem 274:35809–35815

Vet JA, Witjes JA, Marras SA, Hessels D, van der Poel HG, Debruyne FM, Schalken JA (1996) Predictive value of p53 mutations analyzed in bladder washings for progression of high-risk superficial bladder cancer. Clin Cancer Res 2:1055–1061

Wallace HM, Caslake R (2001) Polyamines and colon cancer. Eur J Gastroenterol Hepatol 13:1033–1039

Wang B, Li L, Yao L, Liu L, Zhu Y (2001) Detection of p53 gene mutations in sputum samples and their implications in the early diagnosis of lung cancer in suspicious patients. Chin Med J (Engl) 114:694–697

Wang XW, Vermeulen W, Coursen JD, Gibson M, Lupold SE, Forrester K, Xu G, Elmore L, Yeh H, Hoeijmakers JH, Harris CC (1996) The XPB and XPD DNA helicases are components of the p53-mediated apoptosis pathway. Genes Dev 10:1219–1232

Watanabe K, Kawamori T, Nakatsugi S, Wakabayashi K (2000) COX-2 and iNOS, good targets for chemoprevention of colon cancer. Biofactors 12:129–133

Weston A, Ling-Cawley HM, Caporaso NE, Bowman ED, Hoover RN, Trump BF, Harris CC (1994) Determination of the allelic frequencies of an L-myc and a p53 polymorphism in human lung cancer. Carcinogenesis 15:583–587

Weston A, Perrin LS, Forrester K, Hoover RN, Trump BF, Harris CC, Caporaso NE (1992) Allelic frequency of a p53 polymorphism in human lung cancer. Cancer Epidemiol Biomarkers Prev 1:481–483

Wild CP, Hall AJ (2000) Primary prevention of hepatocellular carcinoma in developing countries. Mutat Res 462:381–393

Wilson JW, Pritchard DM, Hickman JA, Potten CS (1998) Radiation-induced p53 and p21WAF-1/CIP1 expression in the murine intestinal epithelium: apoptosis and cell cycle arrest. Am J Pathol 153:899–909

Wink DA, Kasprzak KS, Maragos CM, Elespuru RK, Misra M, Dunams TM, Cebula TA, Koch WH, Andrews AW, Allen JS, . (1991) DNA deaminating ability and genotoxicity of nitric oxide and its progenitors. Science 254:1001–1003

Xu X, Stower MJ, Reid IN, Garner RC, Burns PA (1996) Molecular screening of multifocal transitional cell carcinoma of the bladder using p53 mutations as biomarkers. Clin Cancer Res 2:1795–1800

Yang A, Schweitzer R, Sun D, Kaghad M, Walker N, Bronson RT, Tabin C, Sharpe A, Caput D, Crum C, McKeon F (1999) p63 is essential for regenerative proliferation in limb, craniofacial and epithelial development. Nature 398:714–718

Yang A, Walker N, Bronson R, Kaghad M, Oosterwegel M, Bonnin J, Vagner C, Bonnet H, Dikkes P, Sharpe A, McKeon F, Caput D (2000) p73-deficient mice have neurological, pheromonal and inflammatory defects but lack spontaneous tumors. Nature 404:99–103

Yang AS, Gonzalgo ML, Zingg JM, Millar RP, Buckley JD, Jones PA (1996) The rate of CpG mutation in Alu repetitive elements within the p53 tumor suppressor gene in the primate germline. J Mol Biol 258:240–250

Yang AS, Shen JC, Zingg JM, Mi S, Jones PA (1995) HhaI and HpaII DNA methyl-transferases bind DNA mismatches, methylate uracil and block DNA repair. Nucleic Acids Res 23:1380–1387

Zhang Y, Xiong Y, Yarbrough WG (1998) ARF promotes MDM 2 degradation and stabilizes p53:ARF-INK4a locus deletion impairs both the Rb and p53 tumor suppression pathways. Cell 92:725–734

CHAPTER 6
Apoptosis

B.W. Stewart

A. Apoptosis and the Genesis of Tumors

Malignant cancers arise as the culmination of a multistage process, and passage through this process may be characterized genetically, morphologically, or biologically. Genetically, tumors are distinguished from normal tissue by alterations in the structure and/or expression of multiple genes, including particular oncogenes and tumor suppressor genes (PONDER 2001). Associated phenotypic change is indicated by the appearance of hyperplastic, benign, invasive, and finally metastatic cell populations, it being recognized that each of these terms is indicative of a spectrum of morphological changes. In terms of biological change, HANAHAN and WEINBERG (HANAHAN and WEINBERG 2000) have suggested that tumors differ from normal tissue by their self-sufficiency in growth signals, resistance to antigrowth signals, evasion of apoptosis, limitless replicative potential, sustained angiogenesis, and tissue invasion and metastasis. Each of these characteristics may be traced back to particular, and not necessarily exclusive, gene sets.

Disordered apoptosis contributes to tumorigenesis. While the more obvious scenario would implicate reduced apoptosis as causing concern, increased cell death may also facilitate malignant transformation by contributing to increased and compensatory proliferative activity (SCHULTE-HERMANN et al. 1997). Thus, growth of some cancers, specifically including breast, has been positively correlated with increasing apoptosis (PARTON et al. 2001a). By comparison with the molecular genetic basis of cell proliferation, genes mediating cell death, and their altered function in malignant as opposed to normal tissue, have been the subject of scrutiny only recently. Within this limited history, initial attention was focused on revealing an immediate genetic basis for the apoptotic phenotype as exemplified by the fragmentation of DNA. Until the mid-1990s, the number of biological parameters considered relevant to progress toward apoptosis, including change in intracellular calcium concentration, was limited and it was practicable to characterize virtually all such changes under particular experimental conditions (STEWART 1994). The opposite is now the case: the number of relevant indicators is sufficient to preclude monitoring all such parameters in any (mammalian) experimental system. Accordingly, mechanisms of apoptosis, as delineated here and in virtually all current publications, are a synthesis predicated upon integration of processes described in a variety of systems, and in particular, in a variety of cell types. The extent to which any particular reaction pathway is operative in a given cell type must be determined directly, although reasonable inferences can be made in many instances on the basis of cell lineage and commonality between species.

While it is true that no single study can be anticipated to include all known biological parameters of apoptosis, it is equally true that no written assessment of the subject can deal with all aspects of this fundamental biological process. This specifically includes the present text, and certain qualifications are appropriate. This chapter is wholly focused on apoptosis in relation to tumorigenesis from both a biological and a medical perspective. It must be noted that apoptosis is being actively researched in other biomedical contexts including developmental biology, immunology, and the pathology of degenerative disease. These endeavors cannot be consciously ignored: insights gained in such fields may prove critical to understanding and/or exploitation of apoptosis in cancer.

B. How Mechanism Has Been Elucidated

Apoptosis is a mode of cell death that was originally characterized as being distinguished from necrosis both morphologically and functionally (WYLLIE 1987). Thus, apoptosis involves single cells rather than areas of tissue and does not provoke inflammation. Tissue homeostasis is dependent on controlled elimination of unwanted cells, often in the context of a continuum in which specialization and maturation is ultimately succeeded by cell death in what may be regarded as the final phase of differentiation. Apart from a physiological context, cells that have been lethally exposed to cytotoxic drugs (HICKMAN 1992) or radiation (LOWE et al. 1993) may be subject to apoptosis. Thus, in response to a variety of stimuli, it was recognized that a particular mode of cell death was marked by condensation and margination of chromatin, a decrease in cell size, blebbing of the cytoplasmic membrane, and sequestration of cell remnants into "apoptotic bodies." Moreover, DNA isolated from such cell populations exhibited a characteristic pattern of fragmentation ("laddering") as a consequence of cleavage at approximately 180-base pair intervals (ARENDS et al. 1990). The latter was characterized as the "hallmark" of apoptosis and perceived as a molecular indicator of loss of viability.

Current understanding of apoptosis marks a transition from a focus of morphological change and DNA laddering to specification of the genes mediating morphological change and, more importantly, regulation of its occurrence. Identification of genes mediating apoptosis in mammalian cells has been critically dependent on definition of the "ced" genes in the nematode *Caenorhabditis elegans*. During ontogeny of the adult hermaphrodite worm, 131 of the 1,090 somatic cells die by apoptosis, leaving an adult

comprised of 959 cells (MEIER et al. 2000). Genes whose loss-of-function inter-
feres with such development, namely ced-9, ced-4, and ced-3, are respectively
homologous to human Bcl-2 (which suppresses apoptosis), Apaf-1 (which
mediates caspase activation), and the caspases themselves (cysteine proteases
which mediate cell death). This paradigm largely encompasses the commonly
recognized phases of apoptosis indicated by the terms "regulation," "effector,"
and "engulfing," respectively (STRASSER et al. 2000). The regulatory phase
includes all the signaling pathways that culminate in commitment to cell death.
Some of these pathways regulate only cell death, but many of them have overlapping roles in the control of cell proliferation, differentiation, responses to
stress, and homeostasis. Critical to apoptosis signaling are the "initiator" caspases (including caspase-8, caspase-9, and caspase-10) whose role is to activate
the more abundant "effector" caspases (including caspase-3 and caspase-7)
which, in turn, brings about the morphological change indicative of apoptosis.
Finally, the engulfing process involves the recognition of cellular "remains"
and their elimination by the engulfing activity of surrounding cells.

C. Apoptosis and Carcinogenesis

Apoptosis, or lack of it, may be critical to tumorigenesis (KAUFMANN and
GORES 2000). At its simplest, tumorigenesis may be perceived as a net local
increase in cell number or, slightly more informatively, an imbalance between
the rate of cell proliferation and the rate of cell death. In terms of cell kinetics, populations of proliferating and dying cells may be identified in a mathe-
matical model of a growing tumor. The occurrence of apoptosis determines
not only which cells are lost but also the period during which particular cell
populations may proliferate (SCHULTE-HERMANN et al. 1999). When this perspective is applied to multistage carcinogenesis, it becomes evident that different subpopulations of cells may be subject to different rates of apoptosis.
Thus, for example, preneoplastic cells may be subject to reduced apoptosis
compared to normal cells (SCHULTE-HERMANN et al. 1999). Accordingly, the
regulation of apoptosis is pivotal to tumor growth. Although approaches to
carcinogenesis are often focused on early stage development, disordered
apoptosis may contribute to late stage carcinogenesis: namely, the growth of
metastases (WONG et al. 2001).

   If apoptosis can be characterized as relevant to tumor development, apoptosis can equally be immediately seen as critical to tumor elimination; that is,
to the goal of cancer treatment and cancer prevention. In respect of treatment,
it is self-evident that radiation or chemotherapy may be effective by increasing the proportion of apoptotic cells. Thus it is asserted that most anticancer
agents now in use induce apoptosis (SCHMITT and LOWE 1999). However, this
represents relatively recent understanding. The notion that cytotoxic drugs
interact with a critical "target" molecule generating a cytotoxic lesion was, and
continues to be, a central focus in molecular pharmacology (CHEN and LIU

1994). However, drug-target interaction is now perceived as the event which initiates apoptosis (DIVE and HICKMAN 1991). On this basis, the efficacy of treatment is consequent upon functionality of the apoptotic process and hence alterations in this process demonstrable in malignant cells are viewed as critical. Less obvious perhaps is the consideration that particular subpopulations, such as those subject to hypoxia, may be subject to a rate of apoptosis different from the rest of the tumor (DENKO et al. 2000).

The understanding that cancer preventive agents may function by inducing apoptosis (LOTAN 1995) may be perceived as having emerged from the study of cytotoxic drugs. Generally, induction of cell death by preventive agents is less marked than that observed using cytotoxic compounds. Nonetheless, results achieved using the latter may have been seen to have provided concepts and models which have been explored in relation to substances which prevent tumor development. Finally, occurrence of apoptosis has been proposed as a susceptibility marker determining carcinogenic risk (ZHAO et al. 2001).

This then is the scope of apoptosis in relation to cancer. While far from encompassing the totality of apoptosis biology, this topic critically includes the relationship between mitogenic and apoptotic pathways, particularly in relation to the consequences of DNA damage. Beyond that, understanding the mechanism of apoptosis is fundamental to defining defective apoptosis in particular tumor cells. Finally, means of perturbing apoptosis are relevant to not only cancer treatment, but also to cancer prevention.

D. Cell Division and Cell Death

I. Interrelationships Between the Mitogenic and Apoptotic Pathways

A relationship between apoptosis and mitosis may be presumed from morphological similarities between the initial stages of both, specifically involving condensation of chromatin. A much more direct and intimate relationship between regulation of growth/mitosis and apoptosis is evident from a variety of relevant signaling pathways which are common to both processes (GUO and HAY 1999). Many differing promoters of cell proliferation have been found to possess proapoptotic activity (CHOISY-ROSSI and YONISH-ROUACH 1998). The activity of the kinase Akt, discussed later in terms of its ability to inhibit the mitochondrial pathway of caspase activation, plays a role in control of cell proliferation (EL DEIRY 2001). The phosphoserine-binding proteins designated 14-3-3 may be characterized as mediating cell cycle progression or apoptosis depending upon the identity of the proteins to which they bind (VAN HEMERT et al. 2001).

An immediate relationship between cell growth and apoptosis was evident from the demonstration by EVAN and colleagues (EVAN et al. 1992) that ectopic expression of the c-myc oncogene (normally associated with proliferative activity) causes apoptosis in cultured cells subjected to serum deprivation (which otherwise prevents proliferation). In common with many such gene products mediating both growth/cell cycle and death functions, discreet signaling pathways may be dissected (PACKHAM et al. 1996) and may be shown to depend on critical interactions with other players. Thus, myc-induced apoptosis can be inhibited by Bcl-2 overexpression (CORY et al. 1999)

Oncogenes that stimulate mitogenesis can also activate apoptosis. These include oncogenic ras, myc, and E2F. The retinoblastoma gene (RB) encodes a 105-kDa nuclear phosphoprotein (pRb) which is critical to the control of the cell cycle, mediating processes essential for the initiation of DNA synthesis: that is progression from G_1 to S phase (KASTEN and GIORDANO 1998) Mutations in E2F that prevent its interaction with pRb accelerate S phase entry and apoptosis (LOGAN et al. 1995). A function of pRb is to suppress apoptosis: pRb-deficient cells seem to be more susceptible to p53-induced apoptosis (HARBOUR and DEAN 2000). In agreement with it being a downstream target of pRB, ectopic expression of E2F (of which there are several family members) results in hyperproliferation and apoptosis. The apoptosis induced by E2F1 is potentiated by p53.

II. Consequences of DNA Damage

Human cells contain 3×10^9 nucleotides which are constantly exposed to an array of DNA damaging agents of environmental origin, such as X-rays, sunlight, and tobacco smoke, as well as damaging agents of endogenous origin, such as reactive oxygen species and spontaneous bond breakage. In most instances, the integrity of the genome is maintained by the repair of such damaged DNA mediated by repair pathways variously relevant to damage of particular types (HOEIJMAKERS 2001). In the immediate term, the adequacy of DNA repair processes will account for the restoration of the original DNA structure; in the longer term it accounts for the avoidance of cancer which is otherwise attributable to the accumulation of gene mutation and other genomic injury. Accordingly, apoptosis might be regarded as the ultimate mode of DNA repair: the death of cells harboring irreparable DNA damage to avoid the possibility of malignant transformation. Not surprisingly, therefore, the interrelationship between processes mediating DNA repair and those bringing about cell death is complex; indeed, the processes are common up to the causation of cell cycle arrest.

A wide variety of agents, specifically including ionizing and nonionizing radiation, genotoxic carcinogens, and most cytotoxic drugs cause apoptotic cell death (GERSCHENSON and ROTELLO 1992; HICKMAN 1992). A distinguishing feature of this route to apoptosis, as distinct from that initiated by certain steroids, antibodies, cell detachment or growth factor receptor antagonists (REED 1999), is the occurrence of cell cycle arrest in response to the initiating agent (RICH et al. 2000). While molecules that sense DNA damage, which may include DNA-dependent protein kinase and poly (ADP-ribose) polymerase, have yet to be fully defined, the necessary signaling of such damage to cause cell cycle arrest is known to be transduced by the ataxia-telangiectasia mutated gene (ATM) and the ATM-rad3-related (ATR) protein (ZHOU and ELLEDGE 2000). Specifically, ATM plays a part in the response to DNA damage caused by ionizing radiation, controlling the initial phosphorylation of key proteins such as p53, Mdm2, BRCA1, Chk2, and Nsb1. ATR/ATM-mediated phosphorylation of human Rad 17 may be a critical early event during checkpoint signaling in DNA-damage cells (BAO et al. 2001). Other phosphorylation targets are being progressively identified (CORTEZ et al. 2001). The sensors of DNA damage may also include mammalian homologues of the PCNA-like yeast proteins Rad1, Rad9, and Hus1. Other specific molecules detect nucleotide mismatch or inappropriate methylation (JONES and GONZALGO 1997).

In their review, ELLEDGE and ZHOU identify a class of effector molecules which, following DNA damage or other replication stress, are the targets of signal transduction and variously mediate cell cycle arrest, DNA repair and apoptosis (ZHOU and ELLEDGE 2000). Foremost amongst such effectors, at least in respect of the principal focus for research, is p53. Others include the checkpoint kinases Chk1 and Chk2 as well as BRCA1, which is an ATM substrate and required for DNA damage-induced homologous recombination. Following exposure of mammalian cells to DNA-damaging agents, p53 is activated by phosphorylation, which greatly increased its stability, and amongst many "targets" upregulated are the cyclin-dependent kinase inhibitor p21/waf1 (which causes G_1 arrest) and Bax (a member of the Bcl-2 family which induces apoptosis). However, these particular responses must be viewed as emblematic of the role of p53 in mediating cycle arrest or apoptosis, it being acknowledged that the actual signaling pathways are more complex. In relation to signaling apoptosis, the ASPP (apoptosis-stimulating protein of p53) family has been described (SAMUELS-LEV et al. 2001). Specific members of this family appear to bind to p53 and enhance transactivation of pro-apoptotic genes, including Bax, but have no effect on relevant cell cycle arrest genes such as mdm2, cyclin G, and p21. While this discussion is necessarily focused on involvement of p53 in apoptosis, with some reference to cell cycle arrest, the role of p53 impinges upon telomere erosion, hypoxia, and angiogenesis and the impact of matrix-related cell survival (EVAN and VOUSDEN 2001).

E. The Regulatory Phase

Activation of caspases is generally regarded to mark irreversible commitment to cell death and to be synonymous with morphological change indicative of such cell death. Accordingly, processes which culminate in apoptosis, or which may circumvent this outcome are categorized as regulating apoptosis primarily on the basis of their occurring "upstream" or prior to caspase activation. Within this concept of the regulatory phase of apoptosis, two major signaling pathways which culminate in caspase activation have been identified in mammalian cells. The "extrinsic" pathway involves the conformational change in certain cell surface receptors following the binding of respective ligands. The "intrinsic" pathway involves mitochondrial function and is initiated by growth factor deprivation and corticosteroids, or by DNA damage and cell cycle arrest induced by radiation or cytotoxic drugs.

I. The Extrinsic Pathway: Death Via Cell Surface Receptors

Apoptosis may be induced by signaling molecules, usually polypeptides such as growth factors or related molecules, which bind to receptors on the cell surface (PETER and KRAMMER 1998). Such cell death was initially investigated in relation to the immune response, but has much wider ramifications. The best characterized receptors belong to the tumor necrosis factor (TNF) receptor gene superfamily, which is defined by similar, cysteine-rich extracellular domains (YEH et al. 1999). In addition, death receptors contain an homologous cytoplasmic sequence, termed the "death domain," to engage the cell's apoptotic machinery. The archetype members of the family are Fas/APO-1/CD95 and TNF 1 receptor (which binds TNFα). The role of Fas was elucidated in the context of the immune response (KRAMMER et al. 1994). Activation of the Fas receptor by its specific ligand (FasL) results in a conformational change such that the death domain interacts with the adapter molecule FADD, which in turn binds procaspase-8/FLICE/MACH (Fig. 1). Upon recruitment by FADD, propcaspase-8 oligermization occurs which drives its activation through self-cleavage. Once TNF is bound, TNFR1 may signal apoptosis in some cell types by protein–protein interactions involving FADD and culminating in caspase 8 activation. Upon binding of TNF, the relevant receptor may also provoke antiapoptotic signaling specifically through activation of NF-κB (ASHKENAZI and DIXIT 1998).

TRAIL (TNF-related apoptosis-inducing ligand, Apo-2L) has 28% amino acid identity to FasL. Unlike expression of FasL, which is restricted mainly to activated T-cells and NK cells, TRAIL is expressed in many tissues. Apoptosis is mediated by a pathway that has not been described with the clarity of that involving either Fas or TNFR1. TRAIL has been characterized as causing cell death in tumorigenic or transformed cells but not in normal cells despite the range of normal tissue in which TRAIL mRNA is detected (GRIFFITH and LYNCH 1998). This paradox may be explained in part by "decoy receptors" (DcRs), which are able to bind the ligand with high affinity but which lack any cytoplasmic death domain critical to the activation of caspases.

Clear and useful distinction can be made between the extrinsic and intrinsic pathways to caspase activation. Thus, p53 may be characterized as not having a role in the extrinsic pathway (O'CONNOR et al. 2000). However, a functional separation is far from absolute as may be indicated by two considerations. Firstly, in some cell types, cytotoxic drug-induced apoptosis is mediated by Fas (FRISEN et al. 1996). This phenomenon appears to be limited (EISCHEN et al. 1997), and may be restricted to certain cell types specifically including

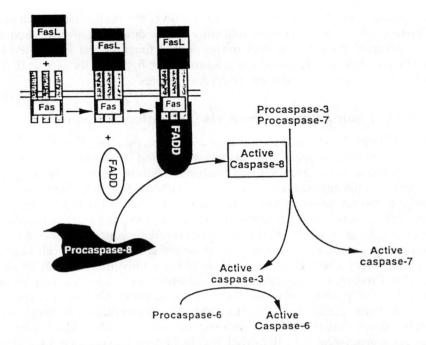

Fig. 1. How Fas functions via the extrinsic pathway to caspase activation. In this simplification, the pathway is indicated in respect of a single species of membrane receptor, namely Fas. Both Fas receptor and signaling molecules such as FADD are single representatives of families of such proteins variously involved in similar patterns of caspase activation. The diagram is an over-simplification to the extent that "communication" with the intrinsic pathway is not directly indicated. (Adapted from KAUFMANN and GORES 2000)

the T-cell lymphoblastoid line CEM. Secondly, activated caspase-8 may, amongst other actions, mediate activation of procaspase-9, which otherwise is key to the intrinsic pathway.

II. The Intrinsic Pathway: The Bcl-2 Family and the Role of Mitochondria

While ced-9 is a single gene with one homolog (EGL-1) in *Caenorhabditis elegans*, its human counterpart, Bcl-2, is but one member of a multigene family related by four conserved Bcl-2 homology (BH) domains designated BH1-4, which correspond to α-helical segments (REED 1997). The respective gene products could be characterized on the basis of whether their exogenous expression suppresses or facilitates apoptosis. The family members including Bcl-2, Bcl-x_L, and Bcl-W suppress apoptosis while others induce apoptosis and may be subdivided on the basis of their ability to dimerize with Bcl-2 and homologous on the basis of BH3 only (Bad, Bik, Bid) or demonstrating BH1, BH2, and BH3 homology (Bax, Bak). Heterodimerization of Bcl-2 family members was discovered on the basis of yeast 2-hydrid systems and the life/death balance mediated by Bcl-2, and Bax was hypothesized as being determined by homodimer/heterodimer balance (OLTVAI et al. 1993). The Bcl-2 gene product was also suggested to suppress apoptosis through its activity as an antioxidant (HOCKENBERY et al. 1993). These explanations are currently perceived as oversimplifications at best, the multiplicity of family members and their respective intracellular locations precluding any simple dimerization model. Thus Bax and Bcl-2 are described as operating independently (KNUDSON and KORSMEYER 1997).

The relationship between p53 and Bcl-2 (and other family members) may be perceived as fundamental to tumorigenesis. Basic observations are that Bcl-2 is able to block p53-mediated apoptosis (CHIOU et al. 1994) and that Bax is a transcription target of p53, the promoter region of Bax containing p53 binding sites (TREVES et al. 1994). Studies on tumorigenesis in appropriate genetically modified animals suggest that deletion of p53 and overexpression of Bcl-2 may be viewed as occurring cooperatively to bring about tumorigenesis. More recently it has been reported that Bax-deficient mice did not display an increased incidence of spontaneous cancers and Bax-deficiency did not further accelerate oncogenesis in mice also deficient in p53 (KNUDSON et al. 2001). Such paradoxical observations are by no means isolated in the field and mitigate against sequential models involving these various genes being adequate to explain all observations made.

While members of the "death receptor" family and their ligands have structural elements in common, agents and stimuli initiating the mitochondrial pathway to apoptosis are diverse (REED 1999). Common to these stimuli, however, is a change in mitochondrial function culminating in release of cytochrome c, a scenario often mediated by members of the Bcl-2 family (GROSS et al. 1999). Following potentially lethal DNA damage by agents such as staurosporine and ultraviolet irradiation, cytosolic and monomeric Bax protein translocates to the mitochondria where it becomes an integral membrane protein mediating release of cytochrome C (WOLTER et al. 1997). Similar insults result in cleavage of Bid and associated alterations in mitochondrial integrity (SLEE et al. 2000); indeed, Bid and Bax may operate together in this context (CROMPTON 2000). Mitochondrial dysfunction is evident from swelling, alkalinization and a fall in the transmembrane potential ($\Psi\Delta m$) constituted by the H^+ gradient integral to the synthesis of ATP, this effect being readily assayed by flow cytometry using an appropriate dye. Loss of transmembrane potential follows cytochrome c release and is dependent on caspase activation (see Sect. F.I.), whereas cytochrome c release is not. Antiapoptotic members of the Bcl-2 family, including Bcl-2 and Bcl-x_L, are found in the outer mitochondria membrane as well as in the endoplasmic reticulum and the nuclear membrane. Processes underlying mitochondrial change coincident with apoptosis have been subject to intense investigation. Bcl-2, Bcl-x_L, and Bax can form ion channels when they are added to synthetic membranes, and this may be related to their impact on mitochondrial biology (Matsuyama et al. 2000). The structural similarity between Bcl-x_L and the pore-forming helices of bacterial toxins has been noted as indicating the Bcl-2 family proteins may possess channel-forming capability (Schendel et al. 1998). However, the exact mechanism whereby antiapoptosis members of the Bcl-2 family function at a mitochondrial level to prevent cell death remains to be established (Strasser et al. 2000).

Generally, cell death mediated by Fas and certain members of the TNF family is not blocked by overexpression of Bcl-2 or other antiapoptotic members of the Bcl-2 family, but this rule is not absolute. In some cells such as Jurkat leukemia, expression of Bcl-2/Bcl-x_L can interfere with the death signal delivered by Fas. Such cell death is not dependent upon activation of caspase 8 but upon mitochondrial dysfunction. Also, after activation of the extrinsic pathway, caspase-8 may cleave the proapoptotic Bcl-2 family member Bid, a fragment of which translocates to the mitochondria and promotes cytochrome c release (Stoka et al. 2001).

In the cytosol after release from mitochondria, cytochrome c activates the caspases through formation of a complex: the vertebrate "apoptosome" (Fig. 2). Cytochrome c binds with the scaffolding protein Apaf-1 (apoptotic-

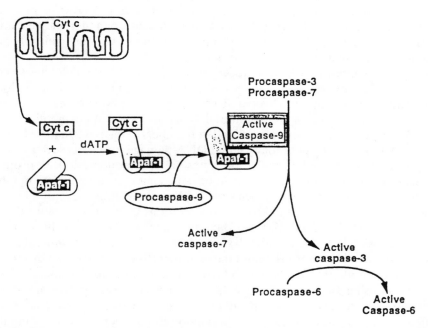

Fig. 2. Components involved in caspase activation by means of the intrinsic pathway. The role that anti- and proapoptotic members of the Bcl-2 family may affect release of cytochrome c from mitochondria in response to a range of stimuli, including irradiation and cytotoxic drugs, is not illustrated and remains to be fully understood. (Adapted from Kaufmann and Gores 2000)

protease activating factor-1), causing an ATP- or dATP-induced conformational change through which procaspase-9 is proteolytically activated (BUDI-HARDJO et al. 1999). Apaf-1 contains a caspase-associated recruitment domain (CARD) which binds specifically to a complementary CARD within the prodomain of procaspase-9. E2F-induced apoptosis, discussed in Sect. D.I., is explicable on the basis of Apaf-1 being a transcriptional target for both E2F and p53 (MORONI et al. 2001).

In the first instance, the machinery of apoptosis is usefully (and inevitably) conceived as a linear relationship between gene products which function either enzymically or as mediating signal transduction to bring about caspase activation and cell death. The difficulty of consistent ordering of observations made concerning apoptosis (or lack of it) resulting from overexpression or deletion of various genes indicates that a network is a more useful, and presumably more valid, means of ordering observations. Moreover, beyond genes identified as mediating apoptosis, there are a range of observations revealing changes in life/death status being critically dependent on specific signaling pathways. Foremost in this category is the role played by the protein kinase Akt (protein kinase B). Akt is activated by phosphorylation through a reaction sequence involving lipid kinase PI3k and 3-phosphoinositide-dependent protein kinases. In common with many other such genes, Akt has a critical role in regulating the cell cycle (EL DEIRY, 2001) as well as apoptosis. The influence exerted by Akt is indicated by the range of its substrates (DATTA et al. 1999). Thus, phosphorylation of Bad protein by Akt (and other kinases) prevents dimerization with Bcl-2 and promotes cell survival. Indeed, Akt is usually described as a survival factor (TESTA and BELLACOSA 2001). It has been shown to exert antiapoptotic activity by preventing release of cytochrome c from mitochondria and inactivating forkhead transcription factors which otherwise induce expression of proapoptotic factors such as FasL. Moreover, Akt activates IκB kinase, a positive regulator of NF-κB, which results in the transcription of antiapoptotic genes. In common with many of the genes regulating apoptosis, various bases for alterations in Akt expression have been described in malignancy, some of which are indicated in Sect. G.

F. The Effector Phase

I. Commitment to Death: Caspase Activation

In mammals, at least 13 proteases homologous to ced-3 have been identified and are designated caspases-1 through -13 (KUMAR 1999). All possess an active site cysteine and cleave substrates after aspartic acid residues. They exist as inactive zymogens, but are activated by different processes which most often involve cleavage of their proforms (designated procaspase-8, etc.) at particular sites, thereby generating subunits which form active proteases consisting of two large and two small subunits. Proteolytic cascades may occur with some caspases operating as upstream initiators (procaspases-8 and -9, which have large N-terminal prodomains and are activated by protein–protein interaction) and others being downstream effectors (procaspases-3, -6 and -7, which are substrates of the initiators). In the context of the extrinsic pathway, affinity labeling suggests caspase-8 activates caspases-3 and -7 and that caspase-3 in turn may activate caspase-6.

With reference to the intrinsic pathway, caspase-9 activates caspase-3 in the first instance. Some interaction between the pathways is evident. Thus, caspase-9 is able to activate caspase-8. Nonetheless, the pathways are separate to the extent that caspase-8 null animals are resistant to Fas- or TNF-induced apoptosis while still susceptible to chemotherapeutic drugs; cells deficient in caspase-9 are sensitive to killing by Fas/TNF but show resistance to drugs and dexamethasone. These findings are indicative of an extensive literature concerning "knockout" of caspases and other components of the cell death pathway (RANGER et al. 2001). Many such knockouts are viable notwithstanding specific defects. Amongst seven caspase knockout phenotypes, for example, only caspase-8 was embryonic lethal. The data are indicative of widespread degeneracy amongst the death signaling pathways: an expression, in itself, of how critical such pathways are.

Caspases-3, -7 and -9 are inactivated by members of the inhibitor of apoptosis proteins (IAPs) family, which include XIAP and survivin, this class of protein being conserved throughout evolution. IAPs suppress apoptosis by preventing activation of procaspases and inhibiting their enzymic activity once activated, thereby mediating another network of control (DEVERAUX and REED 1999). Thus, in response to potentially lethal injury, Smac (second mitochondria-derived activator of caspases)/DIABLO is released from mitochondria along with cytochrome c and regulates apoptosis by interacting with IAPs and thereby enhancing caspase-3 activation (CHAI et al. 2000). Smac also affects the efficacy with which XIAP inhibits caspase-9, suggesting that the ability of caspase-9 and caspase-3 to bring about cell death is dependent upon the stoichiometry of XIAP and its antagonist Smac (SRINIVASULA et al. 2001).

II. Caspase Substrates and Late Stages of Apoptosis

Apoptosis was initially defined by reference to specific morphological change. In fact, both mitosis and apoptosis are characterized by a loss of substrate attachment, condensation of chromatin and phosphorylation and disassembly of nuclear lamins. These changes are now attributable to caspase activation and its consequences.

Most of the more than 60 known caspase substrates are specifically cleaved by caspase-3 and caspase-3 can process procaspases 2, 6, 7, and 9 (PORTER and JANICKE 1999). Despite the multiplicity of substrates, protease activity mediated by caspases is specific and seems likely to account for much of the morphological change associated with apoptosis. Caspases cleave key components of the cytoskeleton, including actin as well as nuclear lamins and other structural proteins. Thus, caspase-3 cleaves the Rho-activated serine/threonine kinase ROCK-1, it being shown that expression of the truncated form of ROCK-1 is sufficient to induce cell contraction and membrane blebbing (COLEMAN et al. 2001). Classes of enzymes cleaved by caspases cover proteins involved in DNA metabolism and repair exemplified by poly(ADP-ribose) polymerase and DNA-dependent protein kinase. Other classes of substrates include various kinases, proteins in signal transduction pathways and proteins involved in cell cycle control, as exemplified by pRb. Cleavage of some substrates is cell type specific.

Caspase activity accounts for internucleosomal cleavage of DNA, one of the first characterized biochemical indicators of apoptosis. ICAD/DFF-45 is a binding partner and inhibitor of the CAD (caspase-activated DNAase) endonuclease, and cleavage of ICAD by capase-3 relieves the inhibition and promotes the endonuclease activity of CAD (NAGATA 2000). Another candidate nuclease has been identified. Mitochondrial proteins released in response to Bid include endonuclease-G, which also generates a DNA "ladder" after incubation with isolated nuclei (LI et al. 2001).

G. Subverting Apoptosis: The Road to Malignancy

The complexity of malignant disease is implicit in its multifaceted nature and the multidirectional approaches that can be taken to either describe the development of cancer or the basis of therapy. The multifaceted nature of the problem is implicit in the multiple chapters of the present volume and it will be readily apparent from these that few exist in total isolation. Rather, these facets are interdependent and their definition – which is necessary for ordering the data available – is somewhat arbitrary. Malignant cells differ from normal cells across a spectrum of parameters, specifically including the apoptotic process. As REED has indicated (REED 1999), mechanisms of apoptosis avoidance are fundamental to cancer development. The issue may be approached by reference to a specific tumor type. Numerous reviews from this perspective are available (PARTON et al. 2001b; LIN 2001; JOHNSON and HAMDY 1998; VOUTSADAKIS 2000; WICKREMASINGHE and HOFFBRAND 1999). The present discussion is a more generic approach in which reference is made to different components of apoptosis as a framework for outlining change observed in various tumor types (Table 1).

The significance of p53 biology to carcinogenesis is readily indicated by this gene being the subject of a separate chapter in the present volume. The role of p53 in cancer is not adequately addressed by its being simply categorized as a cell cycle gene or an apoptosis gene (EVAN and VOUSDEN 2001). On the other hand, consideration of how apoptosis is disrupted in carcinogenesis and in cancer cannot avoid the consideration that this gene is critical to apoptosis and is mutated in most human malignancy (HAINAUT and HOLLSTEIN 2000). The detail of disrupted p53 function in human tumors is not pursued here. However, it should be noted that the manner in which mutation of

Table 1. Apoptosis subverted in cancer cells

Mechanism	Process affected	Tumor type
Deregulation of the link between cell cycle control apoptosis	Mutation of p53	A proportion (sometimes more than 50%) of most human cancer including esophageal, lung, pancreas, colorectum, bladder tumors
Increased cell survival	Overexpression of Bcl-2/Bcl-X$_L$	Follicular lymphoma: t(14,18) AML and prostate, breast, lung, colorectal tumors
Suppression of apoptosis	Mutation or downregulation of Bax	Leukemias; colon, stomach, and breast tumors
Subverting apoptosis otherwise mediated by the immune response	Overexpression of FasL	Leukemias; solid tumors, including head and neck tumors
Subverting the extrinsic pathway	Mutation or downregulation of TRAIL-receptor	Metastatic breast cancer; melanoma
Altered signal transduction	Amplification or upregulation of Akt	Many tumor types including stomach, pancreas, ovarian tumors
	Overexpression of survivin	Many cancers including colorectum, lung
	Upregulation of NF-κB	Breast cancer, lymphoma
Alterations at effector stage	Mutation or reduced expression	Mutation of caspases in some lines
		Altered expression in prostate cancer, neuroblastoma

Of necessity, this table involves an overview. It must be noted that reference to tumor types is indicative of reports that some, as distinct from all, of the malignancies specified exhibit the process in question. Relevant references are cited in the text.

p53 is, in many instances, relatable to specific carcinogenic factors is a singular consideration. In respect of other genetically-based change delineated in this section, the mutation or other effect is evident in the tumor but not attributable to an environmental factor.

Bcl-2 was discovered at the t(14: 18) chromosomal translocation in low grade B cell non-Hodgkin's lymphoma which thereby exemplify neoplastic cell expansion attributable to decreased cell death rather than rapid proliferation. It is now evident that overexpression of antiapoptotic members of the Bcl-2 family is evident in human cancers (ZHENG 2001) although relevant mechanisms are not clear. Such overexpression is often, but not invariably associated with poor prognosis; specific examples include AML, cancer of prostate, and upper aerodigestive tract. However, Bcl-2 is overexpressed in about 80% of breast cancers and is correlated with expression of steroid receptors and other positive prognostic features and with survival (DAIDONE et al. 1999). The paradoxical result is far from exceptional, in that Bcl-2 expression has been correlated with good prognosis in lung (PEZZELLA et al. 1993) and colorectal cancer (KAKLAMANIS et al. 1998). It would appear that Bcl-2 expression is often correlated with a high rather than a low apoptotic index. In most cases, the summary statements here represent generalizations with respect to studies of which there are multiple examples, often involving other indicators and/or consideration of tumors by stage or other subcategory. There seems little doubt that Bcl-2 expression is modified in many tumors; however, simple correlations are not apparent. A possible explanation for paradoxical findings in relation to Bcl-2 (and p53) and prognosis has been offered on the basis of these proteins not being determinant in cells resistant to apoptosis by other mechanisms (BLAGOSKLONNY 2001).

Bcl-x_L is a potent death suppressor as indicated by relevant transduction studies in a variety of malignant cells. By comparison with Bcl-2, there have been relatively few studies of the status of Bcl-x_L status in clinical tumors, though it is reported to be overexpressed, and correlated with poor prognosis, in pancreatic cancer (FRIESS et al. 1998).

Decreased expression of proapoptotic members of the Bcl-2 family, such as Bax and Bak might be anticipated. Downregulation of Bax by both mutational and nonmutational mechanisms has been described in colon and stomach cancer, as well as in hematological malignancies (YIN et al. 1997). Nonetheless, such mutation is not always observed when examined (STURM et al. 2000). The references cited are only indicative of an extensive literature in which tumors are often assessed in relation to multiple genes, and often in respect of parameters which include responsiveness to chemotherapy. Such studies have not given rise to criteria of general application with respect to genetic alterations indicative either of prognosis or responsiveness to cytotoxic drugs.

Growth of tumors is not only favored by mechanisms which suppress apoptosis in malignant cells, but also by mechanisms which induce apoptosis, specifically in cells mediating the immune response. Initially, tumors of hematopoietic origin, and later many carcinomas, were found to express FasL (WALKER et al. 1998) and the list increases. Thus, expression of FasL on squamous cell carcinomas of the head and neck is consistent with this mechanism mediating escape of such tumor cells from immune destruction (GASTMAN et al. 1999). Otherwise, the extrinsic apoptosis pathway may be modified in malignant populations to prevent their being eliminated by this route to cell death. Broad generalizations in relation to TRAIL-mediated apoptosis with respect to multiple tumor types have not emerged (GRIFFITH and LYNCH 1998), although insight is provided from specific studies. In a study of 57 breast cancer cases, those few exhibiting mutations in TRAIL-receptor were restricted to metastatic disease (SHIN et al. 2001). Melanoma cells may downregulate

TRAIL-receptor to escape apoptosis mediated by that route (Griffith et al. 1998).

Multiple mechanisms are evident through which altered Akt function might disrupt apoptosis. For example, phosphorylation of the Bad gene product by Akt (or other kinases) prevents its dimerization with Bcl-2/Bcl-x_L. Akt is sometimes amplified in gastric, pancreatic, or ovarian cancer (Ruggeri et al. 1998). Akt is, in fact, a family of kinases (Akt1, 2 and 3) and it has been suggested that one or more members of that family may become hyperactive in most human cancer (Di Cristofano and Pandolfi, 2000).

The IAP protein "survivin" is overexpressed in a large proportion of human cancers (Ambrosini et al. 1997), a generalization which appears to be a consistent finding in line with expectation. Thus, survivin expression confers poorer prognosis in colorectal cancer (Kawasaki et al. 1998) and nonsmall cell lung carcinoma (Monzo et al. 1999). NF-κB can suppress cell death by inducing transcription of several antiapoptotic genes including Bcl-x_L and some IAPs. Activated NF-κB has been described in primary breast tumors (Nakshatri et al. 1997) and is required for survival of Hodgkin's disease tumor cells (Bargou et al. 1997). Some, but not all forms of non-Hodgkin's lymphoma rely on constitutively active NF-κB signaling pathway for survival (Davis et al. 2001).

Little is known about the involvement of caspase mutations or modified activation in cancer. Examples of loss of expression or mutational inactivation of specific caspases have been found in human tumor cell lines. Thus, no differences in protein level of procaspases-2, -3, -7, and -9 were detected between the small cell lung carcinoma and the nonsmall cell lung carcinoma cell lines, but a striking difference in procaspase-8 expression was noted (Joseph et al. 1999). Procaspase-8 was undetectable in a majority of neuroblastoma lines, apparently as consequence of gene methylation (Teitz et al. 2000). Studies of clinical material are limited. In childhood acute lymphoblastic leukemia, loss of spontaneous caspase-3 processing was evident at relapse (Prokop et al. 2000). No evidence of difference in mRNA levels for various caspases were evident when prostate tumors were compared to normal tissue, although levels of caspase-1 and caspase-3 proteins were relatively reduced in the malignant tissue (Winter et al. 2001). Clearly such findings are insufficient to establish whether effects on caspases are a primary means by which malignant cells gain an advantage over normal tissue.

H. Therapeutic Implications

The manner in which experimental and clinical cancer responds to cytotoxic drugs, and specifically, the differences in such responses between normal and malignant cells, between different malignancies, or between different cell populations belonging to the same type of malignancy, identifies a huge area of investigation. Such research specifically includes the study of drug-resistant phenotypes. While often, at least under experimental conditions, being attributable to altered structure or expression of genes mediating the transport, metabolism, or elimination of drugs from cells, or defining a biological "target" for the drug in question, such genes also include those mediating apoptosis. The role of p53 as determining the efficacy of cytotoxic drugs exemplifies such studies (Lowe et al. 1994). Likewise, the overexpression of Bcl-2 markedly reduces the sensitivity of cultured cells to a range of cytotoxic drugs and to radiation (Reed et al. 1996). These (and similar) observations have prompted surveys of tumors in an attempt to establish correlations of relevant genetic characteristics with prognosis. The results are far from uniform. Thus, clinical studies have not consistently established that mutation of p53 is predictive of a poor response to chemotherapy. Responses are often tumor specific (Kemp et al. 2001). No attempt is made to review those studies here except to note that anticipated "intuitive" correlations are not often reported. Also, it must be noted that the role of p53 and Bcl-2 in apparently mediating drug resistance may be inferred from cytotoxicity assays but not from clonogenic assays (Brown and Wouters 1999). The following discussion is restricted to studies in which specific components of the apoptotic pathway have been identified as "targets" for putative anticancer agents, rather than the possibly broader body of research concerned with identifying apoptotic processes induced by cytotoxic agents (Makin and Hickman 2000; Mow et al. 2001).

In theory, knowledge of critical signaling or effector pathways which bring about apoptosis provides a basis for therapeutic intervention, perhaps by the development of novel drugs to activate particular pathways. Options for therapy include not only inducing apoptosis with a view to cancer treatment, but also of inhibiting apoptosis to improve management of degenerative diseases (Reed 2002). Only approaches perceived as relevant to cancer are considered here.

The possibility of restoring mutant p53 function, or otherwise using p53 to kill cancer cells is recognized (Vogelstein and Kinzler 2001). Options include introducing normal p53 genes, a small compound to alter mutant p53 protein conformation to normal or a protein that attaches itself to p53 and causes cell death, as well as others. A recent protocol has involved an adenovirus which mimics damaged DNA consequently rendering cells with mutant p53 susceptible to apoptosis (Raj et al. 2001). Likewise, members of the Bcl-2 family may be targeted. One strategy is the use of small molecules that bind to Bcl-2/ Bcl-x$_L$ such that they could not bind to Bax and similar proteins to inhibit their death-inducing activity (Zheng 2001). In a variety of cell culture systems and preclinical animal models, suppression of Bcl-2 by an antisense oligonucleotide has been shown to retard tumor growth sufficiently consistently to justify phase 1 trials in non-Hodgkin's lymphoma (Waters et al. 2000).

In theory, any step in the survival signaling pathway(s) might be inhibited and/or a corresponding step mediating apoptosis might be activated as a means of limiting malignant growth (Nicholson 2000). Antisense oligonucleotides directed at "survivin," an inhibitor of apoptosis (IAP) family member, are being evaluated (Olie et al. 2000). The possibility of using recombinant TRAIL to induce apoptosis in malignant cells is under investigation. Peptides that, once internalized by cells, can cause mitochondrial disruption resulting in release of cytochrome c and apoptosis, have been described (Mai et al. 2001), as has adenovirus-mediated transfer of inducible caspases (Shariat et al. 2001). Obviously, these and similar observations are yet to indicate improved therapy for patients, but the potential is obvious.

Drugs shown to induce apoptosis specifically include chemopreventive agents, exemplified by 4-hydroxyphenylretinamide (Kitareewan et al. 1999). TRAIL is implicated as the basis of *all-trans* retinoic-induced apoptosis of promyelocytic leukemia, suggesting a possible role of recombinant TRAIL in cancer therapy (Altucci et al. 2001). Butyrate, a short-chain fatty acid produced by bacterial fermentation of dietary fiber, inhibits cell growth in vitro and promotes differentiation; it also induces apoptosis (Bonnotte et al. 1998). Both roles may contribute to its prevention of colorectal cancer. Dietary flavones have a similar effect (Wenzel et al. 2000). Moreover, cyclooxygenase enzyme (COX-2) expression may modulate intestinal apoptosis via changes in Bcl-2 expression. Aspirin and similar drugs which inhibit COX-2 may promote apoptosis and prevent tumor formation (Huang et al. 2001).

I. Conclusion

By comparison with the role of DNA damage, or the role of proliferative activity in carcinogenesis, study of the role of cell death in this process is recent. So recent, that certain areas of investigation are "missing." There are no comprehensive structure-activity relationships concerning induction of apoptosis analogous to those which provide a comprehensive data base concerning the impact of chemical carcinogens on normal tissue. However, the understanding of carcinogenesis as a multistage process, and the explanation of this process at a genetic level, includes and accommodates knowledge of apoptotic processes. The processes themselves have provided tools for revealing aspects of malignant transformation. Moreover, this same area of investigation has provided increased understanding of how conventional cytotoxic agents work and how better agents might be developed. At this time, limits to the potential offered are not apparent.

References

Altucci L, Rossin A, Raffelsberger W, Reitmair A, Chomienne C, Gronemeyer H (2001) Retinoic acid-induced apoptosis in leukemia cells is mediated by paracrine action of tumor-selective death ligand TRAIL. Nat Med 7:680–686
Ambrosini G, Adida C, Altieri DC (1997) A novel antiapoptosis gene, survivin, expressed in cancer and lymphoma. Nat Med 3:917–921
Arends MJ, Morris RG, Wyllie AH (1990) Apoptosis: The role of endonuclease. AM J Path 136:593–608

Ashkenazi A, Dixit VM (1998) Death receptors: signaling and modulation. Science 281:1305–1308

Bao S, Tibbetts RS, Brumbaugh KM, Fang Y, Richardson DA, Ali A, Chen SM, Abraham RT, Wang XF (2001) ATR/ATM-mediated phosphorylation of human Rad17 is required for genotoxic stress responses. Nature 411:969–974

Bargou RC, Emmerich F, Krappmann D, Bommert K, Mapara MY, Arnold W, Royer HD, Grinstein E, Greiner A, Scheidereit C, Dorken B (1997) Constitutive nuclear factor-kappaB-RelA activation is required for proliferation and survival of Hodgkin's disease tumor cells. J Clin Invest 100:2961–2969

Blagosklonny MV (2001) Paradox of Bcl-2 (and p53): why may apoptosis-regulating proteins be irrelevant to cell death? BE 23:947–953

Bonnotte B, Favre N, Reveneau S, Micheau O, Droin N, Garrido C, Fontana A, Chauffert B, Solary E, Martin F (1998) Cancer cell sensitization to fas-mediated apoptosis by sodium butyrate. Cell Death Differ 5:480–487

Brown JM, Wouters BG (1999) Apoptosis, p53, and tumor cell sensitivity to anticancer agents. Cancer Res 59:1391–1399 Ref ID: 2887

Budihardjo I, Oliver H, Lutter M, Luo X, Wang X (1999) Biochemical pathways of caspase activation during apoptosis. Annu Rev Cell Dev Biol 15:269–290

Chai J, Du C, Wu JW, Kyin S, Wang X, Shi Y (2000) Structural and biochemical basis of apoptotic activation by Smac/DIABLO. Nature 406:855–862

Chen AY, Liu LF (1994) DNA topoisomerases: essential enzymes and lethal targets. Annu Rev Pharmacol Toxicol 34:191–218

Chiou S-K, Rao L, White E (1994) Bcl-2 blocks p53-dependent apoptosis. Mol Cell Biol 14:2556–2563

Choisy-Rossi C, Yonish-Rouach E (1998) Apoptosis and the cell cycle: the p53 connection. Cell Death Differ 5:129–131

Coleman ML, Sahai EA, Yeo M, Bosch M, Dewar A, Olson MF (2001) Membrane blebbing during apoptosis results from caspase-mediated activation of ROCK I. Nat Cell Biol 3:339–345

Cortez D, Guntuku S, Qin J, Elledge SJ (2001) ATR and ATRIP: Partners in Checkpoint Signaling. Science 294:1713–1716

Cory S, Vaux DL, Strasser A, Harris AW, Adams JM (1999) Insights from Bcl-2 and Myc: malignancy involves abrogation of apoptosis as well as sustained proliferation. Cancer Res 59:1685s–1692s

Crompton M (2000) Bax, Bid and the permeabilization of the mitochondrial outer membrane in apoptosis. Curr Opin Cell Biol 12:414–419

Daidone MG, Luisi A, Veneroni S, Benini E, Silvestrini R (1999) Clinical studies of Bcl-2 and treatment benefit in breast cancer patients. Endocr Relat Cancer 6:61–68

Datta SR, Brunet A, Greenberg ME (1999) Cellular survival: a play in three Akts. Genes Dev 13:2905–2927

Davis RE, Brown KD, Siebenlist U, Staudt LM (2001) Constitutive Nuclear Factor kappaB Activity Is Required for Survival of Activated B Cell-like Diffuse Large B Cell Lymphoma Cells. J Exp Med 194:1861–1874

Denko N, Schindler C, Koong A, Laderoute K, Green C, Giaccia A (2000) Epigenetic regulation of gene expression in cervical cancer cells by the tumor microenvironment. Clin Cancer Res 6:480–487

Deveraux QL, Reed JC (1999) IAP family proteins–suppressors of apoptosis. Genes Dev 13:239–252

Di Cristofano A, Pandolfi PP (2000) The multiple roles of PTEN in tumor suppression. Cell 100:387–390

Dive C, Hickman JA (1991) Drug-target interactions: only the first step in the commitment to a programmed cell death? Br J Cancer 64:192–196

Eischen CM, Kottke TJ, Martins LM, Basi GS, Tung JS, Earnshaw WC, Leibson PJ, Kaufmann SH (1997) Comparison of apoptosis in wild-type and fas-resistant cells: Chemotherapy-induced apoptosis is not dependent on fas/fas ligand interactions. Blood 90:935–943

El Deiry WS (2001) Akt takes centre stage in cell-cycle deregulation. Nat Cell Biol 3:E71–E73

Evan GI, Vousden KH (2001) Proliferation, cell cycle and apoptosis in cancer. Nature 411:342–348

Evan GI, Wyllie AH, Gilbert CS, Littlewood TD, Land H, Brooks M, Waters CM, Penn LZ, Hancock DC (1992) Induction of apoptosis in fibroblasts by c-myc protein. Cell 69:119–128

Friess H, Lu Z, Andren-Sandberg A, Berberat P, Zimmermann A, Adler G, Schmid R, Buchler MW (1998) Moderate activation of the apoptosis inhibitor bcl-xL worsens the prognosis in pancreatic cancer. Ann Surg 228:780–787

Frisen C, Herr I, Krammer PH, Debatin K-M (1996) Involvement of the CD95 (APO-1/Fas) receptor/ligand system in drug-induced apoptosis in leukaemia cells. Nature Med 2:574–577

Gastman BR, Atarshi Y, Reichert TE, Saito T, Balkir L, Rabinowich H, Whiteside TL (1999) Fas ligand is expressed on human squamous cell carcinomas of the head and neck, and it promotes apoptosis of T lymphocytes. Cancer Res 59: 5356–5364

Gerschenson LE, Rotello RJ (1992) Apoptosis: A different type of cell death. FASEB 6:2450–2455

Griffith TS, Chin WA, Jackson GC, Lynch DH, Kubin MZ (1998) Intracellular regulation of TRAIL-induced apoptosis in human melanoma cells. J Immunol 161: 2833–2840

Griffith TS, Lynch DH (1998) TRAIL: a molecule with multiple receptors and control mechanisms. Curr Opin Immunol 10:559–563

Gross A, McDonnell JM, Korsmeyer SJ (1999) BCL-2 family members and the mitochondria in apoptosis. Genes Dev 13:1899–1911

Guo M, Hay BA (1999) Cell proliferation and apoptosis. Curr Opin Cell Biol 11: 745–752

Hainaut P, Hollstein M (2000) p53 and human cancer: the first ten thousand mutations. Adv Cancer Res 77:81–137

Hanahan D, Weinberg RA (2000) The hallmarks of cancer. Cell 100:57–70

Harbour JW, Dean DC (2000) Rb function in cell-cycle regulation and apoptosis. Nat Cell Biol 2:E65–E67

Hickman JA (1992) Apoptosis induced by anticancer drugs. Cancer Metast Rev 11:121–139

Hockenbery DM, Oltvai ZN, Yin X-M, Milliman CL, Korsmeyer SJ (1993) Bcl-2 functions in an antioxidant pathway to prevent apoptosis. Cell 75:241–251

Hoeijmakers JH (2001) Genome maintenance mechanisms for preventing cancer. Nature 411:366–374

Huang Y, He Q, Hillman MJ, Rong R, Sheikh MS (2001) Sulindac sulfide-induced apoptosis involves death receptor 5 and the caspase 8-dependent pathway in human colon and prostate cancer cells. Cancer Res 61:6918–6924

Johnson MI, Hamdy FC (1998) Apoptosis regulating genes in prostate cancer (review). Oncol Rep 5:553–557

Jones PA, Gonzalgo ML (1997) Altered DNA methylation and genome instability: A new pathway to cancer? Proc Natl Acad Sci USA 94:2103–2105

Joseph B, Ekedahl J, Sirzen F, Lewensohn R, Zhivotovsky B (1999) Differences in expression of procaspases in small cell and nonsmall cell lung carcinoma. Biochem Biophys Res Commun 262:381–387

Kaklamanis L, Savage A, Whitehouse R, Doussis-Anagnostopoulou I, Biddolph S, Tsiotos P, Mortensen N, Gatter KC, Harris AL (1998) Bcl-2 protein expression: association with p53 and prognosis in colorectal cancer. Br J Cancer 77:1864–1869

Kasten MM, Giordano A (1998) pRb and the Cdks in apoptosis and the cell cycle. Cell Death Differ 5:132–140

Kaufmann SH, Gores GJ (2000) Apoptosis in cancer: cause and cure. Bioessays 22: 1007–1017

Kawasaki H, Altieri DC, Lu CD, Toyoda M, Tenjo T, Tanigawa N (1998) Inhibition of apoptosis by survivin predicts shorter survival rates in colorectal cancer. Cancer Res 58:5071–5074

Kemp CJ, Sun S, Gurley KE (2001) p53 induction and apoptosis in response to r. Cancer Res 61:327–332

Kitareewan S, Spinella MJ, Allopenna J, Reczek PR, Dmitrovsky E (1999) 4HPR triggers apoptosis but not differentiation in retinoid sensitive and resistant human embryonal carcinoma cells through an RARgamma independent pathway. Oncogene 18:5747–5755

Knudson CM, Johnson GM, Lin Y, Korsmeyer SJ (2001) Bax accelerates tumorigenesis in p53-deficient mice. Cancer Res 61:659–665

Knudson CM, Korsmeyer SJ (1997) Bcl-2 and bax function independently to regulate cell death. Nature Gen 16:358–363

Krammer PH, Behrmann I, Daniel P, Dhein J, Debatin K-M (1994) Regulation of apoptosis in the immune system. Curr Opin Immunol 6:279–289

Kumar S (1999) Regulation of caspase activation in apoptosis: implications in pathogenesis and treatment of disease. Clin Exp Pharmacol Physiol 26:295–303

Li LY, Luo X, Wang X (2001) Endonuclease G is an apoptotic DNase when released from mitochondria. Nature 412:95–99

Lin JD (2001) The role of apoptosis in autoimmune thyroid disorders and thyroid cancer. Brit Med J 322:1525–1527

Logan TJ, Evans DL, Mercer WE, Bjornsti M-A, Hall DJ (1995) Expression of a deletion mutant of the E2F1 transcription factor in fibroblasts lengthens S phase and increases sensitivity to S phase-specific toxins. Cancer Res 55:2883–2891

Lotan R (1995) Retinoids and apoptosis: Implications for cancer chemoprevention and therapy. J Natl Cancer Inst 87:1655–1657

Lowe SW, Bodis S, McClatchey A, Remington L, Ruley HE, Fisher DE, Housman DE, Jacks T (1994) P53 status and the efficacy of cancer therapy in vivo. Science 266: 807–810

Lowe SW, Schmitt EM, Smith SW, Osborne BA, Jacks T (1993) p53 is required for radiation-induced apoptosis in mouse thymocytes. Nature 362:847–849

Mai JC, Mi Z, Kim SH, Ng B, Robbins PD (2001) A proapoptotic peptide for the treatment of solid tumors. Cancer Res 61:7709–7712

Makin G, Hickman JA (2000) Apoptosis and cancer chemotherapy. Cell Tissue Res 301:143–152

Matsuyama S, Llopis J, Deveraux QL, Tsien RY, Reed JC (2000) Changes in intramitochondrial and cytosolic pH: early events that modulate caspase activation during apoptosis. Nat Cell Biol 2:318–325

Meier P, Finch A, Evan G (2000) Apoptosis in development. Nature 407:796–801

Monzo M, Rosell R, Felip E, Astudillo J, Sanchez JJ, Maestre J, Martin C, Font A, Barnadas A, Abad A (1999) A novel antiapoptosis gene: Re-expression of survivin messenger RNA as a prognosis marker in nonsmall-cell lung cancers. J Clin Oncol 17:2100–2104

Moroni MC, Hickman ES, Denchi EL, Caprara G, Colli E, Cecconi F, Muller H, Helin K (2001) Apaf-1 is a transcriptional target for E2F and p53. Nat Cell Biol 3:552–558

Mow BM, Blajeski AL, Chandra J, Kaufmann SH (2001) Apoptosis and the response to anticancer therapy. Curr Opin Oncol 13:453–462

Nagata S (2000) Apoptotic DNA fragmentation. Exp Cell Res 256:12–18

Nakshatri H, Bhat-Nakshatri P, Martin DA, Goulet RJ, Jr., Sledge GW, Jr. (1997) Constitutive activation of NF-kappaB during progression of breast cancer to hormone-independent growth. Mol Cell Biol 17:3629–3639

Nicholson DW (2000) From bench to clinic with apoptosis-based therapeutic agents. Nature 407:810–816

O'Connor L, Harris AW, Strasser A (2000) CD95 (Fas/APO-1) and p53 signal apoptosis independently in diverse cell types. Cancer Res 60:1217–1220

Olie RA, Simoes-Wust AP, Baumann B, Leech SH, Fabbro D, Stahel RA, Zangemeister-Wittke U (2000) A novel antisense oligonucleotide targeting survivin expression induces apoptosis and sensitizes lung cancer cells to chemotherapy. Cancer Res 60:2805–2809

Oltvai ZN, Milliman CL, Korsmeyer SJ (1993) Bcl-2 heterodimerizes in vivo with a conserved homolog, bax, that accelerates programmed cell death. Cell 74:609–619

Packham G, Porter CW, Cleveland JL (1996) c-myc induces apoptosis and cell cycle progression by separable, yet overlapping, pathways. Oncogene 13:461–469

Parton M, Dowsett M, Smith I (2001a) Studies of apoptosis in breast cancer. Brit Med J 322:1528–1532

Parton M, Dowsett M, Smith I (2001b) Studies of apoptosis in breast cancer. Brit Med J 322:1528–1532

Peter ME, Krammer PH (1998) Mechanisms of CD95 (APO-1/Fas)-mediated apoptosis. Curr Opin Immunol 10:545–551

Pezzella F, Turley H, Kuzu I, Tungekar MF, Dunnill MS, Pierce CB, Harris A, Gatter KC, Mason DY (1993) bcl-2 protein in nonsmall-cell lung carcinoma. N Engl J Med 329:690–694

Ponder BA (2001) Cancer genetics. Nature 411:336–341

Porter AG, Janicke RU (1999) Emerging roles of caspase-3 in apoptosis. Cell Death Differ 6:99–104

Prokop A, Wieder T, Sturm I, Essmann F, Seeger K, Wuchter C, Ludwig WD, Henze G, Dorken B, Daniel PT (2000) Relapse in childhood acute lymphoblastic leukemia is associated with a decrease of the Bax/Bcl-2 ratio and loss of spontaneous caspase-3 processing in vivo. Leukemia 14:1606–1613

Raj K, Ogston P, Beard P (2001) Virus-mediated killing of cells that lack p53 activity. Nature 412:914–917

Ranger AM, Malynn BA, Korsmeyer SJ (2001) Mouse models of cell death. Nat Genet 28:113–118

Reed JC (1997) Double identity for proteins of the bcl-2 family. Nature 387:773–776

Reed JC (1999) Mechanisms of apoptosis avoidance in cancer. Curr Opin Oncol 11:68–75

Reed JC (2002) Apoptosis-based therapies. Nature Reviews Drug Discovery 1:111–121

Reed JC, Miyashita T, Takayama S, Wang HG, Sato T, Krajewski S, Aime-Sempe C, Bodrug S, Kitada S, Hanada M (1996) BCL-2 family proteins: regulators of cell death involved in the pathogenesis of cancer and resistance to therapy. J Cell Biochem 60:23–32

Rich T, Allen RL, Wyllie AH (2000) Defying death after DNA damage. Nature 407:777–783

Ruggeri BA, Huang L, Wood M, Cheng JQ, Testa JR (1998) Amplification and overexpression of the AKT2 oncogene in a subset of human pancreatic ductal adenocarcinomas. Mol Carcinog 21:81–86

Samuels-Lev Y, O'Connor DJ, Bergamaschi D, Trigiante G, Hsieh JK, Zhong S, Campargue I, Naumovski L, Crook T, Lu X (2001) ASPP proteins specifically stimulate the apoptotic function of p53. Mol Cell 8:781–794

Schendel SL, Montal M, Reed JC (1998) Bcl-2 family proteins as ion-channels. Cell Death Differ 5:372–380

Schmitt CA, Lowe SW (1999) Apoptosis and therapy. J Pathol 187:127–137

Schulte-Hermann R, Bursch W, Low-Baselli A, Wagner A, Grasl-Kraupp B (1997) Apoptosis in the liver and its role in hepatocarcinogenesis. Cell Biol Toxicol 13:339–348

Schulte-Hermann R, Marian B, Bursch W (1999) Tumor promotion. In Toxicology, Marquardt H, Schafer S, McClellan R, Welsch F (eds) pp 179–215. Academic Press: San Diego

Shariat SF, Desai S, Song W, Khan T, Zhao J, Nguyen C, Foster BA, Greenberg N, Spencer DM, Slawin KM (2001) Adenovirus-mediated transfer of inducible caspases: a novel "death switch" gene therapeutic approach to prostate cancer. Cancer Res 61:2562–2571

Shin MS, Kim HS, Lee SH, Park WS, Kim SY, Park JY, Lee JH, Lee SK, Lee SN, Jung SS, Han JY, Kim H, Lee JY, Yoo NJ (2001) Mutations of tumor necrosis factor-related apoptosis-inducing ligand receptor 1 (TRAIL-R1) and receptor 2 (TRAIL-R2) genes in metastatic breast cancers. Cancer Res 61:4942–4946

Slee EA, Keogh SA, Martin SJ (2000) Cleavage of BID during cytotoxic drug and UV radiation-induced apoptosis occurs downstream of the point of Bcl-2 action and is catalyzed by caspase-3:a potential feedback loop for amplification of apoptosis-associated mitochondrial cytochrome c release. Cell Death Differ 7:556–565

Srinivasula SM, Hegde R, Saleh A, Datta P, Shiozaki E, Chai J, Lee RA, Robbins PD, Fernandes-Alnemri T, Shi Y, Alnemri ES (2001) A conserved XIAP-interaction motif in caspase-9 and Smac/DIABLO regulates caspase activity and apoptosis. Nature 410:112–116

Stewart BW (1994) Mechanisms of apoptosis: Integration of genetic, biochemical and cellular indicators. J Natl Cancer Inst 86:1286–1296

Stoka V, Turk B, Schendel SL, Kim TH, Cirman T, Snipas SJ, Ellerby LM, Bredesen D, Freeze H, Abrahamson M, Bromme D, Krajewski S, Reed JC, Yin XM, Turk V, Salvesen GS (2001) Lysosomal protease pathways to apoptosis. Cleavage of bid, not pro caspases, is the most likely route. J Biol Chem 276:3149–3157

Strasser A, O'Connor L, Dixit VM (2000) Apoptosis signaling. Annu Rev Biochem 69:217–245

Sturm I, Papadopoulos S, Hillebrand T, Benter T, Luck HJ, Wolff G, Dorken B, Daniel PT (2000) Impaired BAX protein expression in breast cancer: mutational analysis of the BAX and the p53 gene. Int J Cancer 87:517–521

Teitz T, Wei T, Valentine MB, Vanin EF, Grenet J, Valentine VA, Behm FG, Look AT, Lahti JM, Kidd VJ (2000) Caspase 8 is deleted or silenced preferentially in childhood neuroblastomas with amplification of MYCN. Nat Med 6:529–535

Testa JR, Bellacosa A (2001) AKT plays a central role in tumorigenesis. Proc Natl Acad Sci USA 98:10983–10985

Treves S, Trentini PL, Ascanelli M, Bucci G, Di Virgilio F (1994) Apoptosis is dependent on intracellular zinc and independent of intracellular calcium in lymphocytes. Exp Cell Res 211:339–343

van Hemert MJ, Steensma HY, van Heusden GP (2001) 14-3-3 proteins: key regulators of cell division, signalling and apoptosis. BE 23:936–946

Vogelstein B, Kinzler KW (2001) Achilles' heel of cancer? Nature 412:865–866

Voutsadakis IA (2000) Apoptosis and the pathogenesis of lymphoma. Acta Oncol 39:151–156

Walker PR, Saas P, Dietrich PY (1998) Tumor expression of Fas ligand (CD95L) and the consequences. Curr Opin Immunol 10:564–572

Waters JS, Webb A, Cunningham D, Clarke PA, Raynaud F, di Stefano F, Cotter FE (2000) Phase I clinical and pharmacokinetic study of bcl-2 antisense oligonucleotide therapy in patients with non-Hodgkin's lymphoma. J Clin Oncol 18:1812–1823

Wenzel U, Kuntz S, Brendel MD, Daniel H (2000) Dietary flavone is a potent apoptosis inducer in human colon carcinoma cells. Cancer Res 60:3823–3831

Wickremasinghe RG, Hoffbrand AV (1999) Biochemical and genetic control of apoptosis: relevance to normal hematopoiesis and hematological malignancies. Blood 93:3587–3600

Winter RN, Kramer A, Borkowski A, Kyprianou N (2001) Loss of caspase-1 and caspase-3 protein expression in human prostate cancer. Cancer Res 61:1227–1232

Wolter KG, Hsu YT, Smith CL, Nechushtan A, Xi XG, Youle RJ (1997) Movement of Bax from the cytosol to mitochondria during apoptosis. J Cell Biol 139:1281–1292

Wong CW, Lee A, Shientag L, Yu J, Dong Y, Kao G, Al Mehdi AB, Bernhard EJ, Muschel RJ (2001) Apoptosis: an early event in metastatic inefficiency. Cancer Res 61:333–338

Wyllie AH (1987) Cell death. Internat Rev Cytol 17:755–785

Yeh WC, Hakem R, Woo M, Mak TW (1999) Gene targeting in the analysis of mammalian apoptosis and TNF receptor superfamily signaling. Immunol Rev 169:283–302

Yin C, Knudson CM, Korsmeyer SJ, Van Dyke T (1997) Bax suppresses tumorigenesis and stimulates apoptosis in vivo. Nature 385:637–640

Zhao H, Spitz MR, Tomlinson GE, Zhang H, Minna JD, Wu X (2001) Gamma-radiation-induced G2 delay, apoptosis, and p53 response as potential susceptibility markers for lung cancer. Cancer Res 61:7819–7824

Zheng TS (2001) Death by design: the big debut of small molecules. Nat Cell Biol 3:E43–E46

Zhou BB, Elledge SJ (2000) The DNA damage response: putting checkpoints in perspective. Nature 408:433–439

CHAPTER 7

Deficient DNA Mismatch Repair in Carcinogenesis

P. PELTOMÄKI

A. DNA Mismatch Repair System in Man

The postreplicative DNA mismatch repair (MMR) system maintains genome integrity by recognizing and repairing mismatched nucleotides that result from misincorporation during DNA synthesis. The genes coding for MMR proteins are highly conserved throughout evolution. The human proteins that correspond to the bacterial MutS proteins and participate in MMR include MSH2, MSH3, and MSH6, whereas the human MutL proteins include MLH1, PMS1, PMS2, and MLH3. Characteristics of the human MMR genes are given in Table 1.

Mismatches may represent single-base substitutions, such as G to T transversion, that typically affect nonrepetitive DNA. Alternatively, mismatches may consist of insertion-deletion loops (IDL) that affect repetitive DNA and arise as a consequence of DNA polymerase slippage during DNA replication. In humans, at least six different MMR proteins are required for the correction of mismatches (KOLODNER and MARSISCHKY 1999; BUERMEYER et al. 1999; JIRICNY and NYSTRÖM LAHTI 2000). For mismatch recognition, the MSH2 protein forms a heterodimer with two additional MMR proteins, MSH6 or MSH3 (the resulting complexes are called hMutSα and hMutSβ, respectively) depending on whether base–base mispairs or insertion-deletion loops (IDL) are to be repaired (Table 2). In the former case, MSH6 is required, while in the latter case, MSH3 and MSH6 have partially redundant functions (MARSISCHKY et al. 1996; DAS GUPTA and KOLODNER 2000). A heterodimer of MLH1 and PMS2 (hMutLα) coordinates the interplay between the mismatch recognition complex and other proteins necessary for MMR. These additional proteins may include at least proliferating cell nuclear antigen, replication factor C, DNA polymerases δ and ε, exonuclease 1 (EXO1), single-stranded DNA-binding protein, and possibly helicase(s). Besides PMS2, MLH1 may heterodimerize with two additional proteins, MLH3 and PMS1. While the MLH1-PMS2 complex contributes to the correction of both single-base mismatches and insertion-deletion loops, the MLH1-MLH3 complex primarily functions in the repair of insertion-deletion loops (LIPKIN et al. 2000). The role, if any, of the MLH1-PMS1 complex (hMutLβ) in MMR remains to be determined (RÄSCHLE et al. 1999; LEUNG et al. 2000). Two additional human MutS homologues are known: MSH4 (PAQUIS-FLUCKLINGER et al. 1997) and MSH5

Table 1. Human genes whose products participate in DNA mismatch repair (MMR)

Gene	Chromosomal location	Length of cDNA (kb)	Number of exons	Genomic size (kb)	References for structure
MSH2[a]	2p21	2.8	16	73	LEACH et al. (1993), FISHEL et al. (1993), LIU et al. (1994), KOLODNER et al. (1994)
MLH1[a]	3p21–23	2.3	19	58–100	PAPADOPOULOS et al. (1994), BRONNER et al. (1994), KOLODNER et al. (1995), HAN et al. (1995)
MSH6[a]	2p21	4.1	10	~20	PALOMBO et al. (1995), NICOLAIDES et al. (1996), ACHARYA et al. (1996)
PMS2[a]	7p22	2.6	15	16	NICOLAIDES et al. (1994), NICOLAIDES et al. (1995)
MLH3[a]	14q24.3	4.3	12	~37	LIPKIN et al. (2000)
PMS1	2q31-q33	2.8	Not known	Not known	NICOLAIDES et al. (1994)
MSH3	5q11-q12	3.4	24	~134	FUJII and SHIMADA (1988), WATANABE et al. (1996)

[a] Germline mutations cause susceptibility to HNPCC.

(WINAND et al. 1998) that are required for meiotic (and possibly mitotic) recombination but are not presumed to participate in MMR.

B. Clinical Phenotypes Associated with DNA MMR Deficiency

The detection of clonal gains or losses of short repeat units [such as (CA) within microsatellite $(CA)_n$] in tumor DNA, referred to as microsatellite instability (MSI), is a useful indicator of MMR deficiency. This phenomenon typically, but not always, results from the failure to correct insertion-deletion loops

Table 2. Designation of complexes of human MMR proteins and their functions in MMR

Protein components	Designation of heterodimer	Function
MSH2 + MSH6	hMutSα	Recognition of single-base mismatches and insertion-deletion loops
MSH2 + MSH3	hMutSβ	Recognition of insertion-deletion loops
MLH1 + PMS2	hMutLα	Interacts with hMutSα and hMutSβ to recruit additional proteins to the site of repair
MLH1 + MLH3		Interacts with hMutSβ to recruit additional proteins to the site of repair
MLH1 + PMS1	hMutLβ	Not known

that arise during DNA replication. MSI is a hallmark of a hereditary form of colon cancer, HNPCC (hereditary nonpolyposis colon cancer) that is associated with germline mutations in four, possibly five, DNA MMR genes (Table 3). Additionally, 15%–20% of sporadic colon (and other) cancers display the MSI phenotype, reflecting an acquired defect in DNA MMR.

HNPCC-associated mutations are dominant on the pedigree level: the predisposed individuals carry one defective copy and one normal copy of a given MMR gene in all their nonneoplastic cells. On the cellular level, the mutations are recessive, since both copies of the MMR gene need to be inactivated for the development of tumors and MSI. Thus, bulk DNA extracted from nonneoplastic cells from HNPCC patients that has retained one normal copy of the MMR gene in question does not show MSI, whereas that extracted from tumor cells does, reflecting the propagation of a clone with both copies of the MMR gene inactivated. Nonneoplastic DNA diluted to the level of one genome equivalent and amplified by a small pool PCR technique usually does not show MSI either, except for rare circumstances. These exceptions include presumably "dominant negative" mutations (PARSONS et al. 1995; MIYAKI et al. 1997a) and homozygous (or doubly heterozygous) mutations (HACKMAN et al. 1997; WANG et al. 1999; RICCIARDONE et al. 1999; DE ROSA et al. 2000; VILKKI et al. 2001). In sporadic tumors with MSI, two somatic events in a MMR gene are required that may occur independently (such as two somatic mutations) or as a result of a single mechanism (biallelic inactivation of MLH1 by promoter hypermethylation, see Sect. II).

I. Hereditary Nonpolyposis Colon Cancer

In spite of the fact that the presently known human MMR genes have been identified relatively recently (during the last decade), HNPCC as a clinical entity has been known for almost a century (WARTHIN 1913). HNPCC is one

Table 3. Clinical phenotypes associated with MMR deficiency

Phenotype	Clinical hallmarks	Mutated MMR genes (major genes underlined)
I. Hereditary		Germline mutations:
HNPCC	At least 3 relatives should have colon cancer (Amsterdam criteria I) or cancer of the endometrium, small intestine ureter, or renal pelvis (Amsterdam criteria II) Additionally, one patient should be a first-degree relative to the other two, at least two successive generations should be affected, and at least one tumor should be diagnosed before age 50.	<u>MLH1</u>, <u>MSH2</u>, MSH6, PMS2 (MLH3)
Muir-Torre syndrome	Occurrence of sebaceous gland tumors together with HNPCC-type internal malignancy	<u>MSH2</u>, MLH1
Turcot syndrome	Association of primary brain tumors (usually glioblastomas) with multiple colorectal adenomas and carcinomas	<u>MLH1</u>, PMS2[a]
Hereditary site-specific endometrial cancer	Familial endometrial cancer	<u>MSH6</u>[b]
II. Acquired		Somatic inactivation:
Sporadic cancers of the HNPCC spectrum	Sporadic colon cancers with MSI-H: Late onset (60–70 years), proximal location, favorable prognosis, female predominance	<u>MLH1</u>[c], MSH2, other MMR genes

[a] Part of the cases with Turcot syndrome are associated with germline mutations in the APC gene.
[b] The etiology is unknown in most cases with hereditary site-specific endometrial cancer.
[c] Usually inactivated through promoter hypermethylation and not as a consequence of mutations.

of the most common forms, if not *the* most common form, of hereditary cancer. Based on clinical estimates, it may account for up to 13% of the total colorectal cancer burden (Houlston et al. 1992). However, based on the occurrence of MMR gene germline mutations in unselected patients of colorectal cancer, the incidence of HNPCC may not be quite as high (0.3%–3% of the total colorectal cancer burden; Aaltonen et al. 1998; Ravnik-Glavac et al. 2000; Cunningham et al. 2001; Samowitz et al. 2001; Percesepe et al. 2001).

According to the international diagnostic criteria (Amsterdam criteria I), at least three close relatives should be affected with colon cancer in two successive generations and the age at diagnosis should be below 50 years in at least one (VASEN et al. 1991) (Table 3). In addition to colon cancer, HNPCC patients often have excess of extracolonic cancers, notably endometrial cancer, and to a lesser extent other cancers, including cancers of the small bowel, ureter and renal pelvis. The diagnostic criteria were recently revised to take these extracolonic cancers into account (Amsterdam criteria II) (VASEN et al. 1999). Variant forms of HNPCC include the Muir-Torre syndrome and Turcot syndrome. Additionally, part of familial site-specific endometrial cancer may be associated with inherited mutations in MMR genes, especially MSH6.

The International Collaborative Group on HNPCC maintains a database of HNPCC-associated mutations (http://www.nfdht.nl). To date, the database contains information of more than 400 different predisposing mutations that occur in over 600 HNPCC families from all parts of the world (PELTOMÄKI et al. 1997 and http://www.nfdht.nl). A majority of the mutations affect two genes, MLH1 (~50% of mutations) and MSH2 (~40%), whose protein products are indispensable for MMR. These mutations commonly impair the necessary protein–protein or protein--DNA interactions. MSH2 and MLH1 mutations often (but not always) give rise to "classical" HNPCC families that fulfill the Amsterdam criteria I and have high degree of MSI in tumors (for "grading" of MSI, see Sect. II., "Sporadic Colon Cancers with MSI"). MSH6 accounts for a lower, but significant number of mutations (~10%). MSH6 mutations often occur in clinically less typical HNPCC families with one or more of the following features: late onset, frequent occurrence of endometrial cancer, and low degree of microsatellite instability in tumor tissue (AKIYAMA et al. 1997; MIYAKI et al. 1997b; WIJNEN et al. 1999; WU et al. 1999; KOLODNER et al. 1999).

Only a few germline mutations in PMS2 have been described. These occur mainly in the context of Turcot syndrome, and for the manifestation of the disease two defective copies may be necessary already in the germline, which would be compatible with recessive, rather than dominant, inheritance (HAMILTON et al. 1995; MIYAKI et al. 1997a; DE ROSA et al. 2000). Thus far, no such HNPCC families have been identified in which colon cancer susceptibility would be associated with inherited mutations in MSH3 (HUANG et al. 2001) or PMS1 (LIU et al. 2001). Finally, certain germline variants of the MMR gene MLH3 (WU et al. 2001a) and the EXO1 gene encoding a 5'-3' exonuclease (WU et al. 2001b) may be associated with atypical HNPCC displaying variable degree of MSI in tumor tissue as a suggestion of MMR deficiency.

II. Sporadic Colon Cancer with MSI

MSI, the hallmark of HNPCC, occurs in approximately 15%–20% of sporadic tumors from the colorectum and other organs as well (Table 3). According to international criteria, high-degree of MSI (MSI-H) is defined as instability at ≥2/5 loci, or ≥30%–40% of all microsatellite loci studied, whereas instability at fewer loci is referred to as MSI-low (MSI-L) (BOLAND et al. 1998). Sporadic counterparts of tumors of the HNPCC spectrum, for example, endometrial and gastric cancer, typically show high degree of instability, but an MSI-L subset also exists. MSI-L, as defined by the low involvement of the dinucleotide and mononucleotide repeat markers belonging to the consensus panel (BOLAND et al. 1998), is a predominant pattern in tumors not belonging to the HNPCC spectrum.

From the clinicopathological point of view, colorectal cancers with MSI-H define a group of tumors with predilection in the proximal colon, diploid DNA content, high grade, better survival, and association with female gender (KIM et al. 1994; SANKILA et al. 1996; GRYFE et al. 2000; MALKHOSYAN et al. 2000). These features distinguish MSI-H tumors from those without widespread MSI, i.e., MSI-L or microsatellite-stable (MSS) tumors. The reasons for the observed good prognosis despite aggressive histological features are poorly understood, but plausible explanations include reduced cell viability (SHIBATA et al. 1994) or enhanced immune response (DOLCETTI et al. 1999) due to the accumulation of mutations in critical genes. Low incidence of p53 mutations may also contribute to the favorable outcome (KIM et al. 1994). Estrogens have been offered as an explanation to the sex-specific differences in the incidence of MSI-positive colon tumors. Based on a large population-based series, it was found that estrogens reduce and withdrawal of estrogens increase the risk for MSI-positive colon cancer and that the excess of MSI-positive tumors in women was primarily explained by the excess of MSI-positive tumors at older ages (SLATTERY et al. 2001). Based on these findings the authors suggested that MMR genes may be estrogen responsive, a hypothesis that remains to be verified.

A majority of MSI-H colon cancers is due to inactivation of MLH1, which mostly results from promoter hypermethylation rather than somatic mutations or loss of heterozygosity that are significant mechanisms of MMR gene inactivation in HNPCC tumors (KUISMANEN et al. 2000). MLH1 inactivation by promoter hypermethylation appears to underlie a majority of sporadic MSI-positive endometrial cancers as well (ESTELLER et al. 1998). Studies on cell lines have shown that promoter hypermethylation is often biallelic (VEIGL et al. 1998). This DNA methylation disorder, the mechanism of which is unknown, is present already in nonneoplastic colorectal mucosa and colorectal adenomas and has several other gene targets besides MLH1 (AHUJA et al. 1998; TOYOTA et al. 1999; KUISMANEN et al. 1999; NAKAGAWA et al. 2001). As will be further discussed below, the genetic signature of sporadic MSI-positive tumors may consist of a combination of genetic ("the mutator phenotype" due to MMR deficiency) and epigenetic alterations (hypermethylation tendency).

In the MSI-L subset of colon cancers, immunohistochemical and mutation studies have found no involvement of MLH1, MSH2, MSH6, or MSH3

(THIBODEAU et al. 1998; PERCESEPE et al. 1998; CUNNINGHAM et al. 2001). Given that the clinicopathological features do not seem to distinguish this group from MSS colon cancers, either (THIBODEAU et al. 1998), it has been a subject of debate whether or not MSI-L tumors should be considered separate from MSS tumors. Recent observations, however, have provided important distinguishing features. According to JASS et al. (1999) the early stages of neoplastic evolution in MSI-L tumors might depend on K-ras mutations, rather than APC mutations that characterize the classical adenoma-carcinoma sequence giving rise to MSS tumors. The infrequent occurrence of MSI-H in sporadic adenomas, contrary to adenomas from HNPCC patients, led JASS et al. (2000a) to further hypothesize that a significant proportion of sporadic MSI-H cancers, too, might develop through an alternative pathway not involving the traditional adenoma. It was proposed that neoplastic transformation in this alternative pathway might start within hyperplastic polyps that could progress into MSI-H or MSI-L cancer depending on the presence vs. absence of inactivation of the MMR gene MLH1 (JASS et al. 2000b). WHITEHALL et al. (2001) extended these findings by showing that frequent epigenetic silencing of the O-6-methylguanine DNA methyltransferase (MGMT), whose function is to remove mutagenic adducts from the O^6 position of guanine, may predispose MSI-L tumors to mutations, including those in K-ras. These findings together supported the idea that DNA methylation may play an important role in the determination of MSI-H vs. MSI-L phenotype through selective inactivation of MLH1 vs. MGMT, respectively. KAMBARA et al. (2001) identified loss of heterozygosity at 1p32 and 8p12–22 as further characteristics of the tumorigenic pathway in MSI-L colorectal cancers and showed that MSI-L phenotype was especially common in early colorectal cancers with invasion limited to the submucosa. The results of WHITEHALL et al. (2001) and KAMBARA et al. (2001) also implied a worse outcome for MSI-L colon cancers as compared to the other instability phenotypes, which could be attributed to K-ras mutations or loss of the as yet unidentified colon cancer-associated loci on 1p and 8p. Taken together, the available evidence suggests that tumorigenesis in the MSI-L group may indeed be distinct from that in either the MSI-H or MSS group.

C. Mechanisms of Cancer Development in Tumors with MMR Gene Defects

I. Mutation Frequencies in Normal and Pathological Conditions

The spontaneous mutation rate in normal somatic human cells is estimated to be about 1.4×10^{-10} mutations/bp/cell division (LOEB 1991), which (given the size of the human genome of 3×10^9 bp) would account for less than one mutation in each daughter cell. The mutation rates in cancer are much higher. Using a technique called inter-SSR PCR that monitors nonrepeat sequences between simple sequence repeat elements, STOLER et al. (1999) estimated that at least 11,000 mutation events are likely to occur in each colon cancer cell. STOLER et al. (1999) studied consecutive sporadic colon cancers, most of which are MSI-negative (MMR-proficient). In MMR-deficient cancer cells, the mutation rates are at least 100 times higher than in their MMR-proficient counterparts, as estimated from studies of selectable loci, such as hprt (BHATTACHARYYA et al. 1994; ESHLEMAN et al. 1995) or certain types of short tandem repeats (PARSONS et al. 1993). Using the AP-PCR technique, an unbiased DNA fingerprinting method that takes advantage of primers whose nucleotide sequence is arbitrarily chosen, IONOV et al. (1993) estimated that colon cancer cells may carry more than 100,000 deletion mutations. This accumulation of mutations that is especially characteristic of cells with deficient MMR is termed as "mutator phenotype" and it leads us to more closely examine the important role of the MMR system in mutation avoidance.

II. MMR System in Mutation Avoidance: Generation of the "Mutator Phenotype"

The "mutator phenotype" in MMR-deficient cells is typically a combined consequence of enhanced mutagenesis, inefficient repair, and clonal selection. The mutations may be spontaneous (such as C to T transition generated by spontaneous deamination of 5-methylcytosine), may represent biosynthetic errors (for example, insertion–deletion mismatches generated by DNA polymerase slippage), or be induced by various endogenous or exogenous agents. As discussed above, instability at short tandem repeats, microsatellites, is a useful indicator of MMR deficiency. Studies of disorders with genetic instability, including colon cancers, have shown that several factors influence the stability/instability of microsatellite sequences. First, the number of repeat units plays a role (proneness to instability increases with the increasing number of repeat units, EICHLER et al. 1994). Second, the presence of sequence interruptions stabilizes the repeats (BACON et al. 2000). Third, the type of repeat is important: for example, $(G)_8$ is more mutable than $(A)_8$ (ZHANG et al. 2001), and the background mutation rates of tetranucleotide repeats are higher than those of dinucleotide repeats (WEBER and WONG 1993). Fourth, the sequence context or surrounding chromatin structure may influence the stability of the repeat (ZHANG et al. 2001). Even repeat tracts composed of an identical number of the same nucleotide may show drastically different mutation frequencies in tumors, and if the tracts are part of functionally relevant genes, selection is a likely explanation.

Mutations may confer selective advantage by several mechanisms, but most importantly, by allowing the cells to overcome host-mediated restrictions to viability and expansion (JANIN 2000; LOEB 2001; FISHEL 2001). Table 4 lists a number of genes containing "hypermutable" tracts as part of their coding sequence, whose mutations appear to be selected for in MSI-positive tumors. The affected functions include signal transduction, tumor suppressor activity,

Table 4. Mutational targets of MMR deficiency. The coding DNA of all genes listed below contains a microsatellite repeat whose mutations are selected for in tumors

Functional goal of mutations	Examples of genes	References
Induction of growth-stimulatory signal	TCF4, AXIN2	Duval et al. (1999), Liu et al. (2000)
Loss of tumor suppression	TGFβRII, IGFIIR, PTEN, RIZ	Markowitz et al. (1995), Parsons et al. (1995b), Souza et al. (1996), Guanti et al. (2000), Chadwick et al. (2000), Piao et al. (2000)
Prevention of apoptosis	BAX, caspase-5	Rampino et al. (1997), Schwartz et al. (1999)
Decrease of genomic stability	MSH3, MSH6, MSH2, MBD4	Malkhosyan et al. (1996), Bader et al. (1999), Riccio et al. (1999), Chadwick et al. (2001)
Evasion of host immune reaction	β₂-Microglobulin	Bicknell et al. (1994)

apoptosis, genomic stability, and immune response. Different functions/genes are critical in the development of different tumors, and tissue-specific selection of the mutations might in part explain the characteristic organ involvement in HNPCC ("HNPCC tumor spectrum"). Thus, frameshift mutations in the TGFβRII (Myeroff et al. 1995) and TCF4 (Duval et al. 1999) appear to be strongly selected for in gastrointestinal malignancies but not in endometrial cancer. On the other hand, loss of PTEN function is an early event in endometrial tumorigenesis, but appears less important in colorectal tumorigenesis. Consequently, PTEN is inactivated in 90% of MSI-positive endometrial adenocarcinomas by mutation or other mechanisms (Mutter et al. 2000) and 85% of endometrial tumors from HNPCC patients show PTEN frameshift mutations (Zhou et al. 2002), whereas the repetitive tracts of PTEN are unstable in only some 20% of MSI-positive colon cancers (Guanti et al. 2000).

In the classical adenoma-carcinoma sequence of colorectal tumorigenesis, inactivation of the APC gene is one of the earliest events (Vogelstein et al. 1988). According to a simplified model (Kinzler and Vogelstein 1996), colon tumors from patients with HNPCC go through a similar (but not identical) series of mutations in a process that MMR deficiency speeds up. The spectrum of APC mutations has been used to evaluate the relative order of APC and MMR gene mutations in this process. An excess of APC mutations of the frameshift type, typical of a MMR defect, in MSI-positive colon cancers suggested that genetic instability precedes and is responsible for APC mutation in colorectal tumorigenesis (HUANG et al. 1996). In accordance with the above findings, studies on mice with constitutional defects of both the Apc and Msh2 genes demonstrated that the mechanism of inactivation of the wild-type Apc allele in tumors depended on the Msh2 status (REITMAIR et al. 1996). Thus, in the presence of a functional Msh2 (Apc$^{+/-}$/Msh2$^{+/+}$ or Apc$^{+/-}$/Msh2$^{+/-}$) all tumors displayed loss of heterozygosity at the Apc locus, whereas in the absence of a functional Msh2 (Apc$^{+/-}$/Msh2$^{-/-}$), somatic mutations appeared to be the major mechanism of Apc inactivation. Subsequent mouse studies have confirmed and extended the observations of REITMAIR et al. (1996) by showing that Msh2 or Mlh1 deficiency results in a change in the prevailing mechanism of Apc inactivation from allelic loss to somatic mutation in tumors (SMITS et al. 2000; KURAGUCHI et al. 2000). However, results pointing to an opposite direction were reported by HOMFRAY et al. (1998) who found no difference in the APC mutation spectra between sporadic microsatellite-unstable and -stable colon cancers, suggesting that APC mutations, rather than genomic instability, initiated tumorigenesis in sporadic colorectal cancers. These conflicting results may in part be attributable to the different experimental systems used or characteristics of the tumor series studied (hereditary vs. sporadic). As discussed in Sect. II., widespread hypermethylation of DNA underlies most cases of sporadic (but not hereditary) MSI-positive colon cancers through MLH1 inactivation, and this hypermethylation may affect the APC gene as well (HILTUNEN et al. 1997; ESTELLER et al. 2000). Being an early event, hypermethylation provides a possible mechanism for an early and concurrent inactivation of both APC and MLH1.

As the "mutator phenotype" in the original nontransformed cell is counterselective, mutations blocking apoptosis are among the most vital to "rescue" such a cell to allow malignant transformation as a result of additional mutations to follow (JANIN 2000). One of the most interesting observations made recently is that MMR and apoptosis are directly connected. MMR proteins may function as direct sensors of damage and link signaling pathways that may either incite DNA repair or provoke apoptosis (FISHEL 2001). Thus, mutations in MMR genes can simultaneously provide a selective advantage (owing to mutation to apoptotic resistance) and an increased rate of mutations (resulting from impairment of MMR function). The role of MMR proteins in apoptosis signaling is discussed in greater detail in the next section.

III. Repair of Endogenous and Exogenous DNA Damage

1. Heterocyclic Amine Adducts

Besides biosynthetic errors arising during DNA replication, the MMR system recognizes and corrects several types of chemical DNA damage. As shown by LI et al. (1996), hMutSα can specifically bind to heterocyclic amine adducts, many of which are of dietary origin and may increase the risk of colon cancer (SUGIMURA 1988). Enzymes that metabolize these compounds, including the

N-acetyltransferases 1 and 2 and the glutathione S- and T- transferases show polymorphic variation in the population and may modify the age at onset, tumor site, and cancer risk in MMR gene mutation carriers (MOISIO et al. 1998; HEINIMANN et al. 1999; FRAZIER et al. 2001). Besides being substrates for MMR proteins, whose defects give rise to MSI, heterocyclic amines have recently been implicated in the induction of another type of instability, CIN (gross chromosomal instability, LENGAUER et al. 1998). The molecular mechanisms of CIN are poorly understood. According to recent findings (BARDELLI et al. 2001), specific carcinogens can select for tumor cells with distinct forms of genetic instability: PhIP (an abundant heterocyclic amine in a typical Western diet) selects for cells with CIN, whereas the methylating agent MNNG (N-methyl-N'-nitro-N-nitrosoguanidine) selects for cells with MSI. Both categories of instability, MSI and CIN, exist among colon (and other) cancers (LENGAUER et al. 1998) and carcinogen exposure may thus contribute to the type of genetic instability in tumors.

2. Oxidative Damage

The MMR system also recognizes and eliminates oxidative damage. Oxidation of guanine (8-oxo-G) is a mutagenic lesion that may lead to misincorporation of adenine to the opposite position. In *Saccharomyces cerevisiae*, mutations in MSH2 or MSH6 caused a synergistic increase in mutation rates in combination with mutations in OGG1 (encoding an oxidative damage-specific DNA glycosylase) and the MSH2-MSH6 complex bound to 8-oxo-G:A mispairs with high affinity and specificity (NI et al. 1999). The results indicated that MSH2-MSH6-dependent MMR was the major mechanism correcting this type of error in the yeast. Mouse embryonic stem cells carrying one or two defective copies of Msh2 were shown to survive promutagenic lesions accompanying oxidative stress inflicted by low-level radiation (DE WEESE et al. 1998), which could increase the risk of neoplastic transformation in such cells. Both human epithelial cell and mouse embryo fibroblast cell lines lacking the MLH1 protein were found to display increased resistance to oxidative stress and might possess a selective growth advantage under oxidative stress via dysregulation of apoptosis (HARDMAN et al. 2001). It was also shown that oxidative DNA damage induced MSI in MMR-deficient *Escherichia coli* cells, possibly by increasing strand misalignment during DNA replication or through inefficient repair of the specific lesions (JACKSON et al. 1998). Based on these findings, it was postulated that endogenous production of oxygen-free radicals might be a major source in promoting instability at microsatellite sequences in tumor cells. Reactive oxygen species arise in most cells during normal metabolic processes (AMES et al. 1995); additionally, chronic oxidative stress may be induced in colonic cells, for example, by the cyclo-oxygenase 2 enzyme or in the uterine endometrium by estrogen. Failure of the removal of oxidative damage may therefore play an important role in the elevated colon and endometrial cancer risk in HNPCC.

3. Alkylation Damage

Long before the identification of human MMR genes, resistance to alkylating agents was described as a feature of MMR-deficient *E. coli* cells (JONES and WAGNER 1981; KARRAN and MARINUS 1982). Methylating agents induce a variety of base adducts, including O^6-methylguanine (O^6-meG) that is cyto-toxic in normal cells. In MMR-deficient cells, however, these lesions are allowed to persist ("alkylation tolerance"). Methylation tolerance has been associated with both hMutSα (DE WIND et al. 1995; PAPADOPOULOS et al. 1995) and hMutLα defects (BRANCH et al. 1995) in cancer cells. Even nonneoplastic tissues from MMR-mutation carriers may exhibit methylation tolerance, as demonstrated by MARRA et al. (2001) who suggested that tolerance of human $MSH2^{+/-}$ (but not $MLH1^{+/-}$) lymphoblastoid cells to the methylating agent temozolomide (a widely used chemotherapeutic agent) may distinguish asymptomatic carriers of such mutations. As demonstrated by YAMADA et al. (1997), hMutSα recognizes cisplatin-DNA adducts in a specific manner. Recent studies that will be described in detail below suggest that the alkyla-tion tolerance of MMR-deficient cells specifically results from their failure to induce apoptosis.

Independent observations from several research groups suggest a direct link between the MMR system and apoptosis. O^6-meG lesions, in which the damaged base is paired with either T or C, are subject to excision repair in a reaction that depends on a functional MMR system (DUCKETT et al. 1999). The authors further observed a hMutSα and hMutLα-dependent activation of protein kinases that phosphorylate the p53 tumor suppressor protein in response to DNA methylation damage. Studies on Msh2 null mice showed that Msh2-deficient animals had higher basal levels of mutation in the small intestine and they failed to initiate apoptosis after treatment with temozolo-mide (TOFT et al. 1999). This suggested that apart from impaired repair of DNA lesions, failure to engage apoptosis might contribute to cancer predisposition in Msh2-deficient animals. Further experiments with mice mutant for both Msh2 and p53 indicated the Msh2-dependent apoptosis was primarily medi-ated through a p53-dependent pathway (TOFT et al. 1999). According to HICKMAN et al. (1999), the hMutSα branch, but not the hMutSβ branch, was absolutely required for signaling apoptosis in response to O^6-meG, and the apoptotic response could also be executed in p53-independent manner. The differential involvement of the individual MMR genes in apoptosis signaling could offer an explanation to the observation that mutations in certain MMR genes are more prevalent than others in HNPCC families (FISHEL 2001; see Table 3).

IV. Role of MMR Proteins in Genetic Recombination

A further mechanism by which the MMR proteins promote genomic stability is by suppressing recombination between interspersed, diverged (homeolo-gous) sequences (RHYU 1996). Gene targeting assays in embryonic stem cells conducted by DE WIND et al. (1995) revealed loss of heterology-dependent suppression of recombination in Msh2$^{-/-}$ mice, suggesting that MSH2 deficiency might enhance carcinogenesis by elevating the rate of chromosomal rearrangements. Whereas the comparative genomic hybridization method revealed only a few losses and no gains of DNA sequences in MSI-positive colon carcinomas (SCHLEGEL et al. 1995), spectral karyotyping studies on colon cancer cell lines turned out more informative (ABDEL-RAHMAN et al. 2001). While MSI-positive cell lines generally showed few chromosome abnormalities, two cell lines (LoVo and HCA7) showed a novel pattern of multiple reciprocal translocations, with little numerical change or variability. LoVo is associated with a MSH2 defect and HCA7 with a MLH1 defect (WHEELER et al. 1999), and it is possible that these defects promoted the observed translocation events. Furthermore, the protein products of MLH1, PMS2, MSH4, and MSH5 are known to play a role in meiotic recombination, and their defects lead to infertility in mice (BAKER et al. 1995; BAKER et al. 1996; EDELMANN et al. 1999) and may lead to aneuploidy in the sperm from HNPCC patients (MARTIN et al. 2000).

E. Concluding Remarks

Discoveries made in the characterization of the MMR system provide one of the most illustrative examples of a fruitful synergy between different independent lines of research. Here, the study of different organisms (bacteria, yeast, mice, humans) using different approaches (genetic, biochemical, clinical) has resulted in a better understanding of some fundamental phenomena (basic biology of MMR, carcinogenesis, human disease). Although the picture still remains incomplete in many respects, the acquired information already has immediate clinical applications in mutation diagnostics, and cancer prevention and treatment. Most importantly, these applications are not restricted to patients with hereditary cancer (HNPCC) only, but are relevant for the MSI-positive subset of sporadic cases of cancer as well (in essence, covering 15%–20% of all cancers). Such combined approaches will be necessary also in future studies on the MMR system. For example, no human homologues for a number of MMR genes that are known to exist in prokaryotes have yet been identified. At the same time, not all families that meet the clinical criteria of HNPCC have revealed detectable defects in the presently known MMR genes, not to mention the large number of atypical families, in which the MMR system might or might not be involved. Moreover, even in families with known predisposing mutations, the mechanisms that translate HNPCC genotype into its clinical phenotype remain poorly understood. A more complete understanding may come from the possible detection of additional functions for known MMR genes or from the identification of novel components of the MMR system or other genes that interact with the MMR system to modulate carcinogenesis driven by deficient MMR.

Acknowledgments. The author's research receives grant support from the Sigrid Juselius Foundation, Academy of Finland, Finnish Cancer Foundation, and the National Institutes of Health/National Cancer Institute (CA82282).

References

Aaltonen LA, Salovaara R, Kristo P, Canzian F, Hemminki A, Peltomäki P, Chadwick RB, Percesepe A, Kääriäinen H, Ahtola H, Eskelinen M, Härkönen N, Julkunen R, Kangas E, Ojala S, Tulikoura J, Valkamo E, Järvinen H, Mecklin J-P, de la Chapelle A (1998) Incidence of hereditary nonpolyposis colorectal cancer and molecular screening for the disease. N Engl J Med 338:1481–1487

Abdel-Rahman WM, Katsura K, Rens W, Gorman PA, Sheer D, Bicknell D, Bodmer WF, Arends MJ, Wyllie AH, Edwards PAW (2001) Spectral karyotyping suggests new subsets of colorectal cancers characterized by pattern of chromosome rearrangement. Proc Natl Acad Sci USA 98:2538–2543

Acharya S, Wilson T, Gradia S, Kane MF, Guerrette S, Marsischky GT, Kolodner R, Fishel R (1996) hMSH2 forms specific mispair-binding complexes with hMSH3 and hMSH6. Proc Natl Acad Sci USA 93:13629–13634

Ahuja N, Li Q, Mohan AL, Baylin SB, Issa J-PJ (1998) Aging and DNA methylation in colorectal mucosa and cancer. Cancer Res 58:5489–5494

Akiyama Y, Sato H, Yamada T, Nagasaki H, Tsuchiya A, Abe R, Yuasa Y (1997) Germ-line mutation of the hMSH6/GTBP gene in an atypical hereditary nonpolyposis colorectal cancer kindred. Cancer Res 57:3920–3923

Ames BN, Gold LS, Willett WC (1995). The causes and prevention of cancer. Proc Natl Acad Sci USA 92:5258–5265

Bacon AL, Farrington SM, Dunlop M (2000) Sequence interruptions confer differential stability at microsatellite alleles in mismatch repair deficient cells. Hum Mol Genet 9:2707–2713

Bader S, Walker M, Hendrich B, Bird A, Bird C, Hooper M, Wyllie A (1999) Somatic frameshift mutations in the MBD4 gene of sporadic colon cancers with mismatch repair deficiency. Oncogene 18:8044–8047

Baker SM, Bronner CE, Zhang L, Plug AW, Robatez M, Warren G, Elliott EA, Yu J, Ashley T, Arnheim N, Bradley N, Flavell RA, Liskay RM (1995) Male defective in the DNA mismatch repair gene PMS2 exhibit abnormal chromosome synapsis in meiosis. Cell 82:309–319

Baker SM, Plug AW, Prolla TA, Bronner CE, Harris AC, Yao X, Christie D-M, Monell C, Arnheim N, Bradley A, Ashley T, Liskay RM (1996) Involvement of mouse Mlh1 in DNA mismatch repair and meiotic crossing over. Nat Genet 13:336–342

Bardelli A, Cahill DP, Lederer G, Speicher MR, Kinzler KW, Vogelstein B, Lengauer C (2001) Carcinogen-specific induction of genetic instability. Proc Natl Acad Sci USA 98:5770–5775

Bhattacharyya NP, Skandalis A, Ganesh A, Groden J, Meuth M (1994) Mutator phenotypes in human colorectal carcinoma cell lines. Proc Natl Acad Sci USA 91:6319–6323

Bicknell DC, Rowan A, Bodmer WF. β_2-microglobulin gene mutations: A study of established colorectal cell lines and fresh tumors (1994). Proc Natl Acad Sci USA 91:4751–4755

Boland CR, Thibodeau SN, Hamilton SR, Sidransky D, Eshleman JR, Burt RW, Meltzer SJ, Rodriguez-Bigas MA, Fodde R, Ranzani GN, Srivastava S (1998) A National Cancer Institute workshop on microsatellite instability for cancer detection and familial predisposition: Development of international criteria for the determination of microsatellite instability in colorectal cancer. Cancer Res 58:5248–5257

Branch P, Hampson R, Karran P (1995) DNA mismatch binding defects, DNA damage tolerance, and mutator phenotypes in human colorectal carcinoma cell lines. Cancer Res 55:2304–2309

Bronner CE, Baker SM, Morrison PT, Warren G, Smith LG, Lescoe MK, Kane M, Earabino C, Lipford J, Lindblom A, Tannergård P, Bollag RJ, Godwin AR, Ward DC, Nordenskjold M, Fishel R, Kolodner R, Liskay RM (1994) Mutation in the DNA mismatch repair gene homologue hMLH1 is associated with hereditary nonpolyposis colon cancer. Nature 368:258–261

Buermeyer AB, Deschenes SM, Baker SM, Liskay RM (1999) Mammalian DNA mismatch repair. Annu Rev Genet 33:533–564

Chadwick RB, Jiang G-L, Bennington GA, Yuan B, Johnson CK, Stevens MW, Niemann TH, Peltomäki P, Huang S, de la Chapelle A (2000) Candidate tumor suppressor RIZ is frequently involved in colorectal carcinogenesis. Proc Natl Acad Sci USA 97:2662–2667

Chadwick RB, Pyatt RE, Niemann TH, Richards SK, Johnson CK, Stevens MW, Meek JE, Hampel H, Prior TW, de la Chapelle A (2001) Hereditary and somatic DNA mismatch repair gene mutations in sporadic endometrial carcinoma. J Med Genet 38:461–466

Cunningham JM, Kim C-Y, Christensen ER, Tester DJ, Parc Y, Burgart LJ, Halling KC, McDonnell SK, Schaid DJ, Vockley CW, Kubly V, Nelson H, Michels VV, Thibodeau SN (2001) The frequency of hereditary defective mismatch repair in a prospective series of unselected colorectal carcinomas. Am J Hum Genet 69:780–790

Das Gupta R, Kolodner RD (2000) Novel dominant mutations in *Saccharomyces cerevisiae* MSH6. Nat Genet 24:53–56

De Rosa M, Fasano C, Panariello L, Scarano MI, Belli G, Iannelli A, Ciciliano F, Izzo P (2000) Evidence for a recessive inheritance of Turcot's syndrome caused by compound heterozygous mutations within the PMS2 gene. Oncogene 19:1719–1723

de Wind N, Dekker M, Berns A, Radman M, Riele HT (1995) Inactivation of the mouse Msh2 results in mismatch repair deficiency, methylation tolerance, hyperrecombination, and predisposition to cancer. Cell 82:321–300

deWeese TL, Shipman JM, Larrier NA, Buckley NM, Kidd LCR, Groopman JD, Cutler RG, te Riele, H, Nelson WG (1998) Mouse embryonic stem cells carrying one or two defective Msh2 alleles respond abnormally to oxidative stress inflicted by low-level radiation. Proc Natl Acad Sci USA 95:11915–11920

Dolcetti R, Viel A, Doglioni C, Russo A, Guidoboni M, Capozzi E, Vecchiato N, Macri E, Fornasarig M, Boiocchi M (1999). High prevalence of activated intraepithelial cytotoxic T lymphocytes and increased neoplastic cell apoptosis in colorectal carcinomas with microsatellite instability. Am J Pathol 154:1805–1813

Duckett DR, Bronstein SM, Taya Y, Modrich P (1999) hMutSα and hMutLα-dependent phosphorylation of p53 in response to DNA methylator damage. Proc Natl Acad Sci USA 96:12384–12388

Duval A, Iacopetta B, Ranzani GN, Lothe RA, Thomas G, Hamelin R (1999) Variable mutation frequencies in coding repeats of TCF-4 and other target genes in colon, gastric and endometrial carcinoma showing microsatellite instability. Oncogene 18:6806–6809

Edelmann W, Cohen PE, Kneitz B, Winand N, Lia M, Heyer J, Kolodner R, Pollard JW, Kucherlapati R (1999) Mammalian MutS homologue 5 is required for chromosome pairing in meiosis. Nat Genet 21:123–127

Eichler EE, Holden JJ, Popovich BV, Reiss AL, Snow K, Thibodeau SN, Richards CS, Ward PA, Nelson DL (1994) Length of uninterrupted CGG repeats determines instability in the FMR1 gene. Nat Genet 8:88–94

Eshleman JR, Lang EZ, Bowerfind GK, Parsons R, Vogelstein B, Wilson JKV, Veigl ML, Sedwick WD, Markowitz SD (1995) Increased mutation rate at the hprt locus accompanies microsatellite instability in colon cancer. Oncogene 10:33–37

Esteller M, Levine R, Baylin SB, Hedrick Ellenson L, Herman JG (1998) MLH1 promoter hypermethylation is associated with the microsatellite instability phenotype in sporadic endometrial carcinomas. Oncogene 16:2413–2417

Esteller M, Sparks A, Toyota M, Sanchez-Cespedes M, Capella G, Peinado MA, Gonzalez S, Tarafa G, Sidransky D, Meltzer SJ, Baylin SB, Herman JG (2000) Analysis of adenomatous polyposis coli promoter hypermethylation in human cancer. Cancer Res 60:4366–4371

Fishel R, Lescoe MK, Rao MRS, Copeland NG, Jenkins NA, Garber J, Kane M, Kolodner R (1993) The human mutator gene homolog MSH2 and its association with hereditary nonpolyposis colon cancer. Cell 75:1027–1038

Fishel R (2001) The selection for mismatch repair defects in hereditary nonpolyposis colorectal cancer: Revising the mutator hypothesis. Cancer Res 61:7369–7374

Frazier ML, O'Donnell FT, Kong S, Gu X, Campos I, Luthra R, Lynch PM, Amos CI (2001) Age-associated risk of cancer among individuals with N-acetyltransferase 2 (NAT2) mutations and mutations in DNA mismatch repair genes. Cancer Res 61:1269–1271

Fujii H, Shimada T (1989) Isolation and characterization of cDNA clones derived from the divergently transcribed gene in the region upstream from the human dihydrofolate reductase gene. J Biol Chem 264:10057–10064

Gryfe R, Kim H, Hsieh ETK, Aronson MD, Holowaty EJ, Bull SB, Redston M, Gallinger S (2000) Tumor microsatellite instability and clinical outcome in young patients with colorectal cancer. N Engl J Med 342:69–77

Guanti G, Resta N, Simone C, Cariola F, Demma I, Fiorente P, Gentile M (2000) Involvement of PTEN mutations in the genetic pathways of colorectal cancerogenesis. Hum Mol Genet 9:283–287

Hackman P, Tannergård P, Osei-Mensa S, Chen J, Kane MF, Kolodner R, Lambert B, Hellgren D, Lindblom A (1997) A human compound heterozygote for two MLH1 missense mutations. Nat Genet 17:135–136

Hamilton SR, Liu B, Parsons RE, Papadopoulos N, Jen J, Powell SM, Krush AJ, Berk T, Cohen Z, Tetu B, Burger PC, Wood PA, Taqi F, Booker SV, Petersen GM, Offerhaus GJA, Tersmette AC, Giardiello FM, Vogelstein B, Kinzler KW (1995) The molecular basis of Turcot's syndrome. N Engl J Med 332:839–847

Han H-J, Maruyama M, Baba S, Park J-G, Nakamura Y (1995) Genomic structure of human mismatch repair gene, hMLH1, and its mutation analysis in patients with hereditary nonpolyposis colorectal cancer (HNPCC). Hum Mol Genet 4:237–242

Hardman RA, Afshari CA, Barrett JC (2001) Involvement of mammalian MLH1 in the apoptotic response to peroxide-induced oxidative stress. Cancer Res 61:1392–1397

Heinimann K, Scott RJ, Chappuis P, Weber W, Muller H, Dobbie Z, Hutter P (1999) N-acetyltransferase 2 influences cancer prevalence in hMLH1/hMSH2 mutation carriers. Cancer Res 59:3038–3040

Hickman MJ, Samson LD (1999) Role of DNA mismatch repair and p53 in signaling induction of apoptosis by alkylating agents. Proc Natl Acad Sci USA 96:10764–10769

Hiltunen MO, Alhonen L, Koistinaho J, Myöhänen S, Pääkkönen M, Marin S, Kosma V-M, Jänne J (1997) Hypermethylation of the APC (Adenomatous polyposis coli) gene promoter region in human colorectal carcinoma. Int J Cancer 70:644–648

Homfray TFR, Cottrell SE, Ilyas M, Rowan A, Talbot IC, Bodmer WF, Tomlinson IPM (1998) Defects in mismatch repair occur after APC mutations in the pathogenesis of sporadic colorectal tumours. Hum Mut 11:114–120

Houlston RS, Collins A, Slack J, Morton NE (1992) Dominant genes for colorectal cancer are not rare. Ann Hum Genet 56:99–103

Huang J, Papadopoulos N, McKinley AJ, Farrington SM, Curtis LJ, Wyllie AH, Zheng S, Willson JKV, Markowitz SD, Morin P, Kinzler KW, Vogelstein B, Dunlop MG (1996) APC mutations in colorectal tumors with mismatch repair deficiency. Proc Natl Acad Sci USA 93:9049–9054

Huang J, Kuismanen SA, Liu T, Chadwick RB, Johnson CK, Stevens MW, Richards SK, Meek JE, Gao X, Wright FA, Mecklin J-P, Järvinen HJ, Grönberg H, Bisgaard ML,

Lindblom A, Peltomäki P (2001) MSH6 and MSH3 are rarely involved in genetic predisposition to nonpolypotic colon cancer. Cancer Res 61:1619–1623

Ionov Y, Peinado MA, Malkhosyan S, Shibata D, Perucho M (1993) Ubiquitous somatic mutations in simple repeated sequences reveal a new mechanism for colonic carcinogenesis. Nature 363:558–561

Jackson AL, Chen R, Loeb L (1998) Induction of microsatellite instability by oxidative DNA damage. Proc Natl Acad Sci USA 95:12468–12473

Janin N (2000) A simple model for carcinogenesis of colorectal cancers with microsatellite instability. Adv Cancer Res 77:189–221

Jass JR, Biden KG, Cummings MC, Simms LA, Walsh M, Schoch E, Meltzer SJ, Wright C, Searle J, Young J, Leggett BA (1999) Characterisation of a subtype of colorectal cancer combining features of the suppressor and mild mutator pathways. J Clin Pathol 52:455–460

Jass JR, Young J, Leggett BA (2000a) Hyperplastic polyps and DNA microsatellite unstable cancers of the colorectum. Histopathology 37:295–301

Jass JR, Iino H, Ruszkiewicz A, Painter D, Solomon MJ, Koorey DJ, Cohn D, Furlong KL, Walsh MD, Palazzo J, Bocker Edmonston T, Fishel R, Young J, Leggett BA (2000b) Neoplastic progression occurs through mutator pathways in hyperplastic polyposis of the colorectum. Gut 47:43–49

Jiricny J, Nyström-Lahti M (2000) Mismatch repair defects in cancer. Curr Opin Genet Devel 10:157–161

Jones M, Wagner R (1981) N-methyl-N′-nitro-N-nitrosoguanidine sensitivity of *E. coli* mutants deficient in DNA methylation and mismatch repair. Molecular and General Genetics 184:562–563

Kambara T, Matsubara N, Nakagawa H, Notohara K, Nagasaka T, Yoshino T, Isozaki H, Sharp GB, Shimizu K, Jass J, Tanaka N (2001) High frequency of low-level microsatellite instability in early colorectal cancer. Cancer Res 61:7743–7746

Karran P, Marinus MG (1982) Mismatch correction at O⁶-methylguanine residues in *E. coli* DNA. Nature 296:868–869

Kim H, Jen J, Vogelstein B, Hamilton SR (1994) Clinical and pathological characteristics of sporadic colorectal carcinomas with DNA replication errors in microsatellite sequences. Am J Pathol 145:148–156

Kinzler KW, Vogelstein B (1996) Lessons from hereditary colorectal cancer. Cell 87:159–170

Kolodner RD, Hall NR, Lipford J, Kane MF, Rao MRS, Morrison P, Wirth L, Finan PJ, Burn J, Chapman P, Earabino C, Merchant E, Bishop DT (1994) Structure of the human MSH2 locus and analysis of two Muir-Torre kindreds for msh2 mutations. Genomics 24:516–526

Kolodner RD, Hall NR, Lipford J, Kane MF, Morrison PT, Finan PJ, Burn J, Chapman P, Earabino C, Merchant E, Bishop DT (1995) Structure of the human MLH1 locus and analysis of a large hereditary nonpolyposis colorectal carcinoma kindred for mlh1 mutations. Cancer Res 55:242–248

Kolodner RD, Marsischky GT (1999) Eukaryotic mismatch repair. Curr Opin Genet Devel 9:89–96

Kolodner RD, Tytell JD, Schmeits JL, Kane MF, Gupta RD, Weger J, Wahlberg S, Fox EA, Peel D, Ziogas A, Garber JE, Syngal S, Anton-Culver H, Li FP (1999) Germ-line msh6 mutations in colorectal cancer families. Cancer Res 59:5068–5074

Kuismanen SA, Holmberg MT, Salovaara R, Schweizer P, Aaltonen LA, de la Chapelle A, Nyström-Lahti M, Peltomäki P (1999) Epigenetic phenotypes distinguish microsatellite stable and unstable colorectal cancers. Proc Natl Acad Sci USA 96:12661–12666

Kuismanen SA, Holmberg MT, Salovaara R, de la Chapelle A, Peltomäki P (2000) Genetic and epigenetic modification of MLH1 accounts for a major share of microsatellite-unstable colorectal cancers. Am. J. Pathol. 156:1773–1779

Kuraguchi M, Edelmann W, Yang K, Lipkin M, Kucherlapati R, Brown AMC (2000) Tumor-associated Apc mutations in Mlh1$^{-/-}$Apc^{1638N} mice reveal a mutational signature of Mlh1 deficiency. Oncogene 19:5755–5763

Leach FS, Nicolaides NC, Papadopoulos Nl Liu B, Jen J, Parsons R, Peltomäki P, Sistonen P, Aaltonen LA, Nyström-Lahti M, Guan X-Y, Zhang J, Meltzer PS, Yu J-W, Kao F-T, Chen DJ, Cerosaletti KM, Fournier REK, Todd S, Lewis T, Leach RJ, Naylor SL, Weissenbach J, Mecklin J-P, Järvinen H, Petersen GM, Hamilton SR, Green J, Jass J, Watson P, Lynch HT, Trent JM, de la Chapelle A, Kinzler KW, Vogelstein B (1993) Mutations of a MutS homolog in hereditary nonpolyposis colorectal cancer. Cell 75:1215–1225

Lengauer C, Kinzler KW, Vogelstein B (1998) Genetic instabilities in human cancers. Nature 396:643–649

Leung WK, Kim JJ, Wu L, Sepulveda JL, Sepulveda A (2000) Identification of a second MutL DNA mismatch repair complex (hPMS1 and hMLH1) in human epithelial cells. J Biol Chem 275:15728–15732

Li G-M, Wang H, Romano LJ (1996) Human MutSα specifically binds to DNA containing aminofluorene and acetylaminofluorene adducts. J Biol Chem 271: 24084–24088

Lipkin SM, Wang V, Jacoby R, Banerjee-Basu S, Baxevanis AD, Lynch HT, Elliott RM, Collins FS (2000) MLH3:a DNA mismatch repair gene associated with mammalian microsatellite instability. Nat Genet 24:27–35

Liu B, Parsons RE, Hamilton SR, Petersen GM, Lynch HT, Watson P, Markowitz S, Willson JKV, Green J, de la Chapelle A, Kinzler KW, Vogelstein B (1994) hMSH2 mutations in hereditary nonpolyposis colorectal cancer kindreds. Cancer Res 54:4590–4594

Liu W, Dong X, Mai M, Seelan RS, Taniguchi K, Krishnadath KK, Halling KC, Cunningham JM, Qian C, Christensen E, Roche PC, Smith DI, Thibodeau SN (2000) Mutations in AXIN2 cause colorectal cancer with defective mismatch repair by activating β-catenin/TCF signaling. Nat Genet 26:146–147

Liu T, Yan H, Kuismanen S, Percesepe A, Bisgaard M-L, Pedroni M, Benatti P, Kinzler K, Vogelstein B, Ponz de Leon M, Peltomäki P, Lindblom A (2001) The role of hPMS1 and hPMS2 in predisposing to colorectal cancer. Cancer Res 61:7798–7802

Loeb LA (1991) Mutator phenotype may be required for multistage carcinogenesis. Cancer Res 51:3075–3079

Loeb LA (2001) A mutator phenotype in cancer. Cancer Res 61:3230–3239

Malkhosyan S, Rampino N, Yamamoto H, Perucho M (1996) Frameshift mutator mutations. Nature 382:499–500

Malkhosyan SR, Yamamoto H, Piao Z, Perucho M (2000) Late onset and high incidence of colon cancer of the mutator phenotype with hypermethylated hMLH1 gene in women. Gastroenterology 119:598

Markowitz S, Wang J, Myeroff L, Parsons R, Sun L, Lutterbaugh J, Fan RS, Zborowska E, Kinzlein KW, Vogelstein B, Brattain M, Willson JKW (1995) Inactivation of the type II TGF-β receptor in colon cancer cells with microsatellite instability. Science 268:1336–1338

Marra G, D'atri S, Corti C, Bonmassar L, Cattaruzza MS, Schweizer P, Heinimann K, Bartosova Z, Nystöm-Lahti M, Jiricny J (2001) Tolerance of human MSH2$^{+/-}$ lymphoblastoid cells to the methylating agent temozolomide. Proc Natl Acad Sci USA 98:7164–7169

Marsischky GT, Filosi N, Kane MF, Kolodner R (1996) Redundancy of *Saccharomyces cerevisiae* MSH3 and MSH6 in MSH2-dependent mismatch repair. Genes Dev 10:407–420

Martin RH, Green J, Ko E, Barclay L, Rademaker AW (2000) Analysis of aneuploidy frequencies in sperm from patients with hereditary nonpolyposis colon cancer and an hMSH2 mutation. Am J Hum Genet 66:1149–1152

Miyaki M, Nishio J, Konishi M, Kikuchi-Yanoshita R, Tanaka K, Muraoka M, Nagato M, Chong J-M, Koike M, Terada T, Kawahara Y, Fukutome A, Tomiyama J,

Chuganji Y, Momoi M, Utsunomiya J (1997a) Drastic genetic instability of tumors and normal tissues in Turcot syndrome. Oncogene 15:2877–2881

Miyaki M, Konishi M, Tanaka K, Kikuchi-Yanoshita R, Muraoka M, Yasuno M, Igari T, Koike M, Chiba M, Mori T (1997b) Germline mutation of MSH6 as the cause of hereditary nonpolyposis colorectal cancer. Nat Genet 17:271–272

Moisio A-L, Sistonen P, Mecklin J-P, Järvinen H, Peltomäki P (1998) Genetic polymorphisms in carcinogen metabolism and their association to hereditary nonpolyposis colon cancer. Gastroenterology 115:1387–1394

Mutter G, Lin MC, Fitzgerald JT, Kum JB, Baak JPA, Lees JA, Weng LP, Eng C (2000) Altered PTEN expression as a diagnostic marker for the earliest endometrial precancers. J Natl Cancer Inst 92:924–931

Myeroff LL, Parsons R, Kim S-J, Hedrick L, Cho KR, Orth K, Mathis M, Kinzler KW, Lutterbaugh J, Park K, Bang Y-J, Lee HY, Park JG, Lynch HT, Roberts AB, Vogelstein B, Markowitz SD (1995) A transforming growth factor β receptor type II gene mutation common in colon and gastric but rare in endometrial cancers. Cancer Res 55:5545–5547

Nakagawa H, Nuovo GJ, Zervos EE, Martin EW Jr, Salovaara R, Aaltonen LA, de la Chapelle A (2001) Age-related hypermethylation of the 5′ region of MLH1 in normal colonic mucosa is associated with microsatellite-unstable colorectal cancer development. Cancer Res 61:6991–6995

Ni TT, Marsischky GT, Kolodner RD (1999) MSH2 and MSH6 are required for removal of adenine misincorporated opposite 8-oxo-guanine in S. cerevisiae. Mol Cell 4:439–444

Nicolaides NC, Papadopoulos N, Liu B, Wei YF, Carter KC, Ruben SM, Rosen CA, Haseltine WA, Fleischmann RD, Fraser CM, Adams MD, Venter CJ, Dunlop MG, Hamilton SR, Petersen G, de la Chapelle A, Vogelstein B, Kinzler KW (1994) Mutations of two PMS homologs in hereditary nonpolyposis colon cancer. Nature 371:75–80

Nicolaides NC, Carter KC, Shell BK, Papadopoulos N, Vogelstein B, Kinzler KW (1995) Genomic organization of the human PMS2 gene family. Genomics 30:195–206

Nicolaides NC, Palombo F, Kinzler KW, Vogelstein B, Jiricny J (1996) Molecular cloning of the N-terminus of GTBP. Genomics 31:395–397

Palombo F, Gallinari P, Iaccarino I, Lettleri T, Hughes MA, Truong O, Hsuan JJ, Jiricny J (1995) GTBP, a 160-kilodalton protein essential for mismatch-binding activity in human cells. Science 268:1912–1914

Papadopoulos N, Nicolaides NC, Wei Y-F, Ruben SM, Carter KC, Rosen CA, Haseltine WA, Fleischmann RD, Fraser CM, Adams MD, Venter JC, Hamilton SR, Petersen GM, Watson P, Lynch HT, Peltomäki P, Mecklin J-P, de la Chapelle A, Kinzler KW, Vogelstein B (1994) Mutation of a mutL homolog is associated with hereditary colon cancer. Science 263:1625–1629

Papadopoulos N, Nicolaides NC, Liu B, Parsons R, Lengauer C, Palombo F, D'Arrigo A, Markowitz S, Willson JK, Kinzler KW, Jiricny J, Vogelstein B (1995) Mutations of GTBP in genetically unstable cells. Science 268:1915–1917

Paquis-Flucklinger V, Santucci-Darmanin S, Paul R, Saunieres A, Turc-Carel C, Desnuelle C (1997) Cloning and expression analysis of a meiosis-specific MutS homolog: The human MSH4 gene. Genomics 44:188–194

Parsons R, Li GM, Longley MJ, Fang WH, Papadopoulos N, Jen J, de la Chapelle, A, Kinzler KW, Vogelstein B, Modrich P (1993) Hypermutability and mismatch repair deficiency in RER+ tumor cells. Cell 75:1227–1236

Parsons R, Li G-M, Longley M, Modrich P, Liu B, Berk T, Hamilton SR, Kinzler KW, Vogelstein B (1995a) Mismatch repair deficiency in phenotypically normal cells. Science 268:738–740

Parsons R, Myeroff L, Liu B, Willson J, Markowitz S, Kinzler K, Vogelstein B (1995b) Microsatellite instability and mutations of the transforming growth factor β type II receptor gene in colorectal cancer. Cancer Res 55:5548–5550

Peltomäki P, Vasen HFA, the International Collaborative Group on HNPCC (1997) Mutations predisposing to hereditary nonpolyposis colorectal cancer: database and results of a collaborative study. Gastroenterology 113:1146–1158

Percesepe A, Borghi F, Menigatti M, Losi L, Foroni M, Di Gregorio C, Rossi G, Pedroni M, Sala E, Vaccina F, Roncucci L, Benatti P, Viel A, Genuardi M, Marra G, Kristo P, Peltomaki P, Ponz de Leon M (2001) Molecular screening for hereditary nonpolyposis colorectal cancer (HNPCC): a prospective, population-based study. J Clin Oncol 19:3944–3950

Percesepe A, Kristo P, Aaltonen LA, Ponz de Leon M, de la Chapelle A, Peltomäki P (1998) Mismatch repair genes and mononucleotide tracts as mutation targets in colorectal tumors with different degrees of microsatellite instability. Oncogene 17:157–163

Piao Z, Fang W, Malkhosyan S, Kim H, Horii A, Perucho M, Huang S (2000) Frequent frameshift mutations of RIZ in sporadic gastrointestinal and endometrial carcinomas with microsatellite instability. Cancer Res 60:4701–4704

Rampino N, Yamamoto H, Ionov Y, Li Y, Sawai H, Reed JC, Perucho M (1997) Somatic frameshift mutations in the BAX gene in colon cancers of the microsatellite mutator phenotype. Science 275:967–969

Räschle M, Marra G, Nyström-Lahti M, Schar P, Jiricny J (1999) Identification of hMutLβ, a heterodimer of hMLH1 and hPMS1. J. Biol. Chem 5:32368–32375

Ravnik-Glavac M, Uroš P, Glavac D (2000) Incidence of germline hMLH1 and hMSH2 mutations (HNPCC patients) among newly diagnosed colorectal cancers in a Slovenian population. J Med Genet 37:533–536

Reitmair AH, Cai J-C, Bjerknes M, Redston M, Cheng H, Pind MTL, Hay K, Mitri A, Bapat BV, Mak TW, Gallinger S (1996) MSH2 deficiency contributes to accelerated APC-mediated intestinal tumorigenesis. Cancer Res 56:2922–2926

Rhyu MS (1996) Molecular mechanisms underlying hereditary nonpolyposis colorectal carcinoma. J Natl Cancer Inst 88:240–251

Ricciardone MD, Özcelik T, Cevher B, Özdag H, Tuncer M, Gürgey A, Uzunalimoglu Ö, Çetinkaya H, Tanyeli A, Erken E, Özturk M (1999) Human MLH1 deficiency predisposes to hematological malignancy and neurofibromatosis type I. Cancer Res 59:290–293

Riccio A, Aaltonen LA, Godwin AK, Loukola A, Percesepe A, Salovaara R, Masciullo V, Genuardi M, Paravatou-Petsotas M, Bassi DE, Ruggeri BA, Klein-Szanto AJP, Testa JR, Neri G, Bellacosa A (1999) The DNA repair gene MBD4 (MED1) is mutated in human carcinomas with microsatellite instability. Nat Genet 23: 266–268

Samowitz WS, Curtin K, Lin HH, Robertson MA, Schaffer D, Nichols M, Gruenthal K, Leppert MF, Slattery M (2001) The colon cancer burden of genetically defined hereditary nonpolyposis colon cancer. Gastroenterology 121:830–838

Sankila R, Aaltonen LA, Järvinen HJ, Mecklin J-P (1996) Better survival rates in patients with MLH1-associated hereditary colorectal cancer. Gastroenterology 110:682–687

Schlegel J, Stumm G, Scherthan H, Bocker T, Zirngibl H, Rüschoff J, Hofstädter F (1995) Comparative genomic in situ hybridization of colon carcinomas with replication error. Cancer Res 55:6002–6005

Schmutte C, Marinescu RC, Copeland NG, Jenkins NA, Overhauser J, Fishel R (1998) Refined chromosomal localization of the mismatch repair and hereditary nonpolyposis colorectal cancer genes hMSH2 and hMSH6. Cancer Res 58:5023–5026

Schwartz S, Yamamoto H, Navarro M, Maestro M, Reventos J, Perucho M (2000) Frameshift mutations at mononucleotide repeats in caspase-5 and other target genes in endometrial and gastrointestinal cancer of the microsatellite mutator phenotype. Cancer Res 59:2995–3002

Shibata D, Peinado MA, Ionov Y, Malkhosyan S, Perucho M (1994) Genomic instability in repeated sequences is an early somatic event in colorectal tumorigenesis that persists after transformation. Nat Genet 6:273–281

Slattery ML, Potter JD, Curtin K, Edwards S, Ma K-N, Anderson K, Schaffer D, Samowitz WS (2001) Estrogens reduce and withdrawal of estrogens increase risk of microsatellite instability-positive colon cancer. Cancer Res 61:126–130

Smits R, Hofland N, Edelmann W, Geugien M, Jagmohan-Changur S, Albuquerque C, Braeukel C, Kucherlapati R, Kielman MF, Fodde R (2000) Somatic Apc mutations are selected upon their capacity to inactivate the β-catenin downregulating activity. Genes Chrom Cancer 29:229–239

Souza RF, Appel R, Yin J, Wang S, Smolinski KN, Abraham JM, Zou TT, Shi Y-Q, Lei J, Cottrell J, Cymes K, Biden K, Simms L, Leggett B, Lynch PM, Frazier M, Powell SM, Harpaz N, Sugimura H, Young J, Meltzer SJ (1996) The insulin-like growth factor II receptor gene is a target of microsatellite instability in human gastrointestinal tumours. Nat Genet 14:255–257

Stoler DL, Chen N, Basik M, Kahlenberg MS, Rodriguez-Bigas MA, Petrelli NJ, Anderson GR (1999) The onset and extent of genomic instability in sporadic colorectal tumor progression. Proc Natl Acad Sci USA 96:15121–15126

Sugimura T (1988) Successful use of short-term tests for academic purposes: their use in identification of new environmental carcinogens with possible risks for humans. Mutat Res 205:33–39

Thibodeau SN, French AJ, Cunningham JM, Tester D, Burgart LJ, Roche PC, McDonnell SK, Schaid DJ, Vockley CW, Michels VV, Farr GH Jr, O'Connell MJ (1998) Microsatellite instability in colorectal cancer: different mutator phenotypes and the principal involvement of hMLH1. Cancer Res 58:1713–1718

Toft NJ, Winton DJ, Kelly J, Howard LA, Dekker M, te Riele H, Arends MJ, Wyllie AH, Margison GP, Clarke AR (1999) Msh2 status modulates both apoptosis and mutation frequency in the murine small intestine. Proc Natl Acad Sci USA 96: 3911–3915

Toyota M, Ahuja N, Ohe-Toyota M, Herman JG, Baylin SB, Issa J-P (1999) CpG island methylation phenotype in colorectal cancer. Proc Natl Acad Sci USA 96:8681–8686

Vasen HFA, Mecklin J-P, Meera Khan P, Lynch HT (1991) The International Collaborative Group on hereditary nonpolyposis colorectal cancer (ICG-HNPCC). Dis Colon Rectum 34:424–425

Vasen HFA, Watson P, Mecklin J-P, Lynch HT, The International Collaborative Group on HNPCC (1999) New clinical criteria for HNPCC (Lynch syndrome) proposed by the International Collaborative Group on HNPCC. Gastroenterology 116: 1453–1456

Veigl ML, Kasturi L, Olechnowicz J, Ma AH, Lutterbaugh JD, Periyasamy S, Li G-M, Drummond J, Modrich P, Sedwick WD, Markowitz SD (1998) Biallelic inactivation of hMLH1 by epigenetic silencing, a novel mechanism causing human MSI cancers. Proc Natl Acad Sci USA 95:8698–8702

Vilkki S, Tsao J-L, Loukola A, Pöyhönen M, Vierimaa O, Herva R, Aaltonen LA, Shibata D (2001) Extensive somatic microsatellite mutations in normal human tissue. Cancer Res 61:4541–4544

Vogelstein B, Fearon ER, Hamilton SR, Kern SE, Preisinger AC, Leppert M, Nakamura Y, White R, Smits AM, Bos JL (1988) Genetic alterations during colorectal tumor development. N Engl J Med 319:525–532

Wang Q, Lasset C, Desseigne F, Frappaz D, Bergeron C, Navarro C, Ruano E, Puisieux A (1999) Neurofibromatosis and early onset of cancers in hMLH1-deficient children. Cancer Res 59:294–297

Warthin AS (1913) Heredity with reference to carcinoma. Arch Intern Med 12:546–555

Watanabe A, Ikejima M, Suzuki N, Shimada T (1996) Genomic organization and expression of the human MSH3 gene. Genomics 31:311–318

Weber JL, Wong C (1993) Mutation of human short tandem repeats. Hum Mol Genet 2:123–128

Wheeler JMD, Beck NE, Kim HC, Tomlinson IPM, Mortensen NJMcC (1999) Mechanisms of inactivation of mismatch repair genes in human colorectal cancer cell lines: The predominant role of hMLH1. Proc Natl Acad Sci USA 96:10296–10301

Whitehall VLJ, Walsh MD, Young J, Leggett BA and Jass JR (2001) Methylation of O-6-methylguanine DNA methyltransferase characterizes a subset of colorectal cancer with low-level DNA microsatellite instability. Cancer Res 61:827–830

Wijnen J, de Leeuw W, Vasen H, van der Klift H, Møller P, Stormorken A, Meijers-Heijboer H, Lindhout D, Menko F, Vossen S, Möslein G, Tops C, Bröcker-Vriends A, Wu Y, Hofstra R, Sijmons R, Cornelisse C, Morreau H, Fodde R (1999) Familial endometrial cancer in female carriers of MSH6 germline mutations. Nat Genet 23:142–144

Winand NJ, Panzer JA, Kolodner RD (1998) Cloning and characterization of the human and Caenorhabditis elegans homologs of the Saccharomyces cerevisiae MSH5 gene. Genomics 53:69–80

Wu Y, Berends MJW, Mensink RGJ, Kempinga C, Sijmons RH, van der Zee AGJ, Hollema H, Kleibeuker JH, Buys CHCM, Hofstra RMW (1999) Association of hereditary nonpolyposis colorectal cancer-related tumors displaying low microsatellite instability with MSH6 germline mutations. Am J Hum Genet 65:1291–1298

Wu Y, Berends MJW, Post JG, Mensink RGJ, Verlind E, van der Sluis T, Kempinga C, Sijmons RH, van der Zee, AGJ, Hollema H, Kleibeuker JH, Buys CHCM, Hofstra RMW (2001a) Germline mutations of EXO1 gene in patients with hereditary nonpolyposis colorectal cancer (HNPCC) and atypical HNPCC forms. Gastroenterology 120:1580–1587

Wu Y, Berends MJW, Sijmons RH, Mensink RGJ, Verlind E, Kooi KA, van Der Sluis T, Kempinga C, van der Zee AGJ, Hollema H, Buys CHCM, Kleibeuker JH, Hofstra RM (2001b) A role for MLH3 in hereditary nonpolyposis colorectal cancer. Nat Genet 29:137–138

Zhang L, Yu J, Willson JKV, Markowitz SD, Kinzler KW, Vogelstein B (2001) Short mononucleotide repeat sequence variability in mismatch repair-deficient cancers. Cancer Res 61:3801–3805

Zhou X-P, Kuismanen S, Nyström-Lahti M, Peltomäki P, Eng C (2002) Distinct PTEN mutational spectra in hereditary nonpolyposis colon cancer syndrome-related endometrial carcinomas compared to sporadic microsatellite unstable tumours. Hum Mol Genet 11:445–450

Epigenetic Changes, Altered DNA Methylation and Cancer

F. Lyko

It has been known for a long time that tumor development coincides with changes in DNA methylation. Epigenetic mechanisms such as DNA methylation and specialized chromatin structures are capable of stably modulating gene expression over many cell generations. Thus, an epigenetic mutation can have the same effect like a classical, genetic mutation, i.e., loss- or gain-of-function of any given gene. Sensitive methods for the detection of epigenetic mutations have been developed in the past years and have been used to demonstrate a role of epigenetic mechanisms in tumorigenesis. Recent progress in our understanding of these mechanisms also allowed for the development of epigenetic cancer therapies. These concepts have a high potential for increasing the efficiency of conventional chemotherapy.

A. DNA Methylation Systems

Several mechanisms of gene regulation have roles in regulating epigenetic inheritance. These include DNA methylation, establishment of particular chromatin structures, chromatin modification, and posttranscriptional RNA processing. Since little is known about the activity of the latter two mechanisms in cancer or other diseases, the focus of this chapter will be on DNA methylation and the establishment of DNA-methylation-dependent chromatin structures. In humans, DNA methylation mainly occurs at the 5-position of cytosine in the context of cytosine-guanine (CpG) dinucleotides. CpG dinucleotides are clustered in CpG islands, certain regions of the genome with an unusually high CG-content. The methylation reaction is catalyzed by a class of enzymes termed (cytosine-5) DNA methyltransferases (BESTOR 2000). These enzymes specifically recognize their target sequence and covalently modify genomic cytosine residues. It is possible that some of the biological effects of DNA methylation are mediated directly by 5-methylcytosine. For example, it has been shown that DNA methylation can inhibit binding of transcription factors to DNA in vitro (BECKER et al. 1987; IGUCHI-ARIGA and SCHAFFNER 1989). This effect could be due to sterical hindrance or conformational changes induced by DNA methylation.

In vivo, the conversion of DNA methylation signals to biological effects appears to be more complex. There is an increasing number of proteins that specifically bind to methylated DNA and exert regulatory functions from there (HENDRICH and BIRD 1998). These proteins have been termed methyl-DNA binding proteins and they have been shown to engage in intriguing interactions: the majority of methyl-DNA binding proteins not only interact with methylated DNA but also with transcriptional corepressors and histone deacetylases (BALLESTAR and WOLFFE 2001; NG and BIRD 1999).

The interdepending action of DNA methyltransferases and methyl-DNA binding proteins defined a novel paradigm for epigenetic mechanisms. In this concept, the central factors of epigenetic gene regulation are provided by DNA methylation systems (BIRD and WOLFFE 1999). The core components of DNA methylation systems are the DNA methyltransferases and the methyl-DNA binding proteins (Fig. 1). Associated proteins are recruited from the nuclear pool of histone deacetylases, chromatin repressors, and nucleosome remodeling factors (Fig. 1). The sequential assembly of all factors involved results in the establishment and maintenance of stable, repressive chromatin structures. In this fashion, DNA methylation systems ensure the stable inheritance of epigenetic signals.

While a great wealth of information exists about DNA methylation, less is known about epigenetic chromatin. It is noteworthy that epigenetic inheritance can also be regulated independently of DNA methylation. There are several examples for epigenetic phenomena where DNA methylation appears not to be involved and where epigenetic signals are executed directly by chromatin regulation or by chromatin modification (LYKO and PARO 1999; TURNER 2000). These phenomena have been described mostly in model organisms other than mouse or man and their contribution to tumor formation is largely unknown.

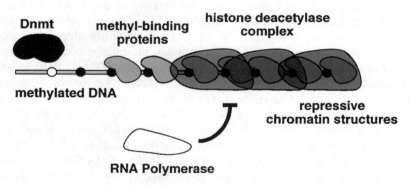

Fig. 1. Epigenetic regulation by DNA methylation systems. DNA methyltransferase (*Dnmt*) site-specifically methylates genomic DNA (*open circles*). Methyl-DNA binding proteins then bind to methylated DNA and function as anchors for corepressors and histone deacetylase complexes. The combined action of all proteins involved results in the establishment of repressive chromatin structures that cannot be accessed by RNA polymerase

The close connection between DNA methylation and chromatin regulation has also been further supported by the identification of methyltransferase interaction partners. These include the retinoblastoma protein, the transcriptional repressor DMAP1, and the histone deacetylases HDAC1 and HDAC2 (FUKS et al. 2000; ROBERTSON et al. 2000; ROUNTREE et al. 2000). Direct interactions between the methyltransferase and chromatin components facilitate the synergistic action of DNA methylation and chromatin networks on epigenetically regulated genes. In addition, the interactions might also target DNA methyltransferases to their site of action. This could be a major factor contributing to the dynamics of DNA methylation.

B. DNA Methylation Changes During Development

For a long time, DNA methylation has been perceived as a stable determinant of epigenetic inheritance. However, it now becomes more and more evident that DNA methylation actually is a dynamic process that undergoes various changes (JAENISCH, 1997). For example, DNA methylation levels change dramatically during mammalian development (Fig. 2). In the zygote, the majority of CpG islands is methylated, but in blastula stage embryos, much of the

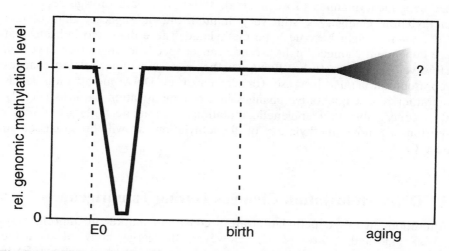

Fig. 2. Dynamic changes in DNA methylation levels during mammalian development. In blastula stage embryos, much of the genome becomes demethylated. Demethylation probably erases the epigenetic program of the zygote and primes the embryonic genome for differentiation processes. During postimplantation development, a wave of global de novo methylation reestablishes embryonic DNA methylation patterns that are then faithfully maintained in differentiated cells. DNA methylation patterns slowly change during aging but very little is known about the nature of these changes

genome becomes demethylated (Kafri et al. 1992; Mayer et al. 2000; Monk et al. 1987; Rougier et al. 1998). Demethylation is the consequence of both active and passive mechanisms and starts with the first embryonic cell division (Mayer et al. 2000; Rougier et al. 1998). The function of early embryonic demethylation remains elusive but it has been hypothesized that the mechanism serves to erase the epigenetic program of the zygote and to allow for the establishment of new programs for embryonic development and differentiation. The low efficiencies in the process of animal cloning can be at least partly attributed to a failure to sufficiently demethylate the embryonic genome (Kang et al. 2001).

After this initial period of demethylation, DNA methylation patterns become reestablished during postimplantation development (Kafri et al. 1992; Monk et al. 1987). During this period, de novo methyltransferases specifically recognize and modify their target sequences. The concomitant increase in genomic methylation levels coincides with cellular differentiation and an increasing commitment of cell lines to certain, specialized functions. In differentiated cells, DNA methylation patterns are maintained by maintenance methyltransferase. This keeps methylation levels stable by simply copying patterns from the parental DNA strand to the daughter strand immediately after replication. The methylation level of a fully differentiated mammalian cell corresponds to 4%–5% of genomic cytosines and about 80% of genomic CpG dinucleotides being methylated.

DNA methylation patterns have also been shown to change in an age-dependent manner (Toyota et al. 1999). The data on age-dependent methylation changes is still very limited but it suggests that certain CpG islands might become hypermethylated. These data also indicate that age-dependent changes might precede cancer-specific changes (see Sect. C.). However, it remains to be shown whether age- and tumor-related changes represent an actual increase (or decrease) in DNA methylation levels or rather reflect qualitative changes in DNA methylation patterns (Fig. 2). It is conceivable that epigenetic mutations accumulate with age through spurious de novo methylation or demethylation, as will be discussed in Sect. C.

C. DNA Methylation Changes During Tumorigenesis

Alterations in DNA methylation are a consistent marker in tumorigenesis (Warnecke and Bestor 2000). However, the large body of available results points into two different, seemingly contradictory directions. Early attempts to detect genome-wide changes by quantification of genomic 5-methylcytosine contents revealed a small but consistent decrease in tumors. Generally, genomic DNA from tumors appeared to contain about 10% less 5-methylcytosine than DNA from control tissues (Bedford and Van Helden 1987; Feinberg et al. 1988; Gama-Sosa et al. 1983). This decrease appeared to be more evident in metastases than in primary tumors (GAMA-SOSA et al. 1983).

Analysis of gene-specific CpG island methylation resulted in a different picture. As soon as genomic Southern blots became commonly established, DNA methylation was analyzed with methylation-sensitive restriction enzymes. Because it was known that methylation of CpG islands is associated with gene silencing, a special focus was put on methylation analysis of CpG islands in the promoter region of tumor suppressor genes. Indeed, several of these CpG islands were found to be hypermethylated, supporting the notion of hypermethylation-induced epigenetic mutations (BAYLIN and HERMAN 2000). More recently, the analysis of CpG island methylation has been extended to the genomic level (COSTELLO et al. 2000; HUANG et al. 1999; TOYOTA et al. 1999). Different strategies were used to obtain a more comprehensive view about alterations in DNA methylation in various tumors. Generally, it was found that about 10% of the CpG islands analyzed were hypermethylated in tumors when compared to healthy control tissue (COSTELLO et al. 2000; HUANG et al. 1999). Thus, there appears to be a tendency towards CpG island hypermethylation as well as genomic hypomethylation. The magnitude of changes might still have been underestimated because the results were derived largely from heterogeneous clinical samples that contain significant amounts of normal cells.

The biological significance of both genomic hypomethylation and CpG island hypermethylation has, to a limited extent, been analyzed in experimental systems. The consequences of genome-wide demethylation were studied in mutant mouse embryonic stem cells lacking the majority of their DNA methyltransferase activity (CHEN et al. 1998). These cells have greatly demethylated DNA and showed a ten-fold increased mutation rate with large-scale chromosomal abnormalities accounting for most of the mutations (CHEN et al. 1998). The results are consistent with decreases in DNA methylation affecting genome stability and concomitantly causing cancer. In contrast, DNA methyltransferase overexpression experiments also appeared to support a role of CpG island hypermethylation in tumorigenesis. Results obtained with transgenic cell lines suggested that DNA methyltransferase overexpression causes both ectopic CpG island hypermethylation and cellular transformation (VERTINO et al. 1996; WU et al. 1993). How this apparent contradiction can be resolved is presently unknown. Possibly, the process is more complex than previously envisaged and involves both an overall decrease in DNA methylation and a redistribution to certain CpG islands. A possible explanation would involve two distinct fractions of genomic 5-methylcytosine, a large fraction in centromeric satellite DNA and a smaller fraction in gene-rich regions of the genome. Genomic DNA hypomethylation could compromise genome stability by reducing the stability of centromeres, whereas hypermethylation could affect gene expression by modulating chromatin structure in gene-rich regions.

D. DNA Methyltransferase Expression in Tumors

The DNA methylation changes during tumorigenesis triggered a considerable interest in DNA methyltransferases. DNA methyltransferases are central factors in epigenetic gene regulation and mammalian methyltransferases have been analyzed extensively. All known (cytosine-5) DNA methyltransferases, from bacteria to man, share a common structure: Their C-terminal domain contains defined catalytic signature motifs that are required for enzymatic methyltransferase function (Kumar et al. 1992). In addition, most eukaryotic DNA methyltransferase also contain an N-terminal, "regulatory" domain that can mediate various functions, mostly by protein–protein interactions.

Presently, there are 4 known human DNA methyltransferases: DNMT1, DNMT2, DNMT3A, and DNMT3B. DNMT1 has been shown to be essential for mammalian development from the onset of cellular differentiation (Li et al. 1992). The enzyme has been analyzed in high detail, both in vitro and in vivo. Most in vivo results are consistent with *DNMT1* encoding a pure maintenance methyltransferase (Lei et al. 1996; Lyko et al. 1999) that is responsible for copying methylation patterns from the parental DNA strand to the newly replicated daughter strand. DNMT1 contains a very large regulatory domain that mediates protein–protein interactions with several factors involved in DNA replication, cell cycle control, and chromatin structure.

Additional human methyltransferases have been discovered more recently and are now being characterized. The function of DNMT2, the second known DNA methyltransferase, is still far from being understood (Okano et al. 1998b; Yoder and Bestor 1998). Unlike most other eukaryotic DNA methyltransferases, DNMT2 does not contain a regulatory domain and therefore looks similar to bacterial methyltransferases. Although the enzyme contains all the catalytic consensus motifs, no enzymatic activity could be detected yet (Okano et al. 1998b). DNMT2 is highly conserved during evolution with known homologs in a variety of diverse organisms such as yeasts, insects, plants, and vertebrates (Dong et al. 2001).

The most recently discovered DNA methyltransferases, DNMT3A and DNMT3B, are two closely related enzymes that have been demonstrated to function as de novo methyltransferases in vitro and in vivo (Hsieh 1999; Lyko et al. 1999; Okano et al. 1999; Okano et al. 1998a). Both enzymes are essential for mammalian development as demonstrated by gene targeting in mice (Okano et al. 1999). While the target genes of DNMT3A are still unknown, the function of DNMT3B appears to be restricted to methylation of centromeric satellite repeats (Okano et al. 1999). This particular sequence specificity also linked DNMT3B to ICF syndrome, a rare autosomal recessive disorder characterized by immunodeficiency, centromeric instability, and facial anomalies. Loss-of-function mutations in the *DNMT3B* gene have now been identified in a considerable number of ICF syndrome patients, thus revealing the molecular origin of the disease (HANSEN et al. 1999; OKANO et al. 1999; XU et al. 1999).

DNA methyltransferase expression has been analyzed in a variety of tumors. While there appears to be a general consensus on methyltransferase upregulation in tumor cells, the significance of the phenomenon is still unclear. Initial reports suggested an up to several-hundred-fold increase of DNMT1 expression in cancer cells (EL-DEIRY et al. 1991), thus suggesting direct consequences for CpG island hypermethylation. Later reports indicated a more modest increase (up to ten-fold) that is not restricted to DNMT1 but appears to also include DNMT2, DNMT3A, and DNMT3B (LIN et al. 2001; ROBERTSON et al. 1999). However, it has also become evident that the magnitude of differences can be influenced by secondary factors: DNA methyltransferase expression was found to be upregulated when compared to actin expression, but not when compared to the proliferation markers PCNA and histone H4 (EADS et al. 1999). Thus, DNA methyltransferase overexpression might simply be a byproduct of tumorigenesis without necessarily affecting epigenetic control of gene expression in tumors (WARNECKE and BESTOR 2000). Indeed, deletion of the *DNMT1* gene in a human colorectal cancer cell line affected methylation of centromeric satellites but not methylation of various other loci, including tumor suppressor genes (RHEE et al. 2000).

E. Epigenetic Mechanisms as a Therapeutic Target

Even though the precise causes of epigenetic changes during tumor progression are unknown, alterations in DNA methylation are undoubtedly involved in tumorigenesis. Apart from the indications for an accumulation of epigenetic mutations (see Sect. C.) there are additional lines of experimentation that provide direct proof for a role of DNA methylation in the development of cancer. For example, it has been shown that genomic demethylation greatly reduces the number of intestinal polyps in the Apc^Min mouse strain (LAIRD et al. 1995). This mouse strain represents an excellent model system for colorectal cancer since it carries a mutation in the *Apc* gene that causes the formation of numerous intestinal polyps and tumors. The incidence of lesions was significantly decreased by either mutational inactivation of the *Dnmt1* gene or by a pharmacological inhibition of DNA methyltransferase or by a combination of both (LAIRD et al. 1995). Genomic demethylation therefore reverted epimutations that normally facilitate the generation of intestinal polyps caused by the *Apc* mutation.

The therapeutic potential of genomic demethylation has also been demonstrated in human cancer cells. Melanoma cells, for example, frequently show a high degree of resistance to conventional chemotherapeutic agents. This chemoresistance could be overcome by treating cells with an inactivator of DNA methyltransferases (SOENGAS et al. 2001). The effect is caused by reversion of the methylation-induced silencing of the apoptosis effector gene

Apaf-1. Experimental demethylation therefore reverted an epigenetic mutation in the apoptosis pathway that had rendered the cells incapable of responding to signals triggered by chemotherapeutic agents.

The significance of epigenetic mutations for cancer therapy lies in their reversibility. In contrast to genetic mutations, that can only be treated by removal of affected tissue, epigenetic mutations can be reverted. Reversion results in epigenetic reprogramming or resetting from the epigenotype of tumor cells to the epigenotype of normal cells. In this respect, inhibitors of DNA methyltransferases have been used with some limited success. The most widely known inhibitor is the cytidine analogue 5-aza-cytidine (Fig. 3) and it has been used in the vast majority of experiments where pharmacological inhibition of methyltransferase activity is involved. The compound gets incorporated into DNA and functions as a suicide analogue for DNA methyltransferases (SANTI et al. 1984). The DNA methyltransferases recognize 5-aza-cytidine as a natural substrate and initiate catalysis. However, with the inhibitor, a covalent reaction intermediate between substrate and enzyme cannot be resolved and the enzyme remains bound to DNA (SANTI et al. 1984). The toxicity of these protein–DNA adducts probably accounts for the highly toxic effects of 5-aza-cytidine (JACKSON-GRUSBY et al. 1997).

The toxicity of 5-aza-cytidine also presented a major obstacle in attempts to use the inhibitor in cancer therapy. Low concentrations have been used in clinical trials (ABELE et al. 1987; LUBBERT 2000; PINTO and ZAGONEL 1993; VAN GROENINGEN et al. 1986) but their success has been rather limited. Several strategies are now being pursued to establish a more effective concept for epi-

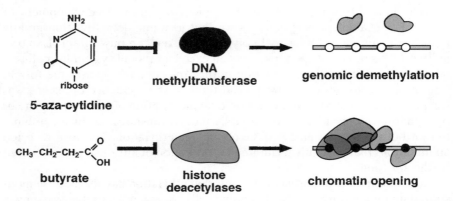

Fig. 3. Pharmacological inhibition of epigenetic factors. 5-aza-cytidine effectively inhibits DNA methyltransferases. This results in genomic demethylation due to ongoing replication. Butyrate inhibits histone deacetylases. This results in the destabilization of repressive chromatin structures. A combination of both strategies acts synergistically and seems to be especially potent in erasing epigenetic signals

genetic cancer therapy. For example, small molecules could be developed that inhibit methyltransferases directly without being incorporated into DNA. This could result in a marked reduction in toxicity. However, screening for methyltransferase inhibitors is a complex task because assays with an easy experimental read-out appear not to be available. An alternative strategy would be to increase the efficiency of low 5-aza-cytidine concentrations. This could be done either by chemical modifications of 5-aza-cytidine or by combining 5-aza-cytidine with a second compound to support synergistic effects. The latter strategy has been applied in experiments to revert epigenetic silencing on the level of both DNA methylation and chromatin structure (CAMERON et al. 1999). While low concentrations of 5-aza-cytidine proved ineffective in many instances, a combination of 5-aza-cytidine with trichostatin A restored gene expression effectively (CAMERON et al. 1999). Similar effects can be achieved with the simpler substance butyrate (BENJAMIN and JOST 2001) (Fig. 3). Both Trichostatin A and butyrate function as inhibitors of histone deacetylases and they can be used to break up the synergistic action of DNA methylation and repressive chromatin structures. Whether this approach can be successfully used for cancer therapy remains to be seen but the general strategy of increasing the effectiveness of 5-aza-cytidine appears to hold some promise for the future.

References

Abele R, Clavel M, Dodion P, Bruntsch U, Gundersen S, Smyth J, Renard J, van Glabbeke M, Pinedo HM (1987) The EORTC Early Clinical Trials Cooperative Group experience with 5-aza- 2'-deoxycytidine (NSC 127716) in patients with colo-rectal, head and neck, renal carcinomas and malignant melanomas. Eur J Cancer Clin Oncol 23:1921–1924

Ballestar E, Wolffe AP (2001) Methyl-CpG-binding proteins. Targeting specific gene repression. Eur J Biochem 268:1–6

Baylin SB, Herman, JG (2000) DNA hypermethylation in tumorigenesis: epigenetics joins genetics. Trends Genet 16:168–174

Becker PB, Ruppert S, Schütz G (1987) Genomic footprinting reveals cell type-specific DNA binding of ubiquitous factors. Cell 51:435–443

Bedford MT, van Helden PD (1987) Hypomethylation of DNA in pathological conditions of the human prostate. Cancer Res 47:5274–5276

Benjamin D, Jost JP (2001) Reversal of methylation-mediated repression with short-chain fatty acids: evidence for an additional mechanism to histone deacetylation. Nucleic Acids Res 29:3603–3610

Bestor TH (2000) The DNA methyltransferases of mammals. Hum Mol Genet 9: 2395–2402

Bird AP, Wolffe, AP (1999) Methylation-induced repression–belts, braces, and chromatin. Cell 99:451–454

Cameron EE, Bachman KE, Myohanen S, Herman JG, Baylin SB (1999) Synergy of demethylation and histone deacetylase inhibition in the re- expression of genes silenced in cancer. Nat Genet 21:103–107

Chen RZ, Pettersson U, Beard C, Jackson-Grusby L, Jaenisch R (1998) DNA hypomethylation leads to elevated mutation rates. Nature 395:89–93

Costello JF et al. (2000) Aberrant CpG-island methylation has nonrandom and tumor-type-specific patterns. Nat Genet 24:132–138

Dong A, Yoder JA, Zhang X, Zhou L, Bestor TH, Cheng X (2001) Structure of human DNMT2, an enigmatic DNA methyltransferase homolog that displays denaturant-resistant binding to DNA. Nucleic Acids Res 29:439–448

Eads CA, Danenberg KD, Kawakami K, Saltz LB, Danenberg PV, Laird PW (1999) CpG island hypermethylation in human colorectal tumors is not associated with DNA methyltransferase overexpression. Cancer Res 59:2302–2306

el-Deiry WS, Nelkin BD, Celano P, Yen RW, Falco JP, Hamilton SR, Baylin SB (1991) High expression of the DNA methyltransferase gene characterizes human neoplastic cells and progression stages of colon cancer. Proc Natl Acad Sci U S A 88:3470–3474

Feinberg AP, Gehrke CW, Kuo KC, Ehrlich M (1988) Reduced genomic 5-methylcytosine content in human colonic neoplasia. Cancer Res 48:1159–1161

Fuks F, Burgers WA, Brehm A, Hughes-Davies L, Kouzarides, T (2000) DNA methyltransferase Dnmt1 associates with histone deacetylase activity. Nat Genet 24:88–91

Gama-Sosa MA, Slagel VA, Trewyn RW, Oxenhandler R, Kuo KC, Gehrke CW, Ehrlich M (1983) The 5-methylcytosine content of DNA from human tumors. Nucleic Acids Res 11:6883–6894

Hansen RS, Wijmenga C, Luo P, Stanek AM, Canfield TK, Weemaes CM, Gartler SM (1999) The *DNMT3B* DNA methyltransferase gene is mutated in the ICF immunodeficiency syndrome. Proc Natl Acad Sci USA 96:14412–14417

Hendrich B, Bird A (1998) Identification and characterization of a family of mammalian methyl-CpG binding proteins. Mol Cell Biol 18:6538–6547

Hsieh CL (1999) In vivo activity of murine de novo methyltransferases, Dnmt3a and Dnmt3b. Mol Cell Biol 19:8211–8218

Huang TH, Perry MR, Laux DE (1999) Methylation profiling of CpG islands in human breast cancer cells. Hum Mol Genet 8:459–470

Iguchi-Ariga SM, Schaffner W (1989) CpG methylation of the cAMP-responsive enhancer/promoter sequence TGACGTCA abolishes specific factor binding as well as transcriptional activation. Genes Dev 3:612–619

Jackson-Grusby L, Laird PW, Magge SN, Moeller BJ, Jaenisch R (1997) Mutagenicity of 5-aza-2'-deoxycytidine is mediated by the mammalian DNA methyltransferase. Proc Natl Acad Sci U S A 94:4681–4685

Jaenisch R (1997) DNA methylation and imprinting: why bother? Trends Genet 13:323–329

Kafri T, Ariel M, Brandeis M, Shemer R, Urven L, McCarrey J, Cedar H, Razin A (1992) Developmental pattern of gene-specific DNA methylation in the mouse embryo and germ line. Genes Dev 6:705–714

Kang YK, Koo DB, Park JS, Choi YH, Chung AS, Lee KK, Han YM (2001) Aberrant methylation of donor genome in cloned bovine embryos. Nat Genet 28:173–177

Kumar S, Cheng X, Pflugrath JW, Roberts RJ (1992) Purification, crystallization, and preliminary X-ray diffraction analysis of an M.HhaI-AdoMet complex. Biochemistry 31:8648–8653

Laird PW, Jackson-Grusby L, Fazeli A, Dickinson SL, Jung WE, Li E, Weinberg RA, and Jaenisch R (1995) Suppression of intestinal neoplasia by DNA hypomethylation. Cell 81:197–205

Lei H, Oh SP, Okano M, Juttermann R, Goss KA, Jaenisch R, Li E (1996) De novo DNA cytosine methyltransferase activities in mouse embryonic stem cells. Development 122:3195–3205

Li E, Bestor TH, Jaenisch R (1992) Targeted mutation of the DNA methyltransferase gene results in embryonic lethality. Cell 69:915–926

Lin CH, Hsieh SY, Sheen IS, Lee WC, Chen TC, Shyu WC, Liaw YF (2001) Genome-wide hypomethylation in hepatocellular carcinogenesis. Cancer Res 61:4238–4243

Lubbert M (2000) DNA methylation inhibitors in the treatment of leukemias, myelodysplastic syndromes and hemoglobinopathies: clinical results and possible mechanisms of action. Curr Top Microbiol Immunol 249:135–164

Lyko F, Paro R (1999) Chromosomal elements conferring epigenetic inheritance. Bioessays 21:824–832

Lyko F, Ramsahoye BH, Kashevsky H, Tudor M, Mastrangelo MA, Orr-Weaver TL, Jaenisch R (1999) Mammalian (cytosine-5) methyltransferases cause genomic DNA methylation and lethality in *Drosophila*. Nat Genet 23:363–366

Mayer W, Niveleau A, Walter J, Fundele R, Haaf T (2000) Demethylation of the zygotic paternal genome. Nature 403:501–502

Monk M, Boubelik M, Lehnert S (1987) Temporal and regional changes in DNA methylation in the embryonic, extraembryonic and germ cell lineages during mouse embryo development. Development 99:371–382

Ng HH, Bird A (1999) DNA methylation and chromatin modification. Curr Opin Genet Dev 9:158–163

Okano M, Bell DW, Haber DA, Li E (1999) DNA methyltransferases Dnmt3a and Dnmt3b are essential for de novo methylation and mammalian development. Cell 99:247–257

Okano M, Xie S, Li E (1998a) Cloning and characterization of a family of novel mammalian DNA (cytosine-5) methyltransferases. Nat Genet 19:219–220

Okano M, Xie S, Li E (1998b) Dnmt2 is not required for de novo and maintenance methylation of viral DNA in embryonic stem cells. Nucleic Acids Res 26:2536–2540

Pinto A, Zagonel V (1993) 5-Aza-2'-deoxycytidine (Decitabine) and 5-azacytidine in the treatment of acute myeloid leukemias and myelodysplastic syndromes: past, present and future trends. Leukemia 7 Suppl 1:51–60

Rhee I, Jair KW, Yen RW, Lengauer C, Herman JG, Kinzler KW, Vogelstein B, Baylin SB, Schuebel KE (2000) CpG methylation is maintained in human cancer cells lacking DNMT1. Nature 404:1003–1007

Robertson KD, Ait-Si-Ali S, Yokochi T, Wade PA, Jones PL, Wolffe AP (2000) DNMT1 forms a complex with Rb, E2F1 and HDAC1 and represses transcription from E2F-responsive promoters. Nat Genet 25:338–342

Robertson KD, Uzvolgyi E, Liang G, Talmadge C, Sumegi J, Gonzales FA, Jones PA (1999) The human DNA methyltransferases (DNMTs) 1, 3a and 3b: coordinate mRNA expression in normal tissues and overexpression in tumors. Nucleic Acids Res 27:2291–2298

Rougier N, Bourc'his D, Gomes DM, Niveleau A, Plachot M, Paldi A, Viegas-Pequignot E (1998) Chromosome methylation patterns during mammalian preimplantation development. Genes Dev 12:2108–2113

Rountree MR, Bachman KE, Baylin SB (2000) DNMT1 binds HDAC2 and a new co-repressor, DMAP1, to form a complex at replication foci. Nat Genet 25:269–277

Santi DV, Norment A, Garrett CE (1984) Covalent bond formation between a DNA-cytosine methyltransferase and DNA containing 5-azacytosine. Proc Natl Acad Sci U S A 81:6993–6997

Soengas MS et al. (2001) Inactivation of the apoptosis effector Apaf-1 in malignant melanoma. Nature 409:207–211

Toyota M, Ahuja N, Ohe-Toyota M, Herman JG, Baylin SB, Issa JP (1999) CpG island methylator phenotype in colorectal cancer. Proc Natl Acad Sci U S A 96:8681–8686

Turner BM (2000) Histone acetylation and an epigenetic code. Bioessays 22:836–845

van Groeningen CJ, Leyva A, O'Brien AM, Gall HE, Pinedo HM (1986) Phase I and pharmacokinetic study of 5-aza-2'-deoxycytidine (NSC 127716) in cancer patients. Cancer Res 46:4831–4836

Vertino PM, Yen RW, Gao J, Baylin SB (1996) De novo methylation of CpG island sequences in human fibroblasts overexpressing DNA (cytosine-5-)-methyltransferase. Mol Cell Biol 16:4555–4565

Warnecke PM, Bestor TH (2000) Cytosine methylation and human cancer. Curr Opin Oncol 12:68–73

Wu J, Issa JP, Herman J, Bassett DE Jr, Nelkin BD, Baylin SB (1993) Expression of an exogenous eukaryotic DNA methyltransferase gene induces transformation of NIH 3T3 cells. Proc Natl Acad Sci U S A 90:8891–8895

Xu GL et al. (1999) Chromosome instability and immunodeficiency syndrome caused by mutations in a DNA methyltransferase gene. Nature 402:187–191

Yoder JA, Bestor TH (1998) A candidate mammalian DNA methyltransferase related to pmt1p of fission yeast. Hum Mol Genet 7:279–284

CHAPTER 9

Hormonal Carcinogenesis

R. Kaaks

Tumor development is a consequence of mutations in proto-oncogenes and tumor suppressor genes that normally control cell proliferation. Such mutations may results from defective DNA repair (Pegg 1999), increased exposures to mutagenic chemical agents either of exogenous origin or of endogenous origin (e.g., oxygen radicals) (Blair and Kazerouni 1997; Cerutti 1985; Loft and Poulsen 1996; Stanley 1995), exposure to radiation (Hall and Angele 1999), and other mechanisms. The occurrence of mutations, and the likelihood that they become fixed by transmission to daughter cells, depends on the rate of cell proliferation, as well as on the failure of cells to undergo apoptosis (programmed death) (Preston-Martin et al. 1990, 1993). In addition, the likelihood of proliferating cells to accumulate mutations may also depend on the pool-size of cells maintained in a relatively undifferentiated state, as only nondifferentiated cells have the potential to divide. Hormones and growth factors have well-documented roles in maintaining a proper balance between cellular differentiation, proliferation, and programmed death (Aaronson 1991; Werner and Leroith 1996). Thus, alterations in the endogenous hormone and growth factor metabolism, or use of exogenous hormones for contraception or postmenopausal replacement therapy, could have effects on the risk of certain types of cancer.

Amongst many classes of hormones, sex steroids (androgens, estrogens, progestogens) have especially received the attention of researchers as factors potentially playing a role in carcinogenesis. Besides their well-documented roles in regulating cellular differentiation, mitosis, and apoptosis, there is abundant evidence from animal experiments and cell or tissue cultures that some of these hormones may favor the selective growth of preneoplastic and neoplastic cells (Dickson and Stancel 2000). Epidemiologists have had a longstanding interest in sex steroids, especially in relation to cancers of steroid-sensitive tissues or organs such as the breast, endometrium, ovary, and prostate (Henderson et al. 1982; Key and Pike 1988a,b).

In addition to the sex steroids, there is increasing interest among molecular biologists, pathologists, and epidemiologists in the possible roles of insulin, IGF-I, and IGF-binding proteins as factors that may favor tumor development (Giovannucci 2001; Kaaks et al. 2000a; Kaaks and Lukanova 2001; Khandwala et al. 2000; Yu and Rohan 2000). Insulin and IGF-I both have mitogenic and antiapoptotic effects in normal and neoplastic cells of various tissue origins (KHANDWALA et al. 2000; WERNER and LEROITH 1996), influence cellular (de-)differentiation, and have been documented to favor neoplastic transformation (KHANDWALA et al. 2000; STEWART and ROTWEIN 1996; WERNER and LEROITH 1996; YU and BERKEL 1999). Insulin and IGF-I exert these trophic effects on a wide variety of tissue types including breast (FOEKENS et al. 1989), endometrium (RUTANEN 1998; WANG and CHARD 1999), ovary (PORETSKY et al. 1999; WANG and CHARD 1999), colon (SINGH and RUBIN 1993), prostate (POLLAK et al. 1998; WONG and WANG 2000), and kidney (HAMMERMAN 1999). In some tissue types (e.g., breast, endometrium, and prostate) the effects of IGF-I have been proven to be synergistic with those of other growth factors and steroids (WESTLEY et al. 1998; YEE and LEE 2000). A further reason for the special interest in insulin and IGF-I in cancer development is that their metabolism is also strongly related to nutrition and energy metabolism. Finally, insulin and IGF-I are key regulators of the synthesis and biological availability of sex steroids, by stimulating steroidogenesis (KAAKS 1996; KAAKS et al. 2000a; PORETSKY et al. 1999) while inhibiting the hepatic synthesis of SHBG (CRAVE et al. 1995; PLYMATE et al. 1988; PUGEAT et al. 1991; SINGH et al. 1990). Circulating levels of insulin and IGF-I are inversely correlated with levels of circulating SHBG, and are directly correlated with total and bioavailable sex steroids in women (PFEILSCHIFTER et al. 1996). Dysregulations in the metabolism of insulin or IGF-I might thus form a metabolic link between a Western lifestyle, characterized by sedentariness and excess energy intake, increased levels of bioavailable androgens and estrogens, and high incidence rates of various forms of cancer that are frequent in industrially developed societies (KAAKS and LUKANOVA 2001).

This chapter will review the epidemiological evidence relating cancer risk to sex steroids (of endogenous or exogenous origin) and to circulating levels of insulin, IGF-I, and IGFBPs. Most of this chapter focuses on cancers of the breast, endometrium, ovary, prostate, and colon, which are all tumors with high incidence rates in the Western, industrially developed world, as compared to developing countries (IARC 1997).

A. Sex Steroids

I. Cancers of the Breast, Endometrium, and Ovary

A number of observations provide indirect evidence that alterations of endogenous sex steroid metabolism can influence the risk of cancer of the breast, endometrium, and ovary. First, the risks of these cancers are related to factors such as early menarche (which marks the onset of ovarian estrogen and progesterone synthesis), late menopause (arrest of ovarian estrogen and progesterone synthesis), age at first full-term pregnancy, and total number of full-term pregnancies experienced lifetime (JOHN et al. 1993; KELSEY et al. 1993; KELSEY and WHITTEMORE 1994; PURDIE and GREEN 2001; SCHILDKRAUT et al. 2001; WHITTEMORE et al. 1992; WHITTEMORE 1994). Second, with increasing age, age-specific incidence rates of cancers of the breast and endometrium rise faster before menopause than after menopause. Third, overweight and obesity increase the risk of breast cancer among postmenopausal women, and of endometrial cancer both before and after menopause. Increased adiposity generally decreases plasma levels of sex hormone-binding globulin (SHBG), due to increase in circulating insulin (see also Sect. B.I.). Among post-menopausal women, increased adiposity augments levels of estrone, and of total and bioavailable estradiol (AUSTIN et al. 1991; KATSOUYANNI et al. 1991; KAYE et al. 1991; KEY et al. 2001). Among premenopausal women, obesity may lead to chronic anovulation and low progesterone levels, especially when women have a predisposition towards the development of ovarian hyperan-drogenism (HAMILTON-FAIRLEY et al. 1992; ROBINSON et al. 1993). Finally (fourth), alterations in endogenous steroid metabolism, and the use of exoge-nous estrogens or progestogens (or combinations) used for contraception or postmenopausal therapy have also been documented to influence risk of mammary, endometrial, and ovarian cancers (see sections below).

1. Breast

Prospective cohort studies have shown increased breast cancer risk among postmenopausal women who have comparatively elevated plasma levels of testosterone and Δ-4 androstenedione, reduced levels of sex hormone-binding globulin (SHBG), and increased levels of total estradiol, and bioavailable estradiol not bound to SHBG (THE ENDOGENOUS HORMONES AND BREAST CANCER COLLABORATIVE GROUP 2002; THOMAS et al. 1997b). Similar observa-tions were made in a number of traditional case-control studies, where blood concentrations of hormones were compared between women who had a diag-nosis of breast cancer and cancer-free control subjects (reviewed in BERNSTEIN and ROSS 1993).

Use of exogenous estrogens for postmenopausal estrogen replacement therapy (ERT) is also associated with an increase in breast cancer risk. Sys-tematic reviews of case-control and cohort studies (IARC 1999), and a pooled analysis of over 50 such studies (COLLABORATIVE GROUP ON HORMONAL FACTORS IN BREAST CANCER 1997), have shown a small increase in breast cancer risk with longer duration of ERT use (5 years or more) in current and recent users. The increase in risk disappears several years after cessation of ERT use. These and other observations support the "estrogen" hypothesis, which postulates that breast cancer risk is increased in women with elevated mammary tissue exposures to estrogens (BERNSTEIN and ROSS 1993; KEY and PIKE 1988a; PIKE et al. 1993). Animal experiments (NANDI et al. 1995) and in vitro studies with tissues and cell lines (CLARKE et al. 1994; DICKSON et al. 1989) have also shown the critical role of estrogens in malignant transformation, and progression and growth of mammary tumors.

An extension of the estrogen excess theory is that, compared to an expo-sure to estrogens alone, breast cancer risk is increased further when women are exposed to the combination of estrogens and progestogens ("estrogen-plus-progestogen" hypothesis) (Key and Pike 1988b). One observation that led to this extended theory is that in premenopausal women breast epithelial proliferation rates are increased during the luteal phase of the menstrual cycle, when progesterone levels are high, as compared to the follicular phase, when progesterone levels are low (Potten et al. 1988). Furthermore, breast cancer incidence rates rise less steeply with age after menopause, when the ovarian synthesis of both estrogens and progesterone ceases, than before. Finally, the estrogen-plus-progestogen hypothesis is supported by recent study results showing that women using combined estrogen-plus-progestogen preparations for postmenopausal replacement therapy (Magnusson et al. 1999) have a greater increase in risk than women using preparations containing only estrogens.

As for breast cancer among premenopausal women, several case-control studies (reviewed in Stoll and Secreto 1992), and at least three prospective studies have been conducted (Helzlsouer et al. 1994; Rosenberg et al. 1994; Thomas et al. 1997a; Wysowski et al. 1987). However, these studies included small numbers of cases, and in general are complicated by the fact that blood levels of sex steroids, especially estrogens and progestogens, vary widely during the menstrual cycle. While suggesting a possible association of breast cancer risk with circulating levels of androgens and total estrogens, the data from these studies are insufficient to allow any firm conclusion at this stage.

In an expert panel review of more than 10 cohort and 50 case-control studies (IARC 1999), it was concluded that use of combined oral contraceptives (OCs), containing both estrogen and progestogen, is associated with a small increase in breast cancer risk. This association, however, did not show any clear difference between types and doses of estrogen/progestogen combinations, and was no longer present 10 years after cessation of OC use. It is possible that the small OC-related increase in breast cancer risk was a result of detection bias, due to increased surveillance of women regularly visiting a physician for OC prescriptions. Conclusions very similar to those of the expert panel review were reached after reanalysis of the pooled, individual-level data of over 50 studies (Collaborative Group on Hormonal Factors in Breast Cancer 1996).

A somewhat paradoxical observation is that obesity is related to a mild reduction in breast cancer risk among premenopausal women (IARC 2002; Ursin et al. 1995), in contrast to the relationship observed in postmenopausal women. This inverse relationship might be explained by the fact that, in premenopausal women, obesity does not lead to any noticeable increase in circulating estradiol (Key et al. 2001), but can, at least in some women with a predisposition towards ovarian hyperandrogenism, lead to chronic anovulation and a decrease in progesterone levels. The inverse relationship of obesity with premenopausal breast cancer risk can therefore also be interpreted as indirect support for the estrogen-plus-progestogen hypothesis.

2. Endometrium

From a histological and molecular pathology perspective, endometrial tumors can be divided into two major types. Type-I tumors, which represent up to about 80% of endometrial cancers, are mostly endometrioid. Type-II tumors are more often serous papillary, clear cell, or squamous carcinomas, and generally develop from the atrophic endometrium in older women. The two types differ also in the pattern of somatic gene mutations: type-I tumors often show mutations in the *ras* proto-oncogene and the *PTEN* tumor suppressor gene, microsatellite instability, but generally no mutations in the *P53* tumor suppressor gene, whereas a majority of serous (type-II) tumors have *P53* mutations, but generally no microsatellite instability, *ras* or *PTEN* mutations (EMONS et al. 2000; SHERMAN 2000). Nutritional lifestyle factors most strongly related to endometrial cancer risk are obesity and lack of physical activity. Together, these two factors may account for up to half of the total incidence of endometrial cancer in Western, industrially developed societies (BERGSTROM et al. 2001; IARC 2002). Most epidemiological studies did not distinguish clearly between type-I and -II tumors, and even when the distinction was made numbers of type-II tumors were usually too small to make clear separate inferences with regard to potential risk factors. Nevertheless, there is evidence that nutritional lifestyle factors such as obesity, and also aspects of hormone metabolism discussed in the following paragraphs, affect mostly the risk of type-I tumors (EMONS et al. 2000).

The predominant theory relating endogenous risk of *endometrial* cancer to endogenous sex steroids is the "unopposed estrogen" hypothesis. This theory stipulates that risk is increased among women who have normal or elevated plasma bioavailable estrogens but low levels of progesterone, so that biological effects of estrogens are insufficiently counterbalanced by those of progesterone (KEY and PIKE 1988a). One observation that led to the unopposed estrogen hypothesis is that mitotic rates of endometrium are higher during the follicular phase of the menstrual cycle when progesterone levels are low, than during the luteal phase (FERENCZY et al. 1979; KEY and PIKE 1988a). Another key observation, confirmed by numerous case-control and cohort studies, is that endometrial cancer risk is increased among postmenopausal women using ERT, with a clear dose-dependence with respect to duration of use, whereas women using combined estrogen-progestogen combinations ("hormone replacement therapy" or HRT) have only a very mild increase in risk compared to women who never used any postmenopausal ERT or HRT (IARC 1999). Results from a few more detailed studies suggest that the increase in risk among HRT users compared to nonusers is present only when progesterone is added for less than 10 days for each (28-day) cycle (IARC 1999; SHAPIRO et al. 1985; VAN LEEUWEN and ROOKUS 1989; WEIDERPASS et al. 1999a). Combination-type OCs that contain both estrogens and progesterone, and that have progestogens for at least 10 days per cycle also reduce risk by approximately 50%, whereas the use of sequential OCs, containing progestogens only in the last 5 days of a cycle, were found to be associated with an increased risk of endometrial cancer (IARC 1999; WEIDERPASS et al. 1999b).

Studies in vitro have shown that estrogens stimulate the proliferation of normal endometrial tissue as well as endometrial tumor cells, and that at least part of this effect may be mediated by an increase in local IGF-I concentrations (GIUDICE et al. 1991; KLEINMAN et al. 1995; MURPHY and GHAHARY 1990; RUTANEN 1998). The estrogen-opposing effects of progestogens, on the other hand, appear to be due largely in part by progesterone's capacity to increase endometrial tissue levels of IGFBP-1. IGFBP-1 is the most abundant IGF-binding protein in endometrial tissue, where it inhibits IGF-I action (GIUDICE et al. 1991; RUTANEN 1998).

In both pre- and postmenopausal women, endometrial cancer risk has been found to be directly related to circulating levels of androstenedione and testosterone (AUSTIN et al. 1991; GIMES et al. 1986; MOLLERSTROM et al. 1993; NAGAMANI et al. 1986; NYHOLM et al. 1993; POTISCHMAN et al. 1996). Premenopausal patients with endometrial cancer often present symptoms or a history of ovarian hyperandrogenic syndromes, such as the polycystic ovary syndrome ((PCOS) COULAM et al. 1983; DAHLGREN et al. 1991; GRADY and ERNSTER 1996; NIWA et al. 2000; SHU et al. 1991) – syndromes that are generally associated with chronic anovulation, and hence with low production of progesterone (EHRMANN et al. 1995). Interestingly, women with PCOS are often obese and insulin resistant, and studies have shown that chronic hyperinsulinemia is at least partially responsible for the ovarian androgen excess in these women (EHRMANN et al. 1995; PORETSKY et al. 1999).

Besides androgens, low circulating levels of sex hormone-binding globulin (SHBG) and elevated total and bioavailable estrogens (estrone, estradiol) have also been associated with increased risk of endometrial cancer, although among postmenopausal women only (ALEEM et al. 1976; AUSTIN et al. 1991; BENJAMIN and DEUTSCH 1976; GIMES et al. 1986; NYHOLM et al. 1993; OETTINGER et al. 1984; PETTERSSON et al. 1986; POTISCHMAN et al. 1996; ZELENIUCH-JACQUOTTE et al. 2001). The elevated estrogen levels can be explained by the fact that many postmenopausal women with endometrial cancer are obese (IARC 2002) and by increased circulating androgen levels. After menopause, the peripheral conversion of circulating androgens within adipose tissue is the major source of estrogens (KEY et al. 2001; SIITERI 1987). Before menopause, risk of endometrial cancer does not appear to be related to circulating levels of estradiol (KEY and PIKE 1988a; POTISCHMAN et al. 1996) and neither are estrogen levels related to body mass index or other measures of obesity (KEY et al. 2001). The high prevalence of both obesity and PCOS among young endometrial cancer patients, but absence of a clear association between premenopausal endometrial cancer risk and circulating estradiol levels, suggest that endometrial cancer risk before the menopause may be due mostly to progesterone deficiency, as a consequence of excess weight, hyperinsulinemia, ovarian androgen excess, and anovulation (KAAKS et al. 2002a; POTISCHMAN et al. 1996).

3. Ovary

The role of hormones in the etiology of *ovarian* cancer is not very well understood. Established epidemiological associations include a reduction in risk among regular users of combined OCs, the reduction being about 50% for women who have used the preparations for at least 5 years (WHITTEMORE 1994; WHITTEMORE et al. 1992; IARC 1999) and a protective effect of high parity. However, there may be a weak (about 20%) increase in ovarian cancer risk in relation to long-term ERT or HRT use (GARG et al. 1998; NEGRI et al. 1999; RODRIGUEZ et al. 2001). Ovarian cancer risk is not clearly related to excess body weight, some studies showing an increase in risk (LEW and GARFINKEL 1979; MOLLER et al. 1994; POLYCHRONOPOULOU et al. 1993; PURDIE et al. 1995; RISCH 1998), whereas others showed no strong relationship (CHEN et al. 1992; KOCH et al. 1988; SHU et al. 1989; SLATTERY et al. 1989) or even a decrease in risk (LUKANOVA et al. 2002e). One cohort study showed a direct association of risk with the waist-to-hip ratio (WHR) (MINK et al. 1996) as a measure of central ("android") obesity, and a similar direct association was observed among premenopausal women in one case-control study (SONNICHSEN et al. 1990).

Two classical hypotheses about the etiopathology of ovarian cancer are the "incessant ovulation" hypothesis, and the "gonadotropin" hypothesis.

The incessant ovulation hypothesis (FATHALLA 1971; RISCH 1998) stipulates that ovarian cancer risk is increased by prolonged periods of uninterrupted ovulatory cycles. Incessant ovulation would increase the formation of ovarian inclusion cysts, which are believed to form as a result of repeated damage and remodeling of the ovarian epithelial surface epithelium induced by regular ovulations. The inclusion cysts would be the origin of epithelial-type ovarian tumors, which constitute about 90% of ovarian malignancies. In an extension of the incessant ovulation hypothesis, it has been proposed that inclusion cysts would gradually transform to tumor cells under the influence of hormonal factors (CRAMER and WELCH 1983; RISCH 1998).

One hormonal factor strongly implicated in the malignant transformation of entrapped epithelium is an excessive stimulation by luteinizing hormone (LH), follicle-stimulating hormone (FSH) or both ["*gonadotropin*" hypothesis (BLAAKAER 1997; CRAMER et al. 1983)]. The gonadotropins might act either directly, through their cognate receptors in ovarian epithelium and activation of gonadotropin-responsive genes, or indirectly, through the stimulation of ovarian production of androgens or estrogens. The gonadotropin hypothesis got its original support from animal experiments, showing enhanced ovarian tumor formation after manipulations that caused excess pituitary gonadotropin secretion.

Several case-control studies have been conducted to examine relationships of ovarian cancer risk with circulating sex steroid levels (RAO and

SLOTMAN 1991). However, these studies were generally small, and their results are difficult to interpret because of possible tumor-induced alterations in ovarian sex steroid secretion. One prospective study, by HELZLSOUER et al., has shown significantly elevated Δ-4-androstenedione levels in prediagnostic blood samples of 13 premenopausal and 18 postmenopausal women who eventually developed ovarian cancer (HELZLSOUER et al. 1995). In a larger prospective study, combining three cohorts in New York (USA), Milan (Italy) and Umeå (northern Sweden), including a total of 132 cases of ovarian cancer cases and 257 controls, ovarian cancer risk showed no statistically significant associations with prediagnostic circulating levels of estrone, androstenedione, and testosterone (LUKANOVA et al. 2002a). However, increased levels of androstenedione measured in women who were premenopausal at recruitment were associated with a modest increase in risk of ovarian cancer [OR = 2.35 (0.81–6.82), $p < 0.12$], although in the second study this association was not statistically significant. Before menopause, about 50% of androstenedione is produced by the ovaries, whereas after menopause the adrenals become the major source. Additional indirect evidence for an association of ovarian production of androstenedione with cancer risk comes from one prospective study showing an increased risk among women who have PCOS, a metabolic disorder that is indeed related to androstenedione excess both from ovaries and adrenals (SCHILDKRAUT et al. 1996). Interestingly, women with PCOS generally also have elevated pituitary luteinizing hormone (LH) secretion. Taken together, these observations suggest an extension of the gonadotropin hypothesis, namely that ovarian tumor development may be enhanced by excess ovarian production of androgens, induced by elevated LH (and possible other regulatory factors, including insulin) (RISCH 1998). This hypothesis requires further investigation.

The incessant ovulation hypothesis is based almost entirely on indirect epidemiological evidence. Ovarian cancer risk is increased in women who have early menarche, late menopause, low parity, and who do not use OCs – factors that all contribute to a woman's lifetime cumulated number of ovulatory cycles. Several of these associations, however, are also in agreement with the gonadotropin/androgen excess hypotheses. In particular, oral contraceptive use causes a suppression of pituitary LH secretion, and is also related to reduced ovarian androgen production in both hyperandrogenic and normoandrogenic women (ADEN et al. 1998; PORCILE and GALLARDO 1991; SOBBRIO et al. 1990; THE ESHRE CAPRI WORKSHOP GROUP 2001; THORNEYCROFT et al. 1999; WIEGRATZ et al. 1995; YAMAMOTO and OKADA 1994).

II. Cancer of the Prostate

Like cancers of the breast, endometrium, and ovary, prostate cancer has also much higher incidence rates in populations with a Western lifestyle than in most parts of the developing world (IARC 1997). In contrast to breast and endometrial cancers, however, prostate cancer risk shows no clear relationship with excess weight (IARC 2002; Kaaks et al. 2000a).

There is substantial indirect evidence for the implication of sex steroids, notably androgens, in prostate tumor development. Surgical or medical castration often dramatically improve the clinical course of prostate cancer patients, and animal studies have also shown increased spontaneous or chemically induced prostatic tumor formation after the administration of testosterone or dihydrotestosterone (DHT) (Bosland 1996). Polymorphisms in the androgen receptor gene causing increased receptor transactivation have also been found to be associated with an increase in prostate cancer risk (Coughlin and Hall 2002; Ross et al. 1998).

The predominant hypothesis is that risk is increased in men who have elevated intraprostatic concentrations of dihydro-testosterone (DHT). DHT is formed within the prostate from testosterone, by the enzyme 5α-reductase type II (SRD5A), and has a higher binding affinity for the androgen receptor and stronger androgenic activity than testosterone. There is some evidence from prospective cohort studies that prostate cancer risk is increased among men who have comparatively elevated circulating levels of androstanediol-glucuronide – a major breakdown product of DHT and a possible marker of intraprostatic androgen (DHT) activity (Eaton et al. 1999; Kaaks et al. 2000a). It is not entirely clear, however, what are the most important determinants of interindividual differences in prostatic DHT concentrations and, especially, how such differences might be related to lifestyle or other environmental factors that are strongly associated with international differences in prostate cancer incidence (Bosland 2000; Kaaks et al. 2000a). Japanese and Chinese immigrants to the USA have lower incidence rates of prostate cancer than men of African or European ancestry, and at the same time have been found to have lower 5-α-reductase activity. Certain polymorphic variants of the SRD5A gene that are associated with increased 5α-reductase activity have also been found to increase prostate cancer risk (Coughlin and Hall 2002; Ross et al. 1998).

Another possible determinant of levels of intraprostatic DHT formation could be levels of bioavailable testosterone in the circulation. This prediction, however, has received only limited support from prospective epidemiological studies (Eaton et al. 1999; Kaaks et al. 2000a). In one study, a multivariate analysis showed a strong trend of increasing prostate cancer risk with increasing levels of plasma testosterone adjusting for SHBG, whereas risk was inversely related to levels of SHBG after adjustment for testosterone (Gann et al. 1996). An association of risk with indicators of bioavailable circulating testosterone, unbound to SHBG, has not been confirmed by at least four other prospective cohort studies and in none of eight cohort studies (reviewed in Bosland 2000; Eaton et al. 1999; Kaaks et al. 2000a), was risk associated with plasma or serum levels of total testosterone. In summary, it remains unclear whether variations in bioavailable testosterone are indeed entirely unrelated to prostate cancer risk, or whether weak associations exist that may have been obscured by, for example, inaccuracies in hormone measurements. Excess weight is not a determinant of increased total and bioavailable testosterone in men (Kaaks et al. 2000a), in contrast to postmenopausal women. Indeed, obesity rather causes a decrease in both total and bioavailable testosterone levels.

Besides androgens, estrogens have also been proposed either to enhance or inhibit prostate cancer development (Bosland 2000; Chang and Prins 1999; Farnsworth 1996) but the lack of any direct association of prostate cancer risk with plasma estrogen levels provides no support to either of these hypotheses (Bosland 2000; Eaton et al. 1999).

B. Insulin, and Insulin-Like Growth Factors

I. Chronic Hyperinsulinemia and Cancer Risk

Epidemiological studies have shown that the risk of a number of cancers that are particularly frequent in Western, industrialized societies is increased by excess body weight (IARC 2002) and lack of physical activity. The associations of risk with excess weight includes cancers of the colon, endometrium, pancreas, and breast (only for tumors diagnosed several years after menopause). Colon cancer risk appears to be associated particularly with increased intra-abdominal body fat stores (i.e., an "androgenic body fat distribution," as measured, for example, by the ratio of waist-to-hip body circumferences) and, possibly for this reason, is stronger among men than among women. Regarding physical activity, there is convincing evidence that it reduces risk of cancers of the breast and colon, and substantial evidence that it may also protect against cancers of the endometrium, and possibly other organ sites (IARC 2002).

Excess weight and lack of physical activity both lead to a diminished sensitivity of tissues (especially skeletal muscle, liver, and adipose tissue) to the physiological actions of insulin. Such insulin resistance is a frequent phenomenon in Western populations. Nutritionally induced insulin resistance can be seen as a metabolic adaptation to increased hepatic and muscular uptake and oxidation of fatty acids, which needs to be compensated by a reduced capacity of these tissues to absorb, store, and metabolize glucose (Kraegen et al. 2001; Randle 1998). The relationship of insulin resistance to excess weight can be explained to a large extent by the constant release of free fatty acids from adipose tissue (especially from intra-abdominal fat stores) into the circulation (Bergman and Ader 2000; Ferrannini et al. 1983). In addition, adipose tissue releases a number of endocrine signalling factors, such as tumor necrosis factor (TNF) α (Hotamisligil 2000) and resistin (Steppan and Lazar 2002), and other molecules (Trayhurn and Beattie 2001) that play a role in regulating insulin sensitivity of liver and skeletal muscle. Physical activity improves insulin sensitivity (Grimm 1999; Raastad et al. 2000; Van Baak and Borghouts 2000). One mechanism through which this may occur is the limitation of weight gain or reduction of excess weight. However, in sedentary subjects, physical activity can improve insulin sensitivity and decrease plasma insulin levels within days, and thus independently of any substantial changes in body weight. Mechanisms that may mediate such effects include reductions of intramuscular triglyceride stores (PAN et al. 1997), increased muscular phosphatidylinositol-3 kinase activity (HOUMARD et al. 1999), and an increased capacity of skeletal muscle to metabolize or store glucose (GOODYEAR and KAHN 1998; HARGREAVES 1998; PERSEGHIN et al. 1996).

In the mid-1990s, MCKEOWN-EYSSEN (1994) and GIOVANNUCCI (1995) formulated the hypothesis that chronically elevated insulin levels might be a causal factor in the etiology of colon cancer. The hypothesis was motivated by the observations of increased colon cancer risk among obese and physical inactive men and women, and among subjects who have low dietary intakes of n-3 polyunsaturated fatty acids, and high intakes of sucrose and other refined and rapidly digestible carbohydrates. These various factors all predispose to the development of insulin resistance and/or lead to elevated postprandial insulinemia. Similar hypotheses have been formulated for breast (KAAKS 1996; STOLL 1999), pancreas (WEIDERPASS et al. 1998) and endometrium (KAAKS et al. 2002a; RUTANEN et al. 1993; RUTANEN 1998). The tumor-enhancing effects of insulin might be either directly mediated by insulin receptors in the (pre)neoplastic target cells, or might be due to related changes in endogenous hormone metabolism, such as increase in IGF-I bioactivity or alterations in sex steroid synthesis and bioavailability.

Indirect evidence that chronic hyperinsulinemia may enhance the development of these various forms of cancer comes from observations that the risk of cancers of the colon (or colorectum) (GIOVANNUCCI 1995; HU et al. 1999; LA VECCHIA et al. 1997; LE MARCHAND et al. 1997; MCKEOWN-EYSSEN 1994; WEIDERPASS et al. 1997a; WILL et al. 1998), endometrium (ADAMI et al. 1991; LA VECCHIA et al. 1994; NIWA et al. 2000; O'MARA et al. 1985; WEIDERPASS et al. 1997b), pancreas (CALLE et al. 1998; EVERHART and WRIGHT 1995; SILVERMAN et al. 1999; WEIDERPASS et al. 1998; WIDEROFF et al. 1997), and kidney (COUGHLIN et al. 1997; LINDBLAD et al. 1999; O'MARA et al. 1985; WIDEROFF et al. 1997) is increased in diabetics. Although a large proportion of studies did not distinguish clearly between diabetes of an early onset (type I) or adult onset (type II), and whether or not the subjects depended on insulin injections, the majority (>80%) of diabetes patients in Western populations is of adult onset and noninsulin dependent. This type of diabetes is usually preceded by a long period of insulin resistance and pancreatic insulin hypersecretion, and even after the onset of diabetic symptoms patients' insulin levels usually remain high for years, until they eventually drop because of pancreatic exhaustion. A large number of epidemiological studies (KAAKS 1996) have not provided any strong evidence for a direct association of diabetes with breast cancer risk. This lack of association could be due to failure to distinguish between pre- and postmenopausal breast cancer. As for obesity, diabetes might have a direct association only with breast cancer risk diagnosed several years after menopause, but not before.

In addition to this indirect evidence, several prospective cohort studies, as well as a few case-control studies, have related cancer risk directly to circulating levels of insulin or C-peptide (a marker of pancreatic insulin secretion), or to metabolic factors that are related to insulin resistance and chronic hyperinsulinemia, such as elevated plasma glucose or triglycerides (Defronzo 1988; Reaven 1988).

With regard to *colorectal* cancer, one recent cohort study of about 6,000 men and women followed for an average of about 7 years, showed significantly elevated levels of fasting and postload (2-h) glucose, as well as of 2-h insulin, for 102 subjects who developed a tumor of the colon or rectum as compared to control subjects who remained cancer-free (Schoen et al. 1999). In another small cohort of more than 14,000 women in New York, which also had 102 incident cases of colorectal cancer (75 for colon, 27 for rectum), risk of colorectal cancer was also significantly increased among women with elevated (nonfasting) C-peptide [odds ratio of 2.92 (95% CI = 1.26–6.75) for highest vs. lowest quintile; $p_{trend} < 0.001$] (Kaaks et al. 2000b). In the latter study, the association of risk with C-peptide levels became stronger when the analysis was focused on colon cancer alone [76 cases; OR 3.96 (1.49–10.50)], while in neither study did adjustment for effects of BMI materially alter the associations of cancer risk with insulin or C-peptide. In both prospective studies, numbers of rectal cancer cases were too small to allow separate risk analysis. Colon cancer tissue has receptors for both insulin and IGF-I (Guo et al. 1992; Macdonald et al. 1993). Signal transduction pathways mediating the effects of insulin on gene expression and mitosis include the activation of the *K-ras* oncogen (Burgering et al. 1989; Burgering et al. 1991), a pathway that is central to colorectal carcinogenesis (Bos 1988; Vogelstein et al. 1988).

The risk of *pancreas* cancer has not been related directly to circulating insulin or C-peptide, so far. However, one prospective study recently showed an increase in the risk of pancreas cancer in men and women who had comparatively elevated plasma glucose levels 2 h after a standard oral glucose dose (Gapstur et al. 2000). Elevated plasma glucose levels are indicative of insulin resistance, and hence of chronically elevated pancreatic insulin production (Defronzo 1988).

For *endometrial* cancer, one case-control study in the USA showed an increase in risk in postmenopausal women with elevated serum levels of C-peptide (Troisi et al. 1997), which did not persist, however, after adjustment for BMI. A much smaller study in Japan, of 23 endometrial cancer patients and 27 healthy control women, showed decreased IGFBP-1 levels in the cases (Ayabe et al. 1997), and another small study in Finland showed increased fasting plasma insulin levels, and decreased expression of the IGFBP-1 gene in endometrial tissue samples, in cancer patients compared to controls (Rutanen et al. 1994). In a pooled prospective study of three cohorts in New

York, Milan and Umeå, which included 166 cases and 315 controls, a strong direct relationship of endometrial cancer risk with serum levels of C-peptide was found (OR = 4.5 (2.0–10.0), 95% CI 2.1–10.7), but no association with levels of IGF-I (Lukanova et al. 2002b).

With respect to *breast* cancer, two case-control studies showed an association of both premenopausal (Bruning et al. 1992; Del Giudice et al. 1998) and postmenopausal risk (Bruning et al. 1992) with measurements of insulin or C-peptide, but this was not confirmed by two prospective studies (Kaaks et al. 2002b; Toniolo et al. 2000).

As mentioned in Sects. A.I and A.II, , there is no clear relationship of *ovarian* and *prostate* cancer risks with excess weight, and neither is there any clear evidence that more central body fat distribution is a risk factor. Furthermore, neither of these two cancer types appears to be related to pre-existing diabetes (Kaaks et al. 2000a; Risch 1998). One prospective cohort study showed no clear relationship of prostate cancer with plasma levels of (fasting) insulin, IGFBP-1, and IGFBP-2 (Stattin et al. 2000).

II. IGF-I, IGFBP-3 and Cancer Risk

IGF-I and at least six different IGF-binding proteins are synthesized in most, perhaps all, organ systems; however, most (>80%) of IGF-I and IGFBPs in the circulation are synthesized in the liver. The biological activity of IGF-I depends on the binding of IGF-I from endocrine (circulation), paracrine, and autocrine sources with cellular receptors. Besides absolute plasma and tissue concentrations of IGF-I, IGF-I bioactivity is strongly modulated by IGFBPs, which control the size of the circulating and tissue IGF-I pools, regulate the efflux of IGF-I from the circulation towards target tissues, and within tissues regulate binding of IGF-I to its tissue receptors (Jones and Clemmons 1995; Wetterau et al. 1999).

More than 90% of IGF-I in the circulation is bound to a ternary complex including IGFBP-3 and another glycoprotein, called acid-labile subunit (ALS). Most of the remainder is bound to IGFBP-5, which also forms a ternary complex with ALS, and to the IGFBPs -1, -2, -4 and -6. Because of the very high affinities of IGFBP-3 and IGFBP-5 for IGF-I, and their large complexes with ALS, IGF-I bound to IGFBP-3 or IGFBP-5 cannot diffuse through the endothelial barrier. The IGFBPs -1, -2, -4 and -6 are smaller (hence can diffuse from the circulation towards the extravascular space), and have lower affinities for IGF-I. At the tissue level, the IGFBPs have been proposed mostly to inhibit binding of IGF-I to its receptor (Jones and Clemmons 1995). Nevertheless, in vitro studies have shown that some IGFBPs may also enhance IGF-I binding to its receptors, depending on the relative concentrations of IGF-I and IGFBPs. These modulating effects of the IGFBPs may be altered by phosphorylation of IGFBPs, or by enzymatic proteolysis (Jones and Clemmons 1995). IGFBP-3 has been shown to exert proapoptotic and anti-mitogenic effects through a specific IGFBP-3 binding site on the membranes of mammary, prostatic, endometrial, or colonic cells (BAXTER 2000; FERRY JR. et al. 1999).

In most tissues, the principal stimulus for the synthesis of IGF-I is provided by growth hormone (GH), although IGF-I synthesis can be modulated by many other physiological factors (LE ROITH et al. 2001). In some tissues, the principal stimulus is not GH; for example, in endometrium the synthesis of IGF-I appears to be mostly under the control of estrogens (GIUDICE et al. 1991; KLEINMAN et al. 1995; MURPHY and GHAHARY 1990; RUTANEN 1998). From a epidemiological and lifestyle perspective, it is important to recognize that nutrition, particularly energy balance, plays a key role in modulating IGF-I synthesis and circulating levels of IGF-I (KAAKS and LUKANOVA 2001). Prolonged fasting and chronic energy undernutrition lead to dramatic reductions in IGF-I (KAAKS and LUKANOVA 2001; THISSEN et al. 1994). A teleological interpretation of this is that IGF-I, as an anabolic factor, can stimulate growth only in the presence of sufficient available energy from diet and body reserves. In well-nourished populations, however, the relationship of IGF-I levels with energy from diet or adipose tissue stores is less clear. Obesity is not associated with any increase in circulating IGF-I, but rather with a small decrease, compared to normally nourished control subjects (KAAKS and LUKANOVA 2001). There is some recent evidence that the relationship of adipose tissue stores with IGF-I may be nonlinear, and that IGF-I may increase with increasing levels of BMI up to about 25–26 kg/m^2, but decrease again thereafter (LUKANOVA et al. 2002d). Apart from energy, IGF-I synthesis depends also on the intake of animal protein (ALLEN et al. 2000; NOGUCHI 2000) and other nutrients (ESTIVARIZ and ZIEGLER 1997; STRAUS 1994; THISSEN et al. 1994). In many developing countries with low incidence rates of cancers of the breast, colon, prostate, and ovary, the average BMI is (or used to be) below 22 kg/m^2 for the vast majority of the population, whereas in industrially developed societies the median BMI may lie around 25 kg/m^2 or above (IARC 2002). Furthermore, low-risk countries have generally much lower intakes of animal protein. Taken together, these data suggest that differences in IGF-I levels may at least partially explain the large differences in cancer risk observed between economically developed and less developed parts of the world.

A substantial number of studies have recently addressed the question whether circulating levels of IGF-I and its major plasmatic binding protein, IGFBP-3, were associated with risk of developing cancer.

With regard to *breast* cancer, four case-control studies (BOHLKE et al. 1998; BRUNING et al. 1995; LI et al. 2001; PEYRAT et al. 1993) and two prospective cohort studies (HANKINSON et al. 1998; TONIOLO et al. 2000) showed an increased risk among women with elevated plasma or serum IGF-I, and especially for breast cancers diagnosed at a young, premenopausal age. However, this finding was not confirmed in a third prospective study, combining two cohorts in northern and southern Sweden (KAAKS et al. 2002b) and in three other case-control studies (DEL GIUDICE et al. 1998; NG et al. 1998; PETRIDOU et al. 2000). In several studies, the association with IGF-I was stronger after adjustment for levels of IGFBP-3 (HANKINSON et al. 1998), or when IGF-I levels were expressed as molar ratios to IGFBP-3 (BRUNING et al. 1995). The latter suggested that risk may be related more strongly to increased bioavailability or bioactivity of IGF-I, due to comparatively low IGFBP-3 levels, or might also point to a direct protective effect of IGFBP-3 through its proper cellular binding sites.

For *colorectal* cancer, epidemiological studies have shown a direct association of colon cancer risk with body stature (height), which may reflect levels of IGF-I during puberty and adolescence. Furthermore, patients with acromegaly – a pathology due to GH excess and associated with elevated IGF-I levels – have an increased risk of developing colonic polyps and colon cancer (CATS et al. 1996; COLAO et al. 1997; GIOVANNUCCI et al. 2000; ITUARTE et al. 1984; JENKINS et al. 1997; ORTEGO et al. 1994). More recently, five cohort studies (GIOVANNUCCI et al. 2000; KAAKS et al. 2000b; MA et al. 1999; PALMQVIST et al. 2002; PROBST-HENSCH et al. 2001) and one case-control study (MANOUSOS et al. 1999) all showed increases in risk either of colon cancer, or of colon and rectal cancers combined. In only one of these studies (PALMQVIST et al. 2002) was the association with absolute circulating levels of IGF-I statistically significant, but for colon cancer only. In two of the five prospective studies (GIOVANNUCCI et al. 2000; MA et al. 1999), the association of colon cancer risk with IGF-I became much stronger, and statistically significant, only after adjustment for IGFBP-3. A similar effect of IGFBP-3 adjustment was seen in studies on other cancer types conducted by the same (Harvard) group (CHAN et al. 1998; HANKINSON et al. 1998). In all of these studies, IGFBP-3 had been measured by an ELISA assay, from DIAGNOSTIC SYSTEMS LABORATORIES (DSL; Webster, Texas). In all other studies (KAAKS et al. 2000b; PALMQVIST et al. 2002; PROBST-HENSCH et al. 2001), IGFBP-3 had been measured by various other assays, and elevated IGFBP-3 was systematically found to be associated with an increased risk of colon cancer. This increase in risk for elevated IGFBP-3, measured by assays other than the DSL-ELISA, has also been observed for other cancer types (STATTIN et al. 2000). In a study in Hawaii, a single nucleotide polymorphism (SNP) ("T1663A" allele) in the growth hormone gene (GH1) was reduced plasma levels of IGF-I, confirming earlier observations of association with reduced GH secretion and adult height (HASEGAWA et al. 2000). The reduced IGF-I levels in the Hawaiian study were thus putatively explained by lower levels of GH. At the same time, the GH1 polymorphism was associated with a reduced risk of colorectal cancer (study of 535 cancer cases and 650 controls), as well as with a reduced risk of colorectal adenomas (139 cases, 202 controls) (LE MARCHAND et al. 2002; WOLK et al. 1998)

With regard to *prostate* cancer, several case-control (MANTZOROS et al. 1997; WOLK et al. 1998) and prospective cohort (CHAN et al. 1998; HARMAN et al. 2000; STATTIN et al. 2000) studies have shown an increase in prostate cancer risk in men with comparatively elevated absolute levels of IGF-I (HARMAN et al. 2000; MANOUSOS et al. 1999; WOLK et al. 1998), or with elevated levels of

IGF-I, either as absolute concentrations or relative to levels of IGFBP-3 (CHAN et al. 1998). At least one recent prospective study did not confirm these findings, however (LACEY, JR. et al. 2001).

One prospective study, based on three pooled cohorts in New York, Milan and Umeå, showed an increase in risk of *ovarian* cancer diagnosed before age 55 [OR = 4.97 (1.22–20.2) for the top versus bottom IGF-I tertile], but no association with risk of ovarian cancer at older ages (LUKANOVA et al. 2002c). This intriguing find, which very much resembles observations for breast cancer, requires confirmation from further prospective studies.

Taken together, it appears that elevated plasma IGF-I, as absolute concentrations or relative to levels of IGFBP-3, may be a risk factor for a number of different tumors that are frequent in Western societies. It is possible that the elevated IGF-I levels in men or women who subsequently develop cancer is due to increased pituitary GH secretion, and further studies are needed to address that question.

C. Concluding Remarks

Epidemiologial studies have shown clear evidence that among post-menopausal women risks of cancers of the breast and endometrium are associated with blood levels of total and bioavailable estrogens, as well androgens. By contrast, blood levels of sex steroids have not been found to be clearly related to the risk of prostate cancer. For premenopausal breast cancer and ovarian cancer there is insufficient evidence to draw any clear conclusions at this stage. Besides the sex steroids, there is increasing evidence from recent studies that elevated blood levels of IGF-I may be associated with increased risks of cancers of the prostate, breast (in young women), colon, and possibly also the ovary, and that elevated insulin levels may be a risk factor for cancers of the colon, endometrium, and possibly pancreas and kidney.

Further studies are needed to confirm the above findings, especially with respect to IGF-I, and to examine possible relationships of cancer risk with premenopausal hormone profiles. In addition, many questions remain about the possible determinants, nutritional, and other lifestyle factors, or genetic background, that may explain the sometimes large interindividual variation in plasma levels of sex steroids, insulin, IGF-I, and IGF-binding proteins.

References

Aaronson SA (1991) Growth factors and cancer. Science 254:1146–1153
Adami HO, McLaughlin J, Ekbom A, Berne C, Silverman D, Hacker D, Persson I (1991) Cancer risk in patients with diabetes mellitus. Cancer Causes Control 2:307–314
Aden U, Jung-Hoffmann C, Kuhl H (1998) A randomized cross-over study on various hormonal parameters of two triphasic oral contraceptives. Contraception 58:75–81
Aleem FA, Moukhtar MA, Hung HC, Romney SL (1976) Plasma estrogen in patients with endometrial hyperplasia and carcinoma. Cancer 38:2101–2104

Allen NE, Appleby PN, Davey GK, Key TJ (2000) Hormones and diet: low insulin-like growth factor-I but normal bioavailable androgens in vegan men. Br J Cancer 83: 95–97

Austin H, Austin JM, Jr., Partridge EE, Hatch KD, Shingleton HM (1991) Endometrial cancer, obesity, and body fat distribution. Cancer Res 51:568–572

Ayabe T, Tsutsumi O, Sakai H, Yoshikawa H, Yano T, Kurimoto F, Taketani Y (1997) Increased circulating levels of insulin-like growth factor-I and decreased circulating levels of insulin-like growth factor binding protein-1 in postmenopausal women with endometrial cancer. Endocr J 44:419–424

Baxter RC (2000) Insulin-like growth factor (IGF)-binding proteins: interactions with IGFs and intrinsic bioactivities. Am J Physiol Endocrinol Metab 278:E967-E976

Benjamin F, Deutsch S (1976) Plasma levels of fractionated estrogens and pituitary hormones in endometrial carcinoma. Am J Obstet Gynecol 126:638–647

Bergman RN, Ader M (2000) Free fatty acids and pathogenesis of type 2 diabetes mellitus. Trends Endocrinol Metab 11:351–356

Bergstrom A, Pisani P, Tenet V, Wolk A, Adami HO (2001) Overweight as an avoidable cause of cancer in Europe. Int J Cancer 91:421–430

Bernstein L, Ross RK (1993) Endogenous hormones and breast cancer risk. Epidemiol Rev 15:48–65

Blaakaer J (1997) The pituitary-gonadal function in postmenopausal women with epithelial ovarian tumors. APMIS Suppl 74:1–27

Blair A, Kazerouni N (1997) Reactive chemicals and cancer. Cancer Causes Control 8:473–490

Bohlke K, Cramer DW, Trichopoulos D, Mantzoros CS (1998) Insulin-like growth factor-I in relation to premenopausal ductal carcinoma in situ of the breast. Epidemiology 9:570–573

Bos JL (1988) The ras gene family and human carcinogenesis. Mutat Res 195:255–271

Bosland MC (1996) Hormonal factors in carcinogenesis of the prostate and testis in humans and in animal models. Prog Clin Biol Res 394:309–352

Bosland MC (2000) The role of steroid hormones in prostate carcinogenesis. J Natl Cancer Inst Monogr 39–66

Bruning PF, Bonfrer JM, van Noord PA, Hart AA, Jong-Bakker M, Nooijen WJ (1992) Insulin resistance and breast-cancer risk. Int J Cancer 52:511–516

Bruning PF, Van Doorn J, Bonfrer JM, van Noord PA, Korse CM, Linders TC, Hart AA (1995) Insulin-like growth-factor-binding protein 3 is decreased in early-stage operable pre-menopausal breast cancer. Int J Cancer 62:266–270

Burgering BM, Medema RH, Maassen JA, van de Wetering ML, van der Eb AJ, McCormick F, Bos JL (1991) Insulin stimulation of gene expression mediated by p21ras activation. EMBO J 10:1103–1109

Burgering BM, Snijders AJ, Maassen JA, van der Eb AJ, Bos JL (1989) Possible involvement of normal p21 H-ras in the insulin/insulin-like growth factor 1 signal transduction pathway. Mol Cell Biol 9:4312–4322

Calle EE, Murphy TK, Rodriguez C, Thun MJ, Heath CW, Jr. (1998) Diabetes mellitus and pancreatic cancer mortality in a prospective cohort of USA adults. Cancer Causes Control 9:403–410

Cats A, Dullaart RP, Kleibeuker JH, Kuipers F, Sluiter WJ, Hardonk MJ, de Vries EG (1996) Increased epithelial cell proliferation in the colon of patients with acromegaly. Cancer Res 56:523–526

Cerutti PA (1985) Prooxidant states and tumor promotion. Science 227:375–381

Chan JM, Stampfer MJ, Giovannucci E, Gann PH, MaJ, Wilkinson P, Hennekens CH, Pollak M (1998) Plasma insulin-like growth factor-I and prostate cancer risk: a prospective study. Science 279:563–566

Chang WY, Prins GS (1999) Estrogen receptor-beta: implications for the prostate gland. Prostate 40:115–124

Chen Y, Wu PC, Lang JH, Ge WJ, Hartge P, Brinton LA (1992) Risk factors for epithelial ovarian cancer in Beijing, China. Int J Epidemiol 21:23–29

Clarke R, Skaar T, Baumann K, Leonessa F, James M, Lippman J, Thompson EW, Freter C, Brunner N (1994) Hormonal carcinogenesis in breast cancer: cellular and molecular studies of malignant progression. Breast Cancer Res Treat 31:237–248

Colao A, Balzano A, Ferone D, Panza N, Grande G, Marzullo P, Bove A, Iodice G, Merola B, Lombardi G (1997) Increased prevalence of colonic polyps and altered lymphocyte subset pattern in the colonic lamina propria in acromegaly. Clin Endocrinol (Oxf) 47:23–28

Collaborative Group on Hormonal Factors in Breast Cancer (1996) Breast cancer and hormonal contraceptives: collaborative reanalysis of individual data on 53 297 women with breast cancer and 100 239 women without breast cancer from 54 epidemiological studies. Lancet 347:1713–1727

Collaborative Group on Hormonal Factors in Breast Cancer (1997) Breast cancer and hormone replacement therapy: collaborative reanalysis of data from 51 epidemiological studies of 52,705 women with breast cancer and 108,411 women without breast cancer. Lancet 350:1047–1059

Coughlin SS, Hall IJ (2002) A review of genetic polymorphisms and prostate cancer risk. Ann Epidemiol 12:182–196

Coughlin SS, Neaton JD, Randall B, Sengupta A (1997) Predictors of mortality from kidney cancer in 332,547 men screened for the Multiple Risk Factor Intervention Trial. Cancer 79:2171–2177

Coulam CB, Annegers JF, Kranz JS (1983) Chronic anovulation syndrome and associated neoplasia. Obstet Gynecol 61:403–407

Cramer DW, Hutchison GB, Welch WR, Scully RE, Ryan KJ (1983) Determinants of ovarian cancer risk. I. Reproductive experiences and family history. J Natl Cancer Inst 71:711–716

Cramer DW, Welch WR (1983) Determinants of ovarian cancer risk. II. Inferences regarding pathogenesis. J Natl Cancer Inst 71:717–721

Crave JC, Lejeune H, Brebant C, Baret C, Pugeat M (1995) Differential effects of insulin and insulin-like growth factor I on the production of plasma steroid-binding globulins by human hepatoblastoma-derived (Hep G2) cells. J Clin Endocrinol Metab 80:1283–1289

Dahlgren E, Friberg LG, Johansson S, Lindstrom B, Oden A, Samsioe G, Janson PO (1991) Endometrial carcinoma; ovarian dysfunction–a risk factor in young women. Eur J Obstet Gynecol Reprod Biol 41:143–150

DeFronzo RA (1988) Lilly lecture 1987. The triumvirate: beta-cell, muscle, liver. A collusion responsible for NIDDM. Diabetes 37:667–687

Del Giudice ME, Fantus IG, Ezzat S, McKeown-Eyssen G, Page D, Goodwin PJ (1998) Insulin and related factors in premenopausal breast cancer risk. Breast Cancer Res Treat 47:111–120

Dickson RB, Stancel GM (2000) Estrogen receptor-mediated processes in normal and cancer cells. J Natl Cancer Inst Monogr 135–145

Dickson RB, Thompson EW, Lippman ME (1989) Hormones and breast cancer in vitro. Hum Cell 2:219–230

Eaton NE, Reeves GK, Appleby PN, Key TJ (1999) Endogenous sex hormones and prostate cancer: a quantitative review of prospective studies. Br J Cancer 80:930–934

Ehrmann DA, Barnes RB, Rosenfield RL (1995) Polycystic ovary syndrome as a form of functional ovarian hyperandrogenism due to dysregulation of androgen secretion. Endocr Rev 16:322–353

Emons G, Fleckenstein G, Hinney B, Huschmand A, Heyl W (2000) Hormonal interactions in endometrial cancer. Endocr Relat Cancer 7:227–242

Estivariz CF, Ziegler TR (1997) Nutrition and the insulin-like growth factor system. Endocrine 7:65–71

Everhart J, Wright D (1995) Diabetes mellitus as a risk factor for pancreatic cancer. A meta-analysis. JAMA 273:1605–1609

Farnsworth WE (1996) Roles of estrogen and SHBG in prostate physiology. Prostate 28:17–23

Fathalla MF (1971) Incessant ovulation–a factor in ovarian neoplasia? Lancet 2:163

Ferenczy A, Bertrand G, Gelfand MM (1979) Proliferation kinetics of human endometrium during the normal menstrual cycle. Am J Obstet Gynecol 133:859–867

Ferrannini E, Barrett EJ, Bevilacqua S, DeFronzo RA (1983) Effect of fatty acids on glucose production and utilization in man. J Clin Invest 72:1737–1747

Ferry RJ, Jr., Katz LE, Grimberg A, Cohen P, Weinzimer SA (1999) Cellular actions of insulin-like growth factor binding proteins. Horm Metab Res 31:192–202

Foekens JA, Portengen H, Janssen M, Klijn JG (1989) Insulin-like growth factor-1 receptors and insulin-like growth factor-1-like activity in human primary breast cancer. Cancer 63:2139–2147

Gann PH, Hennekens CH, Ma J, Longcope C, Stampfer MJ (1996) Prospective study of sex hormone levels and risk of prostate cancer. J Natl Cancer Inst 88:1118–1126

Gapstur SM, Gann PH, Lowe W, Liu K, Colangelo L, Dyer A (2000) Abnormal glucose metabolism and pancreatic cancer mortality. JAMA 283:2552–2558

Garg PP, Kerlikowske K, Subak L, Grady D (1998) Hormone replacement therapy and the risk of epithelial ovarian carcinoma: a meta-analysis. Obstet Gynecol 92:472–479

Gimes G, Szarvas Z, Siklosi G (1986) Endocrine factors in the etiology of endometrial carcinoma. Neoplasma 33:393–397

Giovannucci E (2001) Insulin, insulin-like growth factors and colon cancer: a review of the evidence. J Nutr 131:3109S–3120S

Giovannucci E (1995) Insulin and colon cancer. Cancer Causes Control 6:164–179

Giovannucci E, Pollak MN, Platz EA, Willett WC, Stampfer MJ, Majeed N, Colditz GA, Speizer FE, Hankinson SE (2000) A prospective study of plasma insulin-like growth factor-1 and binding protein-3 and risk of colorectal neoplasia in women. Cancer Epidemiol Biomarkers Prev 9:345–349

Giudice LC, Lamson G, Rosenfeld RG, Irwin JC (1991) Insulin-like growth factor-II (IGF-II) and IGF binding proteins in human endometrium. Ann N Y Acad Sci 626:295–307

Goodyear LJ, Kahn BB (1998) Exercise, glucose transport, and insulin sensitivity. Annu Rev Med 49:235–261

Grady D, Ernster VL (1996) Endometrial Cancer. In: Schottenfeld D, Fraumeni FJ (eds) Cancer Epidemiology and Prevention. Oxford University Press, p 1058

Grimm J J (1999) Interaction of physical activity and diet: implications for insulin-glucose dynamics. Public Health Nutr 2:363–368

Guo YS, Narayan S, Yallampalli C, Singh P (1992) Characterization of insulinlike growth factor I receptors in human colon cancer. Gastroenterology 102:1101–1108

Hall J, Angele S (1999) Radiation, DNA damage and cancer. Mol Med Today 5:157–164

Hamilton-Fairley D, Kiddy D, Watson H, Paterson C, Franks S (1992) Association of moderate obesity with a poor pregnancy outcome in women with polycystic ovary syndrome treated with low dose gonadotrophin. Br J Obstet Gynaecol 99:128–131

Hammerman MR (1999) The growth hormone-insulin-like growth factor axis in kidney re-revisited. Nephrol Dial Transplant 14:1853–1860

Hankinson SE, Willett WC, Colditz GA, Hunter DJ, Michaud DS, Deroo B, Rosner B, Speizer FE, Pollak M (1998) Circulating concentrations of insulin-like growth factor-I and risk of breast cancer. Lancet 351:1393–1396

Hargreaves M (1998) 1997 Sir William Refshauge Lecture. Skeletal muscle glucose metabolism during exercise: implications for health and performance. J Sci Med Sport 1:195–202

Harman SM, Metter EJ, Blackman MR, Landis PK, Carter HB (2000) Serum levels of insulin-like growth factor I (IGF-I), IGF-II, IGF-binding protein-3, and prostate-specific antigen as predictors of clinical prostate cancer. J Clin Endocrinol Metab 85:4258–4265

Hasegawa Y, Fujii K, Yamada M, Igarashi Y, Tachibana K, Tanaka T, Onigata K, Nishi Y, Kato S, Hasegawa T (2000) Identification of novel human GH-1 gene polymorphisms that are associated with growth hormone secretion and height. J Clin Endocrinol Metab 85:1290–1295

Helzlsouer KJ, Alberg AJ, Gordon GB, Longcope C, Bush TL, Hoffman SC, Comstock GW (1995) Serum gonadotropins and steroid hormones and the development of ovarian cancer. JAMA 274:1926–1930

Helzlsouer KJ, Alberg AJ, Bush TL, Longcope C, Gordon GB, Comstock GW (1994) A prospective study of endogenous hormones and breast cancer. Cancer Detect Prev 18:79–85

Henderson BE, Ross RK, Pike MC, Casagrande JT (1982) Endogenous hormones as a major factor in human cancer. Cancer Res 42:3232–3239

Hotamisligil GS (2000) Molecular mechanisms of insulin resistance and the role of the adipocyte. Int J Obes Relat Metab Disord 24 Suppl 4:S23-S27

Houmard JA, Shaw CD, Hickey MS, Tanner CJ (1999) Effect of short-term exercise training on insulin-stimulated PI 3-kinase activity in human skeletal muscle. Am J Physiol 277:E1055-E1060

Hu FB, Manson JE, Liu S, Hunter D, Colditz GA, Michels KB, Speizer FE, Giovannucci E (1999) Prospective study of adult onset diabetes mellitus (type 2) and risk of colorectal cancer in women. J Natl Cancer Inst 91:542–547

IARC (2002) IARC Handbooks of Cancer Prevention, Vol. 6: Weight Control and Physical Activity, International Agency for Research on Cancer, Lyon. pp 1–315

IARC (1997) Cancer incidence in Five continents. Volume VII, Parkin DM, Wheelan SL, Ferlay J, Raymond L, Young J (Eds.) IARC Sci Publ i-1240

IARC (1999) Hormonal contraception and post-menopausal hormonal therapy, IARC Monographs on the Evaluation of Carcinogenic Risks to Humans Vol 72, IARC, Lyon, pp 1–660

Ituarte EA, Petrini J, Hershman JM (1984) Acromegaly and colon cancer. Ann Intern Med 101:627–628

Jenkins PJ, Fairclough PD, Richards T, Lowe DG, Monson J, Grossman A, Wass JA, Besser M (1997) Acromegaly, colonic polyps and carcinoma. Clin Endocrinol (Oxf) 47:17–22

John EM, Whittemore AS, Harris R, Itnyre J (1993) Characteristics relating to ovarian cancer risk: collaborative analysis of seven USA case-control studies. Epithelial ovarian cancer in black women. Collaborative Ovarian Cancer Group. J Natl Cancer Inst 85:142–147

Jones JI, Clemmons DR (1995) Insulin-like growth factors and their binding proteins: biological actions. Endocr Rev 16:3–34

Kaaks R (1996) Nutrition, hormones, and breast cancer: is insulin the missing link? Cancer Causes Control 7:605–625

Kaaks R, Lukanova A (2001) Energy balance and cancer: the role of insulin and insulin-like growth factor-I. Proc Nutr Soc 60:91–106

Kaaks R, Lukanova A, Kurzer M (2002a) Obesity, endogenous hormones, and endometrial cancer risk; a synthetic review., Cancer Epidemiol Biomarkers Prev (in press)

Kaaks R, Lukanova A, Sommersberg B (2000a) Plasma androgens, IGF-I, body size, and prostate cancer risk: a synthetic review. Prostate Cancer & Prostatic Diseases 3:157–172

Kaaks R, Lundin E, Rinaldi S, Manjer J, Biessy C, Soderberg S, Lenner P, Janzon L, Riboli E, Berglund G, Hallmans G (2002b) Prospective study of IGF-I, IGF-binding proteins and breast cancer risk, in Northern and Southern Sweden. Cancer Causes and Control 13:307–316

Kaaks R, Toniolo P, Akhmedkhanov A, Lukanova A, Biessy C, Dechaud H, Rinaldi S, Zeleniuch-Jacquotte A, Shore RE, Riboli E (2000b) Serum C-peptide, insulin-like growth factor (IGF)-I, IGF-binding proteins, and colorectal cancer risk in women. J Natl Cancer Inst 92:1592–1600

Katsouyanni K, Boyle P, Trichopoulos D (1991) Diet and urine estrogens among post-menopausal women. Oncology 48:490–494

Kaye SA, Folsom AR, Soler JT, Prineas RJ, Potter JD (1991) Associations of body mass and fat distribution with sex hormone concentrations in postmenopausal women. Int J Epidemiol 20:151–156

Kelsey JL, Gammon MD, John EM (1993) Reproductive factors and breast cancer. Epidemiol Rev 15:36–47

Kelsey JL, Whittemore AS (1994) Epidemiology and primary prevention of cancers of the breast, endometrium, and ovary. A brief overview. Ann Epidemiol 4:89–95

Key TJ, Allen NE, Verkasalo PK, Banks E (2001) Energy balance and cancer: the role of sex hormones. Proc Nutr Soc 60:81–89

Key TJ, Pike MC (1988a) The dose-effect relationship between "unopposed" oestrogens and endometrial mitotic rate: its central role in explaining and predicting endometrial cancer risk. Br J Cancer 57:205–212

Key TJ, Pike MC (1988b) The role of oestrogens and progestagens in the epidemiology and prevention of breast cancer. Eur J Cancer Clin Oncol 24:29–43

Khandwala HM, McCutcheon IE, Flyvbjerg A, Friend KE (2000) The effects of insulin-like growth factors on tumorigenesis and neoplastic growth. Endocr Rev 21:215–244

Kleinman D, Karas M, Roberts CT, Jr., Leroith D, Phillip M, Segev Y, Levy J, Sharoni Y (1995) Modulation of insulin-like growth factor I (IGF-I) receptors and membrane-associated IGF-binding proteins in endometrial cancer cells by estradiol. Endocrinology 136:2531–2537

Koch M, Jenkins H, Gaedke H (1988) Risk factors of ovarian cancer of epithelial origin: a case control study. Cancer Detect Prev 13:131–136

Kraegen EW, Cooney GJ, Ye J, Thompson AL (2001) Triglycerides, fatty acids and insulin resistance–hyperinsulinemia. Exp Clin Endocrinol Diabetes 109:S516-S526

La Vecchia C, Negri E, Decarli A, Franceschi S (1997) Diabetes mellitus and colorectal cancer risk. Cancer Epidemiol Biomarkers Prev 6:1007–1010

La Vecchia C, Negri E, Franceschi S, D'Avanzo B, Boyle P (1994) A case-control study of diabetes mellitus and cancer risk. Br J Cancer 70:950–953

Lacey JV, Jr., Hsing AW, Fillmore CM, Hoffman S, Helzlsouer KJ, Comstock GW (2001) Null association between insulin-like growth factors, insulin-like growth factor-binding proteins, and prostate cancer in a prospective study. Cancer Epidemiol Biomarkers Prev 10:1101–1102

Le Marchand L, Donlon T, Seifried A, Kaaks R, Rinaldi S, Wilkens LR (2002) Association of a common polymorphism in the human GH1 gene with colorectal neoplasia. J Natl Cancer Inst 94:454–460

Le Marchand L, Wilkens LR, Kolonel LN, Hankin JH, Lyu LC (1997) Associations of sedentary lifestyle, obesity, smoking, alcohol use, and diabetes with the risk of colorectal cancer. Cancer Res 57:4787–4794

Le Roith D, Bondy C, Yakar S, Liu JL, Butler A (2001) The somatomedin hypothesis: 2001. Endocr Rev 22:53–74

Lew EA, Garfinkel L (1979) Variations in mortality by weight among 750,000 men and women. J Chronic Dis 32:563–576

Li BD, Khosravi MJ, Berkel HJ, Diamandi A, Dayton MA, Smith M, Yu H (2001) Free insulin-like growth factor-I and breast cancer risk. Int J Cancer 91:736–739

Lindblad P, Chow WH, Chan J, Bergstrom A, Wolk A, Gridley G, McLaughlin JK, Nyren O, Adami HO (1999) The role of diabetes mellitus in the aetiology of renal cell cancer. Diabetologia 42:107–112

Loft S, Poulsen HE (1996) Cancer risk and oxidative DNA damage in man. J Mol Med 74:297–312

Lukanova A, Lundin E, Akhmedkhanov A, Micheli A, Rinaldi S, Zeleniuch-Jacquotte A, Lenner P, Muti P, Biessy C, Krogh V, Berrino F, Hallmans G, Riboli E, Kaaks

R, Toniolo P (2002a) Circulating levels of sex steroid hormones and risk of ovarian cancer, Int J Cancer (accepted)

Lukanova A, Lundin E, Toniolo P, Micheli A, Akhmedkhanov A, Rinaldi S, Muti P, Biessy C, Krogh V, Zeleniuch-Jacquotte A, Berrino F, Hallmans G, Riboli E, Kaaks R (2002b) Circulating C-peptide, IGF-I, IGF-binding proteins and endometrial cancer: a pooled prospective cohort study., (submitted):

Lukanova A, Lundin E, Toniolo P, Micheli A, Akhmedkhanov A, Rinaldi S, Muti P, Lenner P, Biessy C, Krogh V, Zeleniuch-Jacquotte A, Berrino F, Hallmans G, Riboli E, Kaaks R (2002c) Circulating levels of insulin-like growth factor-I and risk of ovarian cancer, Int J Cancer 101:549–554

Lukanova A, Soderberg S, Stattin P, Palmqvist R, Lundin E, Biessy C, Rinaldi S, Riboli E, Hallmans G, Kaaks R (2002d) Nonlinear relationship of insulin-like growth factor (IGF)-I and IGF-I/IGF-binding protein-3 ratio with indices of adiposity and plasma insulin concentrations, Cancer Causes Control 13:509–516

Lukanova A, Toniolo P, Lundin E, Micheli A, Akhmedkhanov A, Muti P, Zeleniuch-Jacquotte A, Biessy C, Lenner P, Krogh V, Berrino F, Hallmans G, Riboli E, Kaaks R (2002e) Body mass index in relation to ovarian cancer: a multi-centre nested case-control study. Int J Cancer 99:603–608

Ma J, Pollak MN, Giovannucci E, Chan JM, Tao Y, Hennekens CH, Stampfer MJ (1999) Prospective study of colorectal cancer risk in men and plasma levels of insulin-like growth factor (IGF)-I and IGF-binding protein-3. J Natl Cancer Inst 91: 620–625

MacDonald RS, Thornton WH, Jr., Bean TL (1993) Insulin and IGE-1 receptors in a human intestinal adenocarcinoma cell line (CACO-2): regulation of Na+ glucose transport across the brush border. J Recept Res 13:1093–1113

Magnusson C, Baron JA, Correia N, Bergstrom R, Adami HO, Persson I (1999) Breast-cancer risk following long-term oestrogen- and oestrogen-progestin-replacement therapy. Int J Cancer 81:339–344

Manousos O, Souglakos J, Bosetti C, Tzonou A, Chatzidakis V, Trichopoulos D, Adami HO, Mantzoros C (1999) IGF-I and IGF-II in relation to colorectal cancer. Int J Cancer 83:15–17

Mantzoros CS, Tzonou A, Signorello LB, Stampfer M, Trichopoulos D, Adami HO (1997) Insulin-like growth factor 1 in relation to prostate cancer and benign prostatic hyperplasia. Br J Cancer 76:1115–1118

McKeown-Eyssen G (1994) Epidemiology of colorectal cancer revisited: are serum triglycerides and/or plasma glucose associated with risk? Cancer Epidemiol Biomarkers Prev 3:687–695

Mink PJ, Folsom AR, Sellers TA, Kushi LH (1996) Physical activity, waist-to-hip ratio, and other risk factors for ovarian cancer: a follow-up study of older women. Epidemiology 7:38–45

Moller H, Mellemgaard A, Lindvig K, Olsen JH (1994) Obesity and cancer risk: a Danish record-linkage study. Eur J Cancer 30A:344–350

Mollerstrom G, Carlstrom K, Lagrelius A, Einhorn N (1993) Is there an altered steroid profile in patients with endometrial carcinoma? Cancer 72:173–181

Murphy LJ, Ghahary A (1990) Uterine insulin-like growth factor-1: regulation of expression and its role in estrogen-induced uterine proliferation. Endocr Rev 11:443–453

Nagamani M, Hannigan EV, Dillard EA, Jr., Van Dinh T (1986) Ovarian steroid secretion in postmenopausal women with and without endometrial cancer. J Clin Endocrinol Metab 62:508–512

Nandi S, Guzman RC, Yang J (1995) Hormones and mammary carcinogenesis in mice, rats, and humans: a unifying hypothesis. Proc Natl Acad Sci U S A 92:3650–3657

Negri E, Tzonou A, Beral V, Lagiou P, Trichopoulos D, Parazzini F, Franceschi S, Booth M, La Vecchia C (1999) Hormonal therapy for menopause and ovarian cancer in a collaborative re-analysis of European studies. Int J Cancer 80:848–851

Ng EH, Ji CY, Tan PH, Lin V, Soo KC, Lee KO (1998) Altered serum levels of insulin-like growth-factor binding proteins in breast cancer patients. Ann Surg Oncol 5:194–201

Niwa K, Imai A, Hashimoto M, Yokoyama Y, Mori H, Matsuda Y, Tamaya T (2000) A case-control study of uterine endometrial cancer of pre- and post-menopausal women. Oncol Rep 7:89–93

Noguchi T (2000) Protein nutrition and insulin-like growth factor system. Br J Nutr 84 Suppl 2:S241-S244

Nyholm HC, Nielsen AL, Lyndrup J, Dreisler A, Hagen C, Haug E (1993) Plasma oestrogens in postmenopausal women with endometrial cancer. Br J Obstet Gynaecol 100:1115–1119

O'Mara BA, Byers T, Schoenfeld E (1985) Diabetes mellitus and cancer risk: a multi-site case-control study. J Chronic Dis 38:435–441

Oettinger M, Samberg I, Levitan Z, Eibschitz I, Sharf M (1984) Hormonal profile of endometrial cancer. Gynecol Obstet Invest 17:225–235

Ortego J, Vega B, Sampedro J, Escalada J, Boixeda D, Varela C (1994) Neoplastic colonic polyps in acromegaly. Horm Metab Res 26:609–610

Palmqvist R, Hallmans G, Rinaldi S, Biessy C, Stenling R, Riboli E, Kaaks R (2002) Plasma insulin-like growth factor 1, insulin-like growth factor binding protein 3, and risk of colorectal cancer: a prospective study in northern Sweden. Gut 50:642–646

Pan DA, Lillioja S, Kriketos AD, Milner MR, Baur LA, Bogardus C, Jenkins AB, Storlien L H (1997) Skeletal muscle triglyceride levels are inversely related to insulin action. Diabetes 46:983–988

Pegg AE (1999) DNA repair pathways and cancer prevention. Adv Exp Med Biol 472:253–267

Perseghin G, Price TB, Petersen KF, Roden M, Cline GW, Gerow K, Rothman DL, Shulman GI (1996) Increased glucose transport-phosphorylation and muscle glycogen synthesis after exercise training in insulin-resistant subjects. N Engl J Med 335:1357–1362

Petridou E, Papadiamantis Y, Markopoulos C, Spanos E, Dessypris N, Trichopoulos D (2000) Leptin and insulin growth factor I in relation to breast cancer (Greece). Cancer Causes Control 11:383–388

Pettersson B, Bergstrom R, Johansson ED (1986) Serum estrogens and androgens in women with endometrial carcinoma. Gynecol Oncol 25:223–233

Peyrat JP, Bonneterre J, Hecquet B, Vennin P, Louchez MM, Fournier C, Lefebvre J, Demaille A (1993) Plasma insulin-like growth factor-1 (IGF-1) concentrations in human breast cancer. Eur J Cancer 29A:492–497

Pfeilschifter J, Scheidt-Nave C, Leidig-Bruckner G, Woitge HW, Blum WF, Wuster C, Haack D, Ziegler R (1996) Relationship between circulating insulin-like growth factor components and sex hormones in a population-based sample of 50- to 80-year-old men and women. J Clin Endocrinol Metab 81:2534–2540

Pike MC, Spicer DV, Dahmoush L, Press MF (1993) Estrogens, progestogens, normal breast cell proliferation, and breast cancer risk. Epidemiol Rev 15:17–35

Plymate SR, Jones RE, Matej LA, Friedl KE (1988) Regulation of sex hormone binding globulin (SHBG) production in Hep G2 cells by insulin. Steroids 52:339–340

Pollak M, Beamer W, Zhang JC (1998) Insulin-like growth factors and prostate cancer. Cancer Metastasis Rev 17:383–390

Polychronopoulou A, Tzonou A, Hsieh CC, Kaprinis G, Rebelakos A, Toupadaki N, Trichopoulos D (1993) Reproductive variables, tobacco, ethanol, coffee and somatometry as risk factors for ovarian cancer. Int J Cancer 55:402–407

Porcile A, Gallardo E (1991) Long-term treatment of hirsutism: desogestrel compared with cyproterone acetate in oral contraceptives. Fertil Steril 55:877–881

Poretsky L, Cataldo NA, Rosenwaks Z, Giudice LC (1999) The insulin-related ovarian regulatory system in health and disease. Endocr Rev 20:535–582

Potischman N, Hoover RN, Brinton LA, Siiteri P, Dorgan JF, Swanson CA, Berman ML, Mortel R, Twiggs LB, Barrett RJ, Wilbanks GD, Persky V, Lurain JR (1996) Case-control study of endogenous steroid hormones and endometrial cancer. J Natl Cancer Inst 88:1127–1135

Potten CS, Watson RJ, Williams GT, Tickle S, Roberts SA, Harris M, Howell A (1988) The effect of age and menstrual cycle upon proliferative activity of the normal human breast. Br J Cancer 58:163–170

Preston-Martin S, Pike MC, Ross RK, Henderson BE (1993) Epidemiologic evidence for the increased cell proliferation model of carcinogenesis. Environ Health Perspect 101 Suppl 5:137–138

Preston-Martin S, Pike MC, Ross RK, Jones PA, Henderson BE (1990) Increased cell division as a cause of human cancer. Cancer Res 50:7415–7421

Probst-Hensch NM, Yuan JM, Stanczyk FZ, Gao YT, Ross RK, Yu MC (2001) IGF-1, IGF-2 and IGFBP-3 in prediagnostic serum: association with colorectal cancer in a cohort of Chinese men in Shanghai. Br J Cancer 85:1695–1699

Pugeat M, Crave JC, Elmidani M, Nicolas MH, Garoscio-Cholet M, Lejeune H, Dechaud H, Tourniaire J (1991) Pathophysiology of sex hormone binding globulin (SHBG): relation to insulin. J Steroid Biochem Mol Biol 40:841–849

Purdie DM, Green AC (2001) Epidemiology of endometrial cancer. Best Pract Res Clin Obstet Gynaecol 15:341–354

Purdie D, Green A, Bain C, Siskind V, Ward B, Hacker N, Quinn M, Wright G, Russell P, Susil B (1995) Reproductive and other factors and risk of epithelial ovarian cancer: an Australian case-control study. Survey of Women's Health Study Group. Int J Cancer 62:678–684

Raastad T, Bjoro T, Hallen J (2000) Hormonal responses to high- and moderate-intensity strength exercise. Eur J Appl Physiol 82:121–128

Randle PJ (1998) Regulatory interactions between lipids and carbohydrates: the glucose fatty acid cycle after 35 years. Diabetes Metab Rev 14:263–283

Rao BR, Slotman BJ (1991) Endocrine factors in common epithelial ovarian cancer. Endocr Rev 12:14–26

Reaven GM (1988) Banting lecture 1988. Role of insulin resistance in human disease. Diabetes 37:1595–1607

Risch HA (1998) Hormonal etiology of epithelial ovarian cancer, with a hypothesis concerning the role of androgens and progesterone. J Natl Cancer Inst 90:1774–1786

Robinson S, Kiddy D, Gelding SV, Willis D, Niththyananthan R, Bush A, Johnston D G, Franks S (1993) The relationship of insulin insensitivity to menstrual pattern in women with hyperandrogenism and polycystic ovaries. Clin Endocrinol (Oxf) 39:351–355

Rodriguez C, Patel AV, Calle EE, Jacob EJ, Thun MJ (2001) Estrogen replacement therapy and ovarian cancer mortality in a large prospective study of US women. JAMA 285:1460–1465

Rosenberg CR, Pasternack BS, Shore RE, Koenig KL, Toniolo PG (1994) Premenopausal estradiol levels and the risk of breast cancer: a new method of controlling for day of the menstrual cycle. Am J Epidemiol 140:518–525

Ross RK, Pike MC, Coetzee GA, Reichardt JK, Yu MC, Feigelson H, Stanczyk FZ, Kolonel LN, Henderson BE (1998) Androgen metabolism and prostate cancer: establishing a model of genetic susceptibility. Cancer Res 58:4497–4504

Rutanen EM (1998) Insulin-like growth factors in endometrial function. Gynecol Endocrinol 12:399–406

Rutanen EM, Nyman T, Lehtovirta P, Ammala M, Pekonen F (1994) Suppressed expression of insulin-like growth factor binding protein-1 mRNA in the endometrium: a molecular mechanism associating endometrial cancer with its risk factors. Int J Cancer 59:307–312

Rutanen EM, Pekonen F, Nyman T, Wahlstrom T (1993) Insulin-like growth factors and their binding proteins in benign and malignant uterine diseases. Growth Regul 3:74–77

Schildkraut JM, Cooper GS, Halabi S, Calingaert B, Hartge P, Whittemore AS (2001) Age at natural menopause and the risk of epithelial ovarian cancer. Obstet Gynecol 98:85–90

Schildkraut JM, Schwingl PJ, Bastos E, Evanoff A, Hughes C (1996) Epithelial ovarian cancer risk among women with polycystic ovary syndrome. Obstet Gynecol 88:554–559

Schoen RE, Tangen CM, Kuller LH, Burke GL, Cushman M, Tracy RP, Dobs A, Savage PJ (1999) Increased blood glucose and insulin, body size, and incident colorectal cancer. J Natl Cancer Inst 91:1147–1154

Shapiro S, Kelly JP, Rosenberg L, Kaufman DW, Helmrich SP, Rosenshein NB, Lewis JL, Jr., Knapp RC, Stolley PD, Schottenfeld D (1985) Risk of localized and widespread endometrial cancer in relation to recent and discontinued use of conjugated estrogens. N Engl J Med 313:969–972

Sherman ME (2000) Theories of endometrial carcinogenesis: a multidisciplinary approach. Mod Pathol 13:295–308

Shu XO, Brinton LA, Zheng W, Gao YT, Fan J, Fraumeni JF, Jr. (1991) A population-based case-control study of endometrial cancer in Shanghai, China. Int J Cancer 49:38–43

Shu XO, Gao YT, Yuan JM, Ziegler RG, Brinton LA (1989) Dietary factors and epithelial ovarian cancer. Br J Cancer 59:92–96

Siiteri PK (1987) Adipose tissue as a source of hormones. Am J Clin Nutr 45:277–282

Silverman DT, Schiffman M, Everhart J, Goldstein A, Lillemoe KD, Swanson GM, Schwartz AG, Brown LM, Greenberg RS, Schoenberg JB, Pottern LM, Hoover RN, Fraumeni JF, Jr. (1999) Diabetes mellitus, other medical conditions and familial history of cancer as risk factors for pancreatic cancer. Br J Cancer 80:1830–1837

Singh A, Hamilton-Fairley D, Koistinen R, Seppala M, James VH, Franks S, Reed MJ (1990) Effect of insulin-like growth factor-type I (IGF-I) and insulin on the secretion of sex hormone binding globulin and IGF-I binding protein (IBP-I) by human hepatoma cells. J Endocrinol 124:R1-R3

Singh P, Rubin N (1993) Insulin-like growth factors and binding proteins in colon cancer. Gastroenterology 105:1218–1237

Slattery ML, Schuman KL, West DW, French TK, Robison LM (1989) Nutrient intake and ovarian cancer. Am J Epidemiol 130:497–502

Sobbrio GA, Granata A, D'Arrigo F, Arena D, Panacea A, Trimarchi F, Granese D, Pulle C (1990) Treatment of hirsutism related to micropolycystic ovary syndrome (MPCO) with two low-dose estrogen oral contraceptives: a comparative randomized evaluation. Acta Eur Fertil 21:139–141

Sonnichsen AC, Lindlacher U, Richter WO, Schwandt P (1990) Obesity, body fat distribution and the incidence of breast, cervical, endometrial and ovarian carcinomas. Dtsch Med Wochenschr 115:1906–1910

Stanley LA (1995) Molecular aspects of chemical carcinogenesis: the roles of oncogenes and tumor suppressor genes. Toxicology 96:173–194

Stattin P, Bylund A, Rinaldi S, Biessy C, Dechaud H, Stenman UH, Egevad L, Riboli E, Hallmans G, Kaaks R (2000) Plasma insulin-like growth factor-I, insulin-like growth factor-binding proteins, and prostate cancer risk: a prospective study. J Natl Cancer Inst 92:1910–1917

Steppan CM, Lazar MA (2002) Resistin and obesity-associated insulin resistance. Trends Endocrinol Metab 13:18–23

Stewart CE, Rotwein P (1996) Growth, differentiation, and survival: multiple physiological functions for insulin-like growth factors. Physiol Rev 76:1005–1026

Stoll BA (1999) Western nutrition and the insulin resistance syndrome: a link to breast cancer. Eur J Clin Nutr 53:83–87

Stoll BA, Secreto G (1992) New hormone-related markers of high risk to breast cancer. Ann Oncol 3:435–438

Straus DS (1994) Nutritional regulation of hormones and growth factors that control mammalian growth. FASEB J 8:6–12

The Endogenous Hormones and Breast Cancer Collaborative Group (2002) Endoge-
    nous sex hormones and breast cancer in postmenopausal women: reanalysis of
    nine prospective studies. J Natl Cancer Inst 94:606–616
The ESHRE Capri Workshop Group (2001) Ovarian and endometrial function during
    hormonal contraception. Hum Reprod 16:1527–1535
Thissen JP, Ketelslegers JM, Underwood LE (1994) Nutritional regulation of the
    insulin-like growth factors. Endocr Rev 15:80–101
Thomas HV, Key TJ, Allen DS, Moore JW, Dowsett M, Fentiman IS, Wang DY (1997a)
    A prospective study of endogenous serum hormone concentrations and breast
    cancer risk in post-menopausal women on the island of Guernsey. Br J Cancer
    76:401–405
Thomas HV, Reeves GK, Key TJ (1997b) Endogenous estrogen and postmenopausal
    breast cancer: a quantitative review. Cancer Causes Control 8:922–928
Thorneycroft IH, Stanczyk FZ, Bradshaw KD, Ballagh SA, Nichols M, Weber ME
    (1999) Effect of low-dose oral contraceptives on androgenic markers and acne.
    Contraception 60:255–262
Toniolo P, Bruning PF, Akhmedkhanov A, Bonfrer JM, Koenig KL, Lukanova A, Shore
    RE, Zeleniuch-Jacquotte A (2000) Serum insulin-like growth factor-I and breast
    cancer. Int J Cancer 88:828–832
Trayhurn P, Beattie JH (2001) Physiological role of adipose tissue: white adipose tissue
    as an endocrine and secretory organ. Proc Nutr Soc 60:329–339
Troisi R, Potischman N, Hoover RN, Siiteri P, Brinton LA (1997) Insulin and endome-
    trial cancer. Am J Epidemiol 146:476–482
Ursin G, Longnecker MP, Haile RW, Greenland S (1995) A meta-analysis of body
    mass index and risk of premenopausal breast cancer. Epidemiology 6:137–141
van Baak MA, Borghouts LB (2000) Relationships with physical activity. Nutr Rev
    58:S16-S18
van Leeuwen FE, Rookus MA (1989) The role of exogenous hormones in the epi-
    demiology of breast, ovarian and endometrial cancer. Eur J Cancer Clin Oncol
    25:1961–1972
Vogelstein B, Fearon ER, Hamilton SR, Kern SE, Preisinger AC, Leppert M,
    Nakamura Y, White R, Smits AM, Bos JL (1988) Genetic alterations during
    colorectal-tumor development. N Engl J Med 319:525–532
Wang HS, Chard T (1999) IGFs and IGF-binding proteins in the regulation of human
    ovarian and endometrial function. J Endocrinol 161:1–13
Weiderpass E, Adami HO, Baron JA, Magnusson C, Bergstrom R, Lindgren A, Correia
    N, Persson I (1999a) Risk of endometrial cancer following estrogen replacement
    with and without progestins. J Natl Cancer Inst 91:1131–1137
Weiderpass E, Adami HO, Baron JA, Magnusson C, Lindgren A, Persson I (1999b) Use
    of oral contraceptives and endometrial cancer risk (Sweden). Cancer Causes
    Control 10:277–284
Weiderpass E, Partanen T, Kaaks R, Vainio H, Porta M, Kauppinen T, Ojajarvi A,
    Boffetta P, Malats N (1998) Occurrence, trends and environment etiology of
    pancreatic cancer. Scand J Work Environ Health 24:165–174
Weiderpass E, Gridley G, Nyren O, Ekbom A, Persson I, Adami HO (1997a) Diabetes
    mellitus and risk of large bowel cancer. J Natl Cancer Inst 89:660–661
Weiderpass E, Gridley G, Persson I, Nyren O, Ekbom A, Adami HO (1997b) Risk of
    endometrial and breast cancer in patients with diabetes mellitus. Int J Cancer
    71:360–363
Werner H, Leroith D (1996) The role of the insulin-like growth factor system in human
    cancer. Adv Cancer Res 68:183–223
Westley BR, Clayton SJ, Daws MR, Molloy CA, May FE (1998) Interactions between
    the estrogen and insulin-like growth factor signalling pathways in the control of
    breast epithelial cell proliferation. Biochem Soc Symp 63:35–44
Wetterau LA, Moore MG, Lee KW, Shim ML, Cohen P (1999) Novel aspects of the
    insulin-like growth factor binding proteins. Mol Genet Metab 68:161–181

Whittemore AS (1994) Characteristics relating to ovarian cancer risk: implications for prevention and detection. Gynecol Oncol 55:S15-S19

Whittemore AS, Harris R, Itnyre J (1992) Characteristics relating to ovarian cancer risk: collaborative analysis of 12 US case-control studies. IV. The pathogenesis of epithelial ovarian cancer. Collaborative Ovarian Cancer Group. Am J Epidemiol 136:1212–1220

Wideroff L, Gridley G, Mellemkjaer L, Chow WH, Linet M, Keehn S, Borch-Johnsen K, Olsen JH (1997) Cancer incidence in a population-based cohort of patients hospitalized with diabetes mellitus in Denmark. J Natl Cancer Inst 89:1360–1365

Wiegratz I, Jung-Hoffmann C, Kuhl H (1995) Effect of two oral contraceptives containing ethinylestradiol and gestodene or norgestimate upon androgen parameters and serum binding proteins. Contraception 51:341–346

Will JC, Galuska DA, Vinicor F, Calle EE (1998) Colorectal cancer: another complication of diabetes mellitus? Am J Epidemiol 147:816–825

Wolk A, Mantzoros CS, Andersson SO, Bergstrom R, Signorello LB, Lagiou P, Adami HO, Trichopoulos D (1998) Insulin-like growth factor 1 and prostate cancer risk: a population-based, case-control study. J Natl Cancer Inst 90:911–915

Wong YC, Wang YZ (2000) Growth factors and epithelial-stromal interactions in prostate cancer development. Int Rev Cytol 199:65–116

Wysowski DK, Comstock GW, Helsing KJ, Lau HL (1987) Sex hormone levels in serum in relation to the development of breast cancer. Am J Epidemiol 125:791–799

Yamamoto T, Okada H (1994) Clinical usefulness of low-dose oral contraceptives for the treatment of adolescent hyperandrogenemia. Asia Oceania J Obstet Gynaecol 20:225–230

Yee D, Lee AV (2000) Crosstalk between the insulin-like growth factors and estrogens in breast cancer. J Mammary Gland Biol Neoplasia 5:107–115

Yu H, Rohan T (2000) Role of the insulin-like growth factor family in cancer development and progression. J Natl Cancer Inst 92:1472–1489

Yu H, Berkel H (1999) Insulin-like growth factors and cancer. J La State Med Soc 151:218–223

Zeleniuch-Jacquotte A, Akhmedkhanov A, Kato I, Koenig KL, Shore RE, Kim MY, Levitz M, Mittal KR, Raju U, Banerjee S, Toniolo P (2001) Postmenopausal endogenous estrogens and risk of endometrial cancer: results of a prospective study. Br J Cancer 84:975–981

CHAPTER 10

Angiogenesis: A Promising Target for Cancer Prevention

I.U. ALI

The formation of new vasculature proceeds by mechanisms that primarily comprise vasculogenesis and angiogenesis. The process of vasculogenesis, which is mostly confined to early embryonic development, involves de novo differentiation of endothelial cells from mesodermal precursors and their subsequent organization into the vascular capillary network (RISAU and FLAMME 1995; RISAU 1997; PATAN 2000). Angiogenesis, on the other hand, is the process of recruitment of capillaries from preexisting blood vessels by sprouting or sometimes by a nonsprouting mechanism known as intussusception (PATAN et al. 1996). Angiogenesis is required for the supply of oxygen and nutrients to the cells and is therefore essential for cell survival. Although angiogenesis is a key process during embryonic development, the vasculature is usually quiescent in adult life with physiologic angiogenesis occurring only in specific situations such as wound healing, inflammation, and development of corpus luteum during the menstrual cycle. Neovascularization in these situations is tightly regulated and temporally and spatially coordinated.

There is a long list of pathological situations with which angiogenesis is associated, including rheumatoid arthritis, diabetes, various ischemic and inflammatory disorders, and cancer (FOLKMAN 1995; CARMELIET and JAIN 2000). Vascular proliferation is an important aspect of the tumorigenic process (FOLKMAN 1990). Like any developing organ, tumors are angiogenesis-dependent for the acquisition of nutrients and oxygen and hence for their survival and growth. Contrary to the conventional wisdom that angiogenesis is triggered when the tumor reaches a size of approximately 0.2–2mm, i.e., relatively late in the tumorigenic process, evidence is mounting that the angiogenic switch may be an early event in carcinogenesis (FOLKMAN et al. 1989; HANAHAN et al. 1996; HANAHAN and FOLKMAN 1996) and may therefore provide a potential new avenue for cancer prevention. This review will briefly outline the significant steps in angiogenesis, focus on the rationale of using antiangiogenic strategies as a new paradigm for cancer prevention and discuss the potential and problems associated with this approach.

A. Mechanisms of Angiogenesis

Angiogensis is a highly complex process, which, under normal conditions, is exquisitely regulated by the opposing activities of a variety of angiogenic inducers and inhibitors (BOUCK et al. 1996; IRUELA-ARISPE and DVORAK 1997; HANAHAN and WEINBERG 2000). Formation of new vasculature from normally quiescent endothelial cells in itself is an invasive process that comprises well-defined steps involving numerous cellular functions such as degradation of the basement membrane, directed migration of endothelial cells, proliferation, adhesion, and cell–cell and cell–matrix interactions (BOUCK et al. 1996; RISAU 1997). A vast array of cytokines, growth factors, growth factor receptors, adhesion factors, adhesion receptors, proteases, and protease inhibitors participate in multiple steps that occur during neovascularization. Obviously, each of these steps constitutes targets for designing prevention/intervention strategies directed against angiogenesis (EATOCK et al. 2000).

I. Growth Factors and Growth Factor Receptors

There is a long list of growth factors that have mitogenic activity for endothelial cells and act via autocrine or paracrine mechanisms serving as inducers of angiogenesis (FOLKMAN and KLAGSBRUN 1987; LEEK et al. 1994; ZETTER 1998). By far the single most important growth factor, vascular endothelial growth factor or VEGF, is a specific mitogen and a survival factor for endothelial cells (SENGER 1996; FERRARA 2000). VEGF is produced by a wide variety of tumor cells, and plays a central role in angiogenesis (SENGER et al. 1993; FERRARA and ALITALO 1999). It is a bifunctional peptide with vascular permeability and endothelial cell-specific mitogenic activities (SENGER et al. 1983; SENGER et al. 1990; STEPHAN and BROCK 1996). Several biologically active isoforms of VEGF are generated by the alternative splicing of a single gene product (TISCHER et al. 1991). The production of VEGF is often upregulated in tumors by hypoxia partly through the action of the hypoxia-inducible transcription factor, HIF-1 (FORSYTHE et al. 1996). Loss of the tumor suppressor gene, VHL, mutational inactivation of the p53 gene, and the activation of the nuclear factor-kB play an important role in the upregulation of VEGF (KIESER et al. 1994; MUKHOPADHYAY et al. 1997; ROYDS et al. 1998). The activity of VEGF is mediated via two of its receptors, VEGFR-1 and VEGFR-2 belonging to the tyrosine kinase family (VEIKKOLA et al. 2000). VEGFR-2 is expressed predominantly on proliferating endothelial cells (VEIKKOLA et al. 2000). A variety of other proangiogenic cytokines and growth factors regulate angiogenesis by either directly or indirectly modulating VEGF and/or VEGFR signaling.

Another family of angiogenic factors specific for the vascular endothelial cells, named angiopoietins, and endothelial cell-specific tyrosine kinase receptor, Tie-2, have been identified recently and their function elucidated through the use of transgenic and knock-out mice (DAVIS and YANCOPOULOS 1999). It has been demonstrated that the angiopoietin system is crucial for the recruitment of pericytes and smooth muscle cells needed for the stabilization of the developing vasculature and thus in maintaining vascular integrity (PAPAPETROPOULOS et al. 1999).

Besides these endothelial-specific growth factors, numerous other cytokines and growth factors, by virtue of their mitogenic and chemotactic activities on endothelial cells, have been suggested to positively regulate angiogenesis. These include the family of fibroblast growth factors and their receptors, PDGF and its receptor tyrosine kinase, TNFα, IL6 and IL8, HGF/SF (WEBB and VANDE WOUDE 2000), and some members of the CXC chemokine family (BELPERIO et al. 2000; SCHNEIDER et al. 2001).

Although endothelial cell proliferation, stimulated by a variety of growth factors and their receptors, is a critical process during angiogenesis, endothelial cell adhesion events affecting endothelial cell migration, construction and extension of new microvessels, and degradation and remodeling of the extracellular matrix (ECM) are recognized to be essential as well (ELICEIRI and CHERESH 2001). The growth and alignment of endothelial cells and capillary morphogenesis during angiogenesis depend on both cell–cell and cell–ECM adhesions mediated by various adhesion receptors.

II. Cell Adhesion Receptors

Various adhesion receptors expressed either selectively or predominantly on endothelial cells include vascular-endothelial cadherin (VE-cadherin), platelet-endothelial cell adhesion molecule (PECAM-1 or CD31), E- and P-selectins, and integrins (TEDDER et al. 1995; BROOKS 1996; NEWMAN 1997; SHEIBANI and FRAZIER 1999; DEJANA et al. 2001). Endothelial cells interact with a wide variety of ECM components via integrin receptors, which are transmembrane multifunctional proteins and are transducers of biochemical signals between a cell's exterior and interior (GIANCOTTI and RUOSLAHTI 1999; ELICEIRI and CHERESH 2001). The integrin superfamily is composed of at least 16 α and eight β subunits that are expressed in a variety of noncovalently associated heterodimeric combinations (GIANCOTTI and RUOSLAHTI 1999). Endothelial cells, depending on a variety of conditions, express several combinations of these transmembrane heterodimeric receptors (BAZZONI et al. 1999). Two of these integrin receptors, $\alpha v\beta 3$ and $\alpha v\beta 5$, while minimally expressed on quiescent vessels, are highly expressed on new vessels during angiogenesis induced by distinct growth factors (BROOKS et al. 1994). It has been suggested that $\alpha v\beta 3$ integrin receptor provides a survival signal to vascular cells during new blood vessel growth. Preclinical studies have demonstrated that antagonists specific for integrins, including peptidic inhibitors and anti-integrin monoclonal antibodies, inhibit angiogenesis by inducing apoptosis of newly sprouting blood vessels (BROOKS et al. 1994; BROOKS et al. 1995; KUMAR et al. 2001).

III. Proteases and Protease Inhibitors in Extracellular Remodeling

The degradation and remodeling of the extracellular matrix are essential steps in the angiogenic process (BIRKEDAL-HANSEN 1995). A cohort of proteases and protease inhibitors, produced by tumor cells as well as endothelial and nonendothelial cells, mediates these important events. A number of cytokines and growth factors have been shown to regulate the activity of various proteases and protease inhibitors. During the remodeling process, protease cascades, such as plasminogen activator/plasmin system and specific plasmin activator inhibitors and matrix metalloproteinases and their respective tissue inhibitors of metalloproteinases, carry out a controlled degradation of the ECM (PEPPER 2001). Besides remodeling the ECM, interactions between the proteases and the ECM are important at multiple levels. For example, growth factors, many of which have proangiogenic activities, may often be stored in the ECM and finally released by the action of proteases (SAKSELA and RIFKIN 1990; VLODAVSKY et al. 1990). Similarly, ECM components provide substrates for the generation of the inhibitors of angiogenesis by proteolytic cleavage (WEBB and VANDE WOUDE 2000).

IV. Endogenous Inhibitors of Angiogenesis

Naturally occurring endogenous inhibitors of angiogenesis are believed to function in the maintenance of vascular quiescence. The first inhibitor of angiogenesis to be identified was thrombospondin, TSP-1, a member of the family of extracellular proteins with multifunctional domains that participate in cell–cell and cell–matrix communications (LAWLER 2000). The inhibitory effect of TSP-1 on angiogenesis is mediated through its binding to the CD36 transmembrane receptor expressed on microvascular endothelial cells thereby inducing receptor-mediated apoptosis (DAWSON et al. 1997). Many other inhibitors of angiogenesis are generated in vivo by proteolytic degradation of the components of the ECM. Angiostatic activities of angiostatin and endostatin, which are the proteolytic cleavage fragments of plasminogen and collagen XVIII respectively, have been extensively studied (O'REILLY 1997; O'REILLY et al. 1997). It has been suggested that circulating levels of these antiangiogenic fragments, generated by the activity of proteases elaborated by primary tumors, help maintain the distant micrometastases in a dormant state. Several in vitro experiments have shown that similar proteolytic fragments of prolactin, fibronectin, collagen IV, and hepatocyte growth factor/scatter factor inhibit endothelial cell growth suggesting a potential in vivo antiangiogenic role for them as well (FERRARA et al. 1991; CLAPP et al. 1993; JIANG et al. 1999; ELICEIRI and CHERESH 2001). Also, some members of the CXC chemokine family, which are inducible by interferons, have been shown to be potent inhibitors of angiogenesis (BELPERIO et al. 2000; SCHNEIDER et al. 2001).

It is clear that, based upon the molecular details of angiogenesis, prevention/intervention strategies can be directed at multiple steps of this complex process. A variety of antiangiogenic agents are already in clinical trials for the treatment of tumors with high vascularity and other advanced and metastatic cancers (BENCE et al. 2001; TOSETTI et al. 2002). These compounds that block the remodeling of ECM, interfere with the integrin signaling critical for cell survival, and/or inhibit the activity of various proangiogenic growth factors hold great potential for blocking angiogenesis.

B. Angiogenesis as a Component of Precancerous Phenotype

It has long been known that the growth of advanced and metastatic tumors is dependent upon angiogenesis. That angiogenesis may also be a potentially rate-limiting step in the conversion of dormant preinvasive cells to those with the tumorigenic invasive phenotype has been suggested by studies of animal models, experimental assay systems, and analysis of a variety of human premalignant lesions.

I. Animal Models

In multiple transgenic models of tumorigenesis, employing dominant oncogenes and/or null alleles of tumor suppressor genes and modeling the multistage tumor development pathways in human cancers, the angiogenic phenotype is often evident in the premalignant stage prior to tumor formation. The induction of the "angiogenic switch" has been reported in distinct premalignant stages of SV40 T antigen-expressing pancreatic islet cell carcinoma (HANAHAN 1985; FOLKMAN et al. 1989), bovine papillomavirus (BPV-1) oncogene carrying dermal fibrosarcoma (LACEY et al. 1986; HANAHAN et al. 1989), and human papillomavirus (HPV-16) expressing squamous cell carcinoma (ARBEIT et al. 1996; COUSSENS et al.1996). Especially, the pancreatic islet carcinoma model has provided molecular insights into the discrete role of angiogenesis in tumor progression (HANAHAN and FOLKMAN 1996). In this experimental mouse model, although all hyperplastic pancreatic islets express the transgene, SV40 T antigen, only the ones that switch to the angiogenic phenotype, probably by inactivating the angiogenesis suppressor gene thrombospondin, progress to form invasive tumors. Most notably, a study using these mice at different stages of the carcinogenic spectrum provided evidence that distinct antiangiogenic compounds act in a stage-specific manner (BERGERS et al. 1999). Of special interest are the angiogenesis inhibitors that block the progression of premalignant lesions into tumors.

In another example, distinct angiogenic initiation and angiogenic progression switches were reported in the transgenic adenocarcinoma of the mouse prostrate (TRAMP) model. TRAMP mice, expressing the SV40 large T antigen driven by the rat probasin promoter specific for prostate epithelium, develop prostate cancer that displays the entire spectrum of the human disease ranging from mild to severe hyperplasia corresponding to PIN lesions, well-differentiated to poorly-differentiated neoplasia, and finally metastatic tumors (GREENBERG et al. 1995). The two distinct angiogenic switches, the first one corresponding to the tumor initiation phase and another late angiogenic switch coinciding with the progression phase of the tumor development, exhibited distinct molecular profiles of angiogenic markers (HUSS et al. 2001). These findings have significant implications in terms of designing target-specific and stage-specific antiangiogenic therapies.

II. Experimental Systems

The events that precede tumor cell proliferation and neovascularization have been analyzed in an elegant experimental system. When only 20–50 mammary tumor cells were implanted into transparent skin chambers of rats and mice, the earliest event was chemotaxis-like directional migration of tumor cells towards the host vasculature followed by tumor cell proliferation and onset of angiogenesis (LI et al. 2000). At this stage of the onset of neovascularization, the tumor mass contained approximately 100 cells. A fully functional microvasculature was evident when the cluster grew to about 300–400 tumor cells. Most importantly, injection of an angiogenesis inhibitor, a truncated form of the vascular endothelial growth factor receptor, together with tumor cells, not only blocked the initial angiogenesis but also caused tumor cell apoptosis (LI et al. 2000). These experiments clearly demonstrate that the cross talk between tumor cells and the host vasculature resulting in the onset of angiogenesis is the earliest event during tumorigenesis, and that antiangiogenesis agents, when administered early enough, can prevent tumor formation. Since the mammary tumor cells used in the skin chamber assays had a fully invasive and angiogenic genotype, the question arises if premalignant breast epithelial cells depicting the early progression events in human primary breast tumors would also elicit such an early angiogenic response.

Many experimental systems including rodent models and human breast tumor lines xenografted in murine hosts, both in their structural architecture as well as biological behavior, do not truly reflect the complex and heterogeneous characteristics that accompany the progression of human breast disease. In this context, a unique xenograft model using MCF10A cells, derived from the breast tissue of a patient with fibrocystic disease, has been described (MILLER et al. 1993). Ha-ras-transformed derivatives of MCF10A, when xenografted in mice, evolve into proliferative lesions displaying histologic features of the entire spectrum of the human breast disease including mild to moderate hyperplasia, atypical hyperplasia, dysplasia, carcinoma in situ, and invasive carcinoma (DAWSON et al. 1996). Coculturing of MCF10 A cells, which are normal and do not form lesions in immune-deficient mice, and MCFd10AT1-EIII8 cells, which produce preneoplastic lesions, with human umbilical vein endothelial cells in matrigel appears to recapitulate interactions between endothelial cells and breast epithelial cells in vivo (SHEKHAR et al. 2000). Although there is a preferential interaction between the endothelial cells and both normal and premalignant breast epithelial cells, sustained proliferation of endothelial cells occurs only in cocultures of EIII8 premalignant breast epithelial cells. This induction of angiogenesis supported the formation of hyperplastic proliferative ductal alveolar outgrowths with invasive potential suggesting a cause-effect relationship. Furthermore, both processes were enhanced by estrogens and inhibited by antiestrogens (SHEKHAR et al. 2001).

III. Human Cancers

Angiogenesis is detected in early neoplastic lesions associated with a variety of human cancers including ductal carcinoma of breast, cervical carcinoma, prostate cancer, bladder cancer, skin cancer, and probably many other types of cancers. The original histopathological observations using immunostaining to detect microvessel density in premalignant stages have later been substantiated by molecular techniques of profiling angiogenic markers.

1. Breast Cancer

The critical morphological and histological features, suggesting that onset of angiogenesis is a relatively early event in breast carcinogenesis, have been defined much before the advent of molecular characterization (GIMBRONE and GULLINO 1976; BREM et al. 1978). In women with fibrocystic disease, the risk of breast cancer increased with the number and density of microvessels in the hyperplastic lesions (WEIDNER et al. 1992; GUINEBRETIERE et al. 1994). Ductal carcinoma in situ (DCIS) is considered to be the preinvasive version of breast cancer with complete genotypic potential of invasion and malignancy (SILVERSTEIN and MASETTI 1998). Compared with normal breast epithelium, DCIS lesions generally overexpress VEGF (GUIDI et al. 1997). Two distinct patterns of vascularity, a diffuse stromal vascularity between the ducts and a dense rim of microvessels around the ducts, have been defined in the DCIS lesions suggesting the presence of two different angiogenic pathways (ENGELS et al. 1997). An upregulation of the platelet-derived endothelial cell growth factor, also known as thymidine phosphorylase, which is chemotactic for endothelial cells, has been reported in the rimmed version of DCIS (ENGELS et al. 1997).

In various studies, increased vascularity has been reported in preinvasive breast pathologies possibly even before the appearance of defined histopathological changes. Analysis of angiogenic growth factors during the progression through various histopathologies suggests that the regulation of each phenotype may have a complex and distinct angiogenic profile. The growth factors examined and found to be altered include VEGF, bFGF, PD-ECGF, IGF I, and IGF II, which are produced by epithelial, endothelial, and other cell types. Especially, an increase in VEGF, bFGF, and PD-ECGF was reported at the transition from atypical hyperplasia to carcinoma in situ (HEFFELFINGER et al. 1999). It appears that a dynamic balance of several angiogenic factors derived from various cell types regulates the vascularity during the initiation and progression of breast cancer through multiple stages. Analysis of the angiogenic profiles during the early stages of preinvasive breast lesions would provide insights into the multifactorial nature of regulation of angiogenesis and identify stage-specific molecular targets for the development of chemopreventive strategies.

2. Prostate Cancer

Well-defined progressive histopathologic stages can be delineated in prostate cancer ranging from low-grade to high-grade PIN lesions, focal carcinoma, and finally to invasive carcinoma and metastasis (NUPPONEN and VISAKORPI 1999). Although high grade PIN is widely regarded to be the likely precursor of prostate cancer, most of the PIN lesions remain permanently dormant and progression of these lesions to clinical prostate cancer is a rare event (CARTER et al. 1990). Several studies, employing immunohistochemical staining for determining the microvessel density, have suggested that neovascularity is an essential requirement in the progression of prostate carcinoma through various pathologic stages (CAMPBELL 1997; SAKR and GRIGNON 1997). Microvessel density was reported to be of prognostic importance and an independent predictor of pathologic stage as well as of malignant potential of prostate cancer (BRAWER 1996; BORRE et al. 1998). Also, in a xenotransplant model, use of angiogenesis inhibitors such as linomide has been shown to be effective against prostate cancer growth (JOSEPH and ISAACS 1997).

There are numerous reports of the expression of proangiogenic factors such as VEGF, PD-ECGF, IGF-1, IGF-2, and TGFβ in prostate carcinoma (reviewed in (RUSSELL et al. 1998)). Administration of anti-VEGF antibodies targeting neovascularization effectively suppressed the growth of prostate cancer xenografts in nude mice beyond the initial prevascular growth phase as well as the metastasis of established prostate cancer (BORGSTROM et al. 1998; MELNYK et al. 1999).

3. Glial Tumors

Astrocytic neoplasms are believed to progress via independent genetic pathways ultimately giving rise to glioblastoma multiforme (GBM), the most malignant form of the glial tumors. One of the genetic pathways to GBMs involves linear progression of low-grade astrocytomas, which are considered semi-benign primary brain tumors, by acquiring increasing genetic alterations. (KLEIHUES and OHGAKI 1999). The GBMs are endothelial-rich tumors with prominent vascular proliferation, which is mediated by a dynamic balance of angiogenesis inducers and inhibitors (GUERIN and LATERRA 1997). VEGF has been shown to play a significant role in the neovascularity of glial tumors. Various studies have examined angiogenesis in fibrillary low-grade astrocytomas in an attempt to differentiate between tumors with differing propensities for early recurrence and/or malignant transformation. Immunohistochemical staining to assess microvessel density or the expression of various angiogenesis stimulating-growth factors, especially VEGF and its receptor Flk-1, in diffuse fibrillary low-grade astrocytomas indicates that a significant association exists between positive staining for both VEGF and Flk-1 and earlier recurrence and overall shorter survival (Yao et al. 2001).

In another recent study, patients with fibrillary astrocytomas were examined by dynamic susceptibility contrast-enhanced MRI to measure the pretherapeutic cerebral blood volume as a surrogate marker of tumor angiogenesis (Fuss et al. 2001). The observed values were then correlated with clinical outcome subsequent to radiotherapy. The results suggest that based upon the angiogenic activity measured by this technique, low-grade astrocytomas may be categorized into more or less favorable entities in terms of malignant transformation or early local recurrence (Fuss et al. 2001). If born out by future studies, this noninvasive method of measuring the angiogenic activity of low-grade astrocytomas would have far-reaching prognostic and therapeutic consequences.

4. Other Cancers

Other examples of induction of angiogenesis in premalignant phases of oncogenesis include colonic adenomas and dysplastic lesions of the uterine cervix. In colonic adenomas, immunostaining detected increased levels of VEGF as well as microvessel density as compared to normal colonic epithelium (Bossi et al. 1995; Wong et al. 1999). Analysis of VEGF expression by in situ hybridization confirmed its upregulation in adenomas prior to the establishment of the invasive phenotype with a further increase during the development of adenocarcinoma (Wong et al. 1999). Similarly, onset of angiogenesis is an important event in the progression of cervical carcinogenesis. Multiple studies have demonstrated an increase in the VEGF expression as well as in microvessel density in cervical dysplasia or intraepithelial lesions ranging from CIN I to CIN III (Ravazoula et al. 1996; Dellas et al. 1997; Obermair et al. 1997).

In summary, studies of both in vitro and in vivo experimental models and analyses of human cancers have provided compelling evidence that neovascularization ensues at the earliest stage of tumor development and therefore constitutes a critical target for prevention. An understanding of the molecular differences in tumor-specific vasculature would not only be of diagnostic value, but also enhance the prospects of tailored preventive approaches.

C. Molecular Architecture of Normal Versus Tumor-Derived Vasculature

The development of normal vasculature in various tissue types is highly specific and conforms to the environmental and metabolic needs of a specific organ. Vascular remodeling of the endometrium during the menstrual cycle and of the mammary gland during various stages of its life cycle are examples of the highly organized, genetically programmed, and tissue-specific angiogenesis. Tumor vasculature, on the other hand, is known to be abnormal and disorganized, both structurally and functionally (BAISH and JAIN 2000; CARMELIET and JAIN 2000; HASHIZUME et al. 2000), and probably reflects the qualitative and quantitative imbalance in angiogenic stimulators and inhibitors. Studies using the microvascular corrosion casting technique followed by scanning electron microscopy have revealed the differences between the vascular architectures of normal tissues and tumors (KONERDING et al. 1999). The normal vasculature is highly organized and displays uniform patterns of vascular densities, branching, and vessel diameters. In contrast, characteristic features of tumor vessels include heterogeneous vessel densities and significant differences in vessel diameters as well as in intervessel and interbranching distances. Comparison of the colorectal adenomas and carcinomas exhibited architectural similarities although the vascular hierarchy was better maintained in adenomas (KONERDING et al. 2001). Another striking finding of the studies was the presence of tumor-specific microvascular architecture in both xenografted human tumor cell lines in mice as well as in primary human tumors (KONERDING et al. 1992).

Besides these architectural differences in the vasculature, significant molecular differences have been identified between normal and tumor-derived endothelial cells. Recent findings from two studies have furthered our understanding of the molecular aspects of tumor angiogenesis (ST CROIX et al. 2000; CARSON-WALTER et al. 2001). A large number of genes are differentially expressed on tumor endothelial cells and have been designated as tumor endothelial cell markers (TEMs) (ST CROIX et al. 2000). Identification and characterization of some of these TEMs, originally isolated from a colon tumor, demonstrated that (a) the expression of TEMs is largely restricted to the vasculature of tumors derived from a variety of tissue types, (b) although not detectable in adult normal vessels, most of the TEMs are generally expressed during normal angiogenesis such as in the corpus leuteum and healing wounds, and (c) the mouse counterparts of TEMs are also selectively expressed in mouse tumors as well as in the vasculature of the developing mouse embryos (CARSON-WALTER et al. 2001). It is clear that these TEMs render themselves as molecular targets for antiangiogenic therapies. Given the complex heterogeneity of human cancers, it is conceivable that significant qualitative and/or quantitative differences exist in the molecular profiles of vasculatures derived from different tumors. Future investigations would reveal if tumor tissue-specific and/or stage-specific TEMs exist for designing of highly specific prevention/intervention strategies targeting angiogenesis.

D. Angiogenesis as a Target for Chemoprevention – Potential and Challenges

Cancer prevention is fast emerging as a discipline with a very promising potential. The nature of the multistep progression of cancer development provides a strong rationale to develop preventive approaches in the premalignant phase of the disease much before the appearance of clinical symptoms. Carcinogenesis at a premalignant stage can be inhibited or even reversed by dietary and/or pharmacological interventions, a strategy defined as chemoprevention (SPORN 1976; KELLOFF et al. 1994). It is obviously a very challenging terrain for at least two reasons. First, it is very difficult to detect subtle changes that are indicative of the onset of the carcinogenic process and to subsequently follow the efficacy of chemopreventive agents by monitoring these subtle alterations. And second, chronic administration of appropriate chemopreventive agents in mostly healthy individuals must provide a protective effect without toxicity. It is expected that the explosion in molecular information that is providing new mechanistic insights into cellular signaling networks would enable the development of target-selective agents for cancer prevention with low or no toxicity profiles.

Most chemopreventive compounds currently in clinical use probably act via multiple mechanisms, which are often unclear and sometimes controversial. Although certain classes of chemopreventives have a designated central mechanism, for example, scavengers of free radicals, antagonists of hormones, modulators of signal transduction, or differentiation agents, it is difficult to assess the relative contribution of different and probably overlapping mechanisms to their chemopreventive activity as well as their long-term side effects. The chemopreventives used in multiple prevention trials including retinoids, interferons, selenium, linomide, aromatase inhibitors, selective estrogen receptor modulators like tamoxifen, and NSAIDS, especially the COX-2 inhibitor, celecoxib, have been shown to inhibit angiogenesis (NAKAMURA et al. 1996; JOSEPH and ISAACS 1997; LINGEN et al. 1998; TSUJII et al. 1998; JIANG et al. 1999; FATHALLAH-SHAYKH et al. 2000; MARSON et al. 2001; MCNAMARA et al. 2001). The antiangiogenic activity of these compounds probably contributes to their protective and chemopreventive effect. If so, use of specific antiangiogenesis agents, alone as chemopreventives or in combination with other chemopreventive agents, is likely to have several benefits in prevention trials.

The antiangiogenesis approach has some widely recognized advantages over other treatment modalities. First, antiangiogenic therapies targeting new vasculature are expected to be highly tumor specific as 99.99% of the endothelial cells in the normal vasculature are in a state of quiescence (HOBSON and DENEKAMP 1984). Furthermore, endothelial cells involved in angiogenesis can be distinguished via various markers from those in mature quiescent vasculature. Second, the normal endothelial cells of the tumor vasculature are genetically stable and thus the commonly encountered problem of drug-resistance by the tumor cells can be avoided (KERBEL 1997). Finally, the antiangiogenesis agents easily access endothelial cells lining the lumen of blood vessels leading to a better efficacy profile (JAIN 1987).

The utility of angiogenesis, both as a biomarker, especially in cancer prevention trials, and as a chemoprevention target, would clearly be enhanced by the development of molecular technologies. The most commonly used technique to measure tumor angiogenesis is microvessel density determination by immunohistochemical staining of fixed specimens (Fox and HARRIS 1997). This is not a convenient and sensitive endpoint amenable for high-throughput screening in clinical settings. Recently, a sensitive quantitative assay utilizing the real-time PCR technology has been used to develop and validate quantitative molecular profiles associated with angiogenesis in the mouse model of proliferative retinopathy, the TRAMP mouse transgenic model of prostate adenocarcinoma, and a mouse Matrigel model of VEGF-transfected human melanoma cells (ALI et al. 2001; CALVO et al. 2002; SHIH et al. 2002). Such high-throughput and sensitive molecular assays are needed to quantitate tumor-specific angiogenic profiles as biomarkers in clinical specimens both to monitor angiogenesis in early phases of carcinogenesis and to follow the efficacy of various antiangiogenesis treatments.

Angiogenesis, being one of the early changes on the carcinogenic spectrum, certainly qualifies as an important and specific target for chemoprevention. The challenges lie not only in developing a sensitive molecular technique to quantitate subtle changes in angiogenesis in the premalignant lesions, but also in identifying tumor-specific and stage-specific molecular targets. The continually emerging molecular information of this complex process can be exploited for designing highly specific antiangiogenic strategies.

Conceivably, specific antiangiogenic compounds aimed at defined molecular targets will have improved efficacy and reduced toxicity compared with a variety of chemopreventive agents or antiangiogeneic agents currently in use. In the future, molecular profiling of the vascular patterns, especially of precancerous lesions, by using powerful technologies such as expression microarrays and/or proteomics analysis, is expected to identify a panel of markers suitable for developing highly specific preventive strategies. The promising outcomes of antiangiogenic strategies in prevention models predict that, in the foreseeable future, tailored tumor- and stage-specific approaches to curtail angiogenesis may become instrumental in cancer prevention.

Acknowledgments. I am grateful to Drs. Donald Senger and Ronald Lubet for their helpful comments on the manuscript.

References

Ali IU, Senger DR et al. (2001) Angiogenesis as a potential biomarker in prostate cancer chemoprevention trials. Urology 57(4 Suppl 1):143–147

Arbeit JM, Olson DC et al. (1996) Upregulation of fibroblast growth factors and their receptors during multi-stage epidermal carcinogenesis in K14-HPV16 transgenic mice. Oncogene 13(9):1847–1857

Baish JW, Jain RK (2000) Fractals and cancer. Cancer Res 60(14):3683–3688

Bazzoni G, Dejana E et al. (1999) Endothelial adhesion molecules in the development of the vascular tree: the garden of forking paths. Curr Opin Cell Biol 11(5):573–581

Belperio JA, Keane MP et al. (2000) CXC chemokines in angiogenesis. J Leukoc Biol 68(1):1–8

Bence AK, Sheehan JB et al. (2001) Antiangiogenesis agents in clinical trials. J Am Pharm Assoc (Wash) 41(6):893–895

Bergers G, Javaherian K et al. (1999) Effects of angiogenesis inhibitors on multistage carcinogenesis in mice. Science 284(5415):808–812

Birkedal-Hansen H (1995) Proteolytic remodeling of extracellular matrix. Curr Opin Cell Biol 7(5):728–735

Borgstrom P, Bourdon MA et al. (1998) Neutralizing anti-vascular endothelial growth factor antibody completely inhibits angiogenesis and growth of human prostate carcinoma micro tumors in vivo. Prostate 35(1):1–10

Borre M, Offersen BV et al. (1998) Microvessel density predicts survival in prostate cancer patients subjected to watchful waiting. Br J Cancer 78(7):940–944

Bossi P, Viale G et al. (1995) Angiogenesis in colorectal tumors: microvessel quantitation in adenomas and carcinomas with clinicopathological correlations. Cancer Res 55(21):5049–5053

Bouck N, Stellmach V et al. (1996) How tumors become angiogenic. Adv Cancer Res 69:135–174

Brawer MK (1996) Quantitative microvessel density. A staging and prognostic marker for human prostatic carcinoma. Cancer 78(2):345–349

Brem SS, Jensen HM et al. (1978) Angiogenesis as a marker of preneoplastic lesions of the human breast. Cancer 41(1):239–244

Brooks PC (1996) Cell adhesion molecules in angiogenesis. Cancer Metastasis Rev 15(2):187–194

Brooks PC, Clark RA et al. (1994) Requirement of vascular integrin alpha v beta 3 for angiogenesis. Science 264(5158):569–571

Brooks PC, Stromblad S et al. (1995) Antiintegrin alpha v beta 3 blocks human breast cancer growth and angiogenesis in human skin. J Clin Invest 96(4):1815–1822

Calvo A, Smith LE et al. (2002) Inhibition of mammary gland adenocarcinoma angiogenic switch in C3(1)/SV40 transgenic mice by a mutated form of human endostatin. Int J Cancer. 101(3):224–234

Campbell SC (1997) Advances in angiogenesis research: relevance to urological oncology. J Urol 158(5):1663–1674

Carmeliet P, Jain RK (2000) Angiogenesis in cancer and other diseases. Nature 407(6801):249–257

Carson-Walter EB, Watkins DN et al. (2001) Cell surface tumor endothelial markers are conserved in mice and humans. Cancer Res 61(18):6649–6655

Carter HB, Piantadosi S et al. (1990) Clinical evidence for and implications of the multistep development of prostate cancer. J Urol 143(4):742–746

Clapp C, Martial JA et al. (1993) The 16-kilodalton N-terminal fragment of human prolactin is a potent inhibitor of angiogenesis. Endocrinology 133(3):1292–1299

Coussens LM, Hanahan D et al. (1996) Genetic predisposition and parameters of malignant progression in K14-HPV16 transgenic mice. Am J Pathol 149(6): 1899–1917

Davis S, Yancopoulos GD, (1999) The angiopoietins: Yin and Yang in angiogenesis. Curr Top Microbiol Immunol 237:173–185

Dawson DW, Pearce SF et al. (1997) CD36 mediates the In vitro inhibitory effects of thrombospondin-1 on endothelial cells. J Cell Biol 138(3):707–717

Dawson PJ, Wolman SR et al. (1996) MCF10AT: a model for the evolution of cancer from proliferative breast disease. Am J Pathol 148(1):313–319

Dejana E, Spagnuolo R et al. (2001) Interendothelial junctions and their role in the control of angiogenesis, vascular permeability and leukocyte transmigration. Thromb Haemost 86(1):308–315

Dellas A, Moch H et al. (1997) Angiogenesis in cervical neoplasia: microvessel quantitation in precancerous lesions and invasive carcinomas with clinicopathological correlations. Gynecol Oncol 67(1):27–33

Eatock MM, Schatzlein A et al. (2000) Tumour vasculature as a target for anticancer therapy. Cancer Treat Rev 26(3):191–204

Eliceiri BP, Cheresh DA (2001) Adhesion events in angiogenesis. Curr Opin Cell Biol 13(5):563–568

Engels K, Fox SB et al. (1997) Distinct angiogenic patterns are associated with high-grade in situ ductal carcinomas of the breast. J Pathol 181(2):207–212

Engels K, Fox SB et al. (1997) Up-regulation of thymidine phosphorylase expression is associated with a discrete pattern of angiogenesis in ductal carcinomas in situ of the breast. J Pathol 182(4):414–420

Fathallah-Shaykh HM, Zhao LJ et al. (2000) Gene transfer of IFN-gamma into established brain tumors represses growth by antiangiogenesis. J Immunol 164(1):217–222

Ferrara N (2000) VEGF: an update on biological and therapeutic aspects. Curr Opin Biotechnol 11(6):617–624

Ferrara N, Alitalo K (1999) Clinical applications of angiogenic growth factors and their inhibitors. Nat Med 5(12):1359–1364

Ferrara N, Clapp C et al. (1991) The 16 K fragment of prolactin specifically inhibits basal or fibroblast growth factor stimulated growth of capillary endothelial cells. Endocrinology 129(2):896–900

Folkman J (1990) What is the evidence that tumors are angiogenesis dependent? J Natl Cancer Inst 82(1):4–6

Folkman J (1995) Angiogenesis in cancer, vascular, rheumatoid and other disease. Nat Med 1(1):27–31

Folkman J, Klagsbrun M (1987) Angiogenic factors. Science 235(4787):442–447

Folkman J, Watson K et al. (1989) Induction of angiogenesis during the transition from hyperplasia to neoplasia. Nature 339(6219):58–61

Forsythe JA, Jiang BH et al. (1996) Activation of vascular endothelial growth factor gene transcription by hypoxia-inducible factor 1. Mol Cell Biol 16(9):4604–4613

Fox SB, Harris AL (1997) Markers of tumor angiogenesis: clinical applications in prognosis and anti-angiogenic therapy. Invest New Drugs 15(1):15–28

Fuss M, Wenz F et al. (2001) Tumor angiogenesis of low-grade astrocytomas measured by dynamic susceptibility contrast-enhanced MRI (DSC-MRI) is predictive of local tumor control after radiation therapy. Int J Radiat Oncol Biol Phys 51(2):478–482

Giancotti FG, Ruoslahti E (1999) Integrin signaling. Science 285(5430):1028–1032

Gimbrone MA, Gullino Jr PM (1976) Angiogenic capacity of preneoplastic lesions of the murine mammary gland as a marker of neoplastic transformation. Cancer Res 36(7 PT 2):2611–2620

Greenberg NM, DeMayo F et al. (1995) Prostate cancer in a transgenic mouse. Proc Natl Acad Sci U S A 92(8):3439–3443

Guerin C, Laterra J (1997) Regulation of angiogenesis in malignant gliomas. Exs 79:47–64

Guidi AJ, Schnitt SJ et al. (1997) Vascular permeability factor (vascular endothelial growth factor) expression and angiogenesis in patients with ductal carcinoma in situ of the breast. Cancer 80(10):1945–1953

Guinebretiere JM, Le Monique G et al. (1994) Angiogenesis and risk of breast cancer in women with fibrocystic disease. J Natl Cancer Inst 86(8):635–636

Hanahan D (1985) Heritable formation of pancreatic beta-cell tumours in transgenic mice expressing recombinant insulin/simian virus 40 oncogenes. Nature 315(6015):115–122

Hanahan D, Christofori G et al. (1996) Transgenic mouse models of tumour angiogenesis: the angiogenic switch, its molecular controls, and prospects for preclinical therapeutic models. Eur J Cancer 32A(14):2386–2393

Hanahan D, Folkman J (1996) Patterns and emerging mechanisms of the angiogenic switch during tumorigenesis. Cell 86(3):353–364

Hanahan D, Weinberg RA (2000) The hallmarks of cancer. Cell 100(1):57–70

Hanahan D, Wetzel E et al. (1989) Tumorigenic latency and separable stages during fibrosarcoma development in transgenic mice carrying papillomavirus genomes. Princess Takamatsu Symp 20:289–296

Hashizume H, Baluk P et al. (2000) Openings between defective endothelial cells explain tumor vessel leakiness. Am J Pathol 156(4):1363–1380

Heffelfinger SC, Miller MA et al. (1999) Angiogenic growth factors in preinvasive breast disease. Clin Cancer Res 5(10):2867–2876

Hobson B, Denekamp J (1984) Endothelial proliferation in tumours and normal tissues: continuous labelling studies. Br J Cancer 49(4):405–413

Huss WJ, Hanrahan CF et al. (2001) Angiogenesis and prostate cancer: identification of a molecular progression switch. Cancer Res 61(6):2736–2743

Iruela-Arispe ML,Dvorak HF (1997) Angiogenesis: a dynamic balance of stimulators and inhibitors. Thromb Haemost 78(1):672–677

Jain RK (1987) Transport of molecules in the tumor interstitium: a review. Cancer Res 47(12):3039–3051

Jiang C, Jiang W et al. (1999) Selenium-induced inhibition of angiogenesis in mammary cancer at chemopreventive levels of intake. Mol Carcinog 26(4):213–225

Jiang WG, Hiscox SE et al. (1999) Antagonistic effect of NK4, a novel hepatocyte growth factor variant, on in vitro angiogenesis of human vascular endothelial cells. Clin Cancer Res 5(11):3695–3703

Joseph IB, Isaacs JT (1997) Potentiation of the antiangiogenic ability of linomide by androgen ablation involves down-regulation of vascular endothelial growth factor in human androgen-responsive prostatic cancers. Cancer Res 57(6):1054–1057

Kelloff GJ, Boone CW et al. (1994) Progress in cancer chemoprevention: perspectives on agent selection and short-term clinical intervention trials. Cancer Res 54(7 Suppl):2015s–2024s

Kerbel RS (1997) A cancer therapy resistant to resistance. Nature 390(6658):335–336

Kieser A, Weich HA et al. (1994) Mutant p53 potentiates protein kinase C induction of vascular endothelial growth factor expression. Oncogene 9(3):963–969

Kleihues P, Ohgaki H (1999) Primary and secondary glioblastomas: from concept to clinical diagnosis. Neuro-oncol 1(1):44–51

Konerding MA, Fait E et al. (2001) 3D microvascular architecture of precancerous lesions and invasive carcinomas of the colon. Br J Cancer 84(10):1354–1362

Konerding MA, Malkusch W et al. (1999) Evidence for characteristic vascular patterns in solid tumours: quantitative studies using corrosion casts. Br J Cancer 80(5–6): 724–732

Konerding MA, Steinberg F et al. (1992) Vascular patterns of tumors: scanning and transmission electron microscopic studies on human xenografts. Strahlenther Onkol 168(8):444–452

Kumar CC, Malkowski M et al. (2001) Inhibition of angiogenesis and tumor growth by SCH221153, a dual alpha(v)beta3 and alpha(v)beta5 integrin receptor antagonist. Cancer Res 61(5):2232–2238

Lacey M, Alpert S et al. (1986) Bovine papillomavirus genome elicits skin tumours in transgenic mice. Nature 322(6080):609–612

Lawler J (2000) The functions of thrombospondin-1 and -2. Curr Opin Cell Biol 12(5): 634–640

Leek RD, Harris AL et al. (1994) Cytokine networks in solid human tumors: regulation of angiogenesis. J Leukoc Biol 56(4):423–435

Li CY, Shan S et al. (2000) Initial stages of tumor cell-induced angiogenesis: evaluation via skin window chambers in rodent models. J Natl Cancer Inst 92(2): 143–147

Lingen MW, Polverini PJ et al. (1998) Retinoic acid and interferon alpha act synergistically as antiangiogenic and antitumor agents against human head and neck squamous cell carcinoma. Cancer Res 58(23):5551–5558

Marson LP, Kurian KM et al. (2001) The effect of tamoxifen on breast tumour vascularity. Breast Cancer Res Treat 66(1):9–15

184   I.U. ALI

McNamara DA, Harmey J et al. (2001) Tamoxifen inhibits endothelial cell proliferation and attenuates VEGF- mediated angiogenesis and migration in vivo. Eur J Surg Oncol 27(8):714–718

Melnyk O, Zimmerman M et al. (1999) Neutralizing anti-vascular endothelial growth factor antibody inhibits further growth of established prostate cancer and metastases in a pre clinical model. J Urol 161(3):960–963

Miller FR, Soule HD et al. (1993) Xenograft model of progressive human proliferative breast disease. J Natl Cancer Inst 85(21):1725–1732

Mukhopadhyay D, Knebelmann B et al. (1997) The von Hippel-Lindau tumor suppressor gene product interacts with Sp1 to repress vascular endothelial growth factor promoter activity. Mol Cell Biol 17(9):5629–5639

Nakamura J, Savinov A et al. (1996) Estrogen regulates vascular endothelial growth/permeability factor expression in 7,12-dimethylbenz(a)anthracene induced rat mammary tumors. Endocrinology 137(12):5589–5596

Newman PJ (1997) The biology of PECAM-1. J Clin Invest 100(11 Suppl):S25–S29

Nupponen N, Visakorpi T (1999) Molecular biology of progression of prostate cancer. Eur Urol 35(5–6):351–354

O'Reilly MS (1997) Angiostatin: an endogenous inhibitor of angiogenesis and of tumor growth. Exs 79:273–294

O'Reilly MS, Boehm T et al. (1997) Endostatin: an endogenous inhibitor of angiogenesis and tumor growth. Cell 88(2):277–285

Obermair A, Bancher-Todesca D et al. (1997) Correlation of vascular endothelial growth factor expression and microvessel density in cervical intraepithelial neoplasia. J Natl Cancer Inst 89(16):1212–1217

Papapetropoulos A, Garcia-Cardena G et al. (1999) Direct actions of angiopoietin-1 on human endothelium: evidence for network stabilization, cell survival, and interaction with other angiogenic growth factors. Lab Invest 79(2):213–223

Patan S (2000) Vasculogenesis and angiogenesis as mechanisms of vascular network formation, growth and remodeling. J Neurooncol 50(1–2):1–15

Patan S, Munn LL et al. (1996) Intussusceptive microvascular growth in a human colon adenocarcinoma xenograft: a novel mechanism of tumor angiogenesis. Microvasc Res 51(2):260–272

Pepper MS (2001) Role of the Matrix Metalloproteinase and Plasminogen Activator-Plasmin Systems in Angiogenesis. 21(7):1104–1117

Ravazoula P, Zolota V et al. (1996) Assessment of angiogenesis in human cervical lesions. Anticancer Res 16(6B):3861–3864

Risau W (1997) Mechanisms of angiogenesis. Nature 386(6626):671–674

Risau W, Flamme I (1995) Vasculogenesis. Annu Rev Cell Dev Biol 11:73–91

Royds JA, Dower SK et al. (1998) Response of tumour cells to hypoxia: role of p53 and NFkB. Mol Pathol 51(2):55–61

Russell PJ, Bennett S et al. (1998) Growth factor involvement in progression of prostate cancer. Clin Chem 44(4):705–723

Sakr WA, Grignon DJ (1997) Prostate cancer: indicators of aggressiveness. Eur Urol 32(Suppl 3):15–23

Saksela O, Rifkin DB (1990) Release of basic fibroblast growth factor-heparan sulfate complexes from endothelial cells by plasminogen activator-mediated proteolytic activity. J Cell Biol 110(3):767–775

Schneider GP, Salcedo R et al. (2001) The diverse role of chemokines in tumor progression: prospects for intervention (Review) Int J Mol Med 8(3):235–244

Senger DR (1996) Molecular framework for angiogenesis: a complex web of interactions between extravasated plasma proteins and endothelial cell proteins induced by angiogenic cytokines. Am J Pathol 149(1):1–7

Senger DR, Connolly DT et al. (1990) Purification and NH2-terminal amino acid sequence of guinea pig tumor- secreted vascular permeability factor. Cancer Res 50(6):1774–1778

Senger DR, Galli SJ et al. (1983) Tumor cells secrete a vascular permeability factor that promotes accumulation of ascites fluid. Science 219(4587):983–985

Senger DR, Van de Water L et al. (1993) Vascular permeability factor (VPF, VEGF) in tumor biology. Cancer Metastasis Rev 12(3–4):303–324

Sheibani N, Frazier WA (1999) Thrombospondin-1, PECAM-1, and regulation of angiogenesis. Histol Histopathol 14(1):285–294

Shekhar MP, Werdell J et al. (2001) Breast stroma plays a dominant regulatory role in breast epithelial growth and differentiation: implications for tumor development and progression. Cancer Res 61(4):1320–1326

Shekhar MP, Werdell J et al. (2000) Interaction with endothelial cells is a prerequisite for branching ductal-alveolar morphogenesis and hyperplasia of preneoplastic human breast epithelial cells: regulation by estrogen. Cancer Res 60(2):439–449

Shih S-C, Calvo A et al. (2002) Molecular profiling of angiogenesis markers. Am. J. Pathol. 161(1):35–41

Silverstein MJ, Masetti R (1998) Hypothesis and practice: are there several types of treatment for ductal carcinoma in situ of the breast? Recent Results Cancer Res 152:105–122

Sporn MB (1976) Approaches to prevention of epithelial cancer during the preneoplastic period. Cancer Res 36(7 PT 2):2699–2702

St Croix B, Rago C et al. (2000) Genes expressed in human tumor endothelium. Science 289(5482):1197–1202

Stephan CC, Brock TA (1996) Vascular endothelial growth factor, a multifunctional polypeptide. P R Health Sci J 15(3):169–178

Tedder TF, Steeber DA et al. (1995) The selectins: vascular adhesion molecules. Faseb J 9(10):866–873

Tischer E, Mitchell R et al. (1991) The human gene for vascular endothelial growth factor. Multiple protein forms are encoded through alternative exon splicing. J Biol Chem 266(18):11947–1154

Tosetti F, Ferrari N et al. (2002) Angioprevention: angiogenesis is a common and key target for cancer chemopreventive agents. Faseb J 16(1):2–14

Tsujii M, Kawano S et al. (1998) Cyclooxygenase regulates angiogenesis induced by colon cancer cells. Cell 93(5):705–716

Veikkola T, Karkkainen M et al. (2000) Regulation of angiogenesis via vascular endothelial growth factor receptors. Cancer Res 60(2):203–212

Vlodavsky I, Korner G et al. (1990) Extracellular matrix-resident growth factors and enzymes: possible involvement in tumor metastasis and angiogenesis. Cancer Metastasis Rev 9(3):203–226

Webb CP, Vande Woude GF (2000) Genes that regulate metastasis and angiogenesis. J Neurooncol 50(1–2):71–87

Weidner N, Folkman J et al. (1992) Tumor angiogenesis: a new significant and independent prognostic indicator in early-stage breast carcinoma. J Natl Cancer Inst 84(24):1875–1887

Wong MP, Cheung N et al. (1999) Vascular endothelial growth factor is up-regulated in the early pre malignant stage of colorectal tumour progression. Int J Cancer 81(6):845–850

Yao Y, Kubota T et al. (2001) Prognostic value of vascular endothelial growth factor and its receptors Flt-1 and Flk-1 in astrocytic tumours. Acta Neurochir 143(2):159–166

Zetter BR (1998) Angiogenesis and tumor metastasis. Annu Rev Med 49:407–424

CHAPTER 11
Arachidonic Acid Pathway in Cancer Prevention

G.J. KELLOFF and C.C. SIGMAN

A. Arachidonic Acid Metabolic Pathways Provide Molecular Targets for Cancer Preventive Intervention

The potential role of products of arachidonic acid (AA) metabolism in carcinogenesis has been reviewed extensively (KELLOFF et al. 1994; MARNETT 1995; TAKETO 1998a,b; DANNENBERG et al. 2001; FUNK 2001), as have cancer prevention strategies based on modulation of these pathways (LIPPMAN et al. 1998; KELLOFF 2000; GUPTA and DUBOIS 2001; ANDERSON et al. 2002). AA metabolism begins with the intracellular release of AA, mediated by either phospholipase A_2 (PLA_2), or by the combined actions of phospholipase C (PLC) and diacylglycerol kinase or phospholipase D (PLD) and PLA_2 (NEEDLEMAN et al. 1986). In leukocytes, cytokines including IL-1 and TNF can activate PLA_2 by stimulating a phospholipase-activating protein (CLARK et al. 1991). AA is then metabolized to prostaglandins (PGs), thromboxanes, leukotrienes (LTs), and hydroxyeicosatetraenoic acids (HETEs) via oxidative enzymes (FUNK 2001). Activated oxygen species and alkylperoxy species are formed throughout this process; AA metabolism is increased during inflammation. The major pathways of AA metabolism, PG synthesis and LT synthesis, are associated strongly with carcinogenesis; both are inhibited by antioxidants and anti-inflammatory agents. Evidence also suggests that direct modulation of cellular AA levels may affect carcinogenesis.

I. Prostaglandin Synthetic Pathway

The first step in the PG synthetic pathway is mediated by the enzyme prostaglandin H synthase (PHS). This enzyme has two activities – cyclooxygenase (COX), which catalyzes the formation of prostaglandin G_2 (PGG_2) from arachidonic acid, and hydroperoxidase, which catalyzes the reduction of PGG_2 to PGH_2 (SMITH et al. 1991; FITZGERALD and PATRONO 2001; FUNK 2001). To return to its native state, the hydroperoxidase requires a reducing cosubstrate; procarcinogens, for example arylamino and arylnitro compounds, are such substrates. According to the model proposed, the procarcinogens are activated (oxidized) during catalysis to free radicals and electrophiles that can form adducts with DNA and initiate carcinogenesis. PGH_2 is further metabolized to form PGs (PGE_2, $PGF_{2\alpha}$, PGD_2), thromboxanes, and prostacyclin. The

specific products formed are tissue and cell type dependent, and these products in turn are autocrine and paracrine signal transduction mediators via a
family of cell- and ligand-specific G-protein coupled receptors. Most significant for carcinogenesis, PGE_2 acts through receptor subtypes EP_1–EP_4 (FUNK
2001). PGs may also interact with other cellular receptors to modulate signal
transduction. For example, PGE_2 transactivates epidermal growth factor
receptor (EGFR) (PAI et al. 2001). Additionally, PGH_2 itself breaks down to
form a known direct-acting mutagen, malondialdehyde (MARNETT 1992). This
process can be stopped five ways: (1) at formation of PGG_2 via inhibition of
COX, (2) by inhibition of peroxidase activity, (3) by prevention of formation
of reactive intermediates, (4) by scavenging reactive intermediates (e.g., by
GSH conjugation), and (5) blocking PG receptors. Of these, inhibition of COX
has been explored most extensively, particularly using nonsteroidal anti-
inflammatory drugs (NSAIDs) which derive their pharmacological activity
specifically from COX inhibition.

However, the multiple tissue specific activities of PGs and other PHS
products, both beneficial and deleterious, have challenged the development
of COX inhibitors as cancer preventive drugs (WOLFE et al. 1999; KULKARNI
et al. 2000; FITZGERALD and PATRONO 2001). For example, PGE_2 in the gut promotes protective mucosal secretions; lowered gut PG levels resulting from
NSAID administration are associated with one of the major side effects
of long-term NSAID treatment, gastrointestinal ulceration and bleeding
(e.g., WOLFE et al. 1999). Likewise, PGs in the kidney and thromboxanes in
platelets are important to normal physiological function. Their loss is associated with renal tubule toxicity and excessive bleeding, respectively
(FITZGERALD and PATRONO 2001). The discovery of an inducible form of COX
(COX-2), which predominates at inflammation sites, in macrophages and in
synoviocytes, and is strongly associated with carcinogenesis has provided a feasible approach to minimizing the toxicity of COX inhibition. The constitutive
COX-1 isoform predominates in the sites of potential toxicity: stomach,
gastrointestinal tract, platelets, and kidney. Drugs which selectively inhibit
COX-2 activity at pharmacological doses (e.g., celecoxib, rofecoxib) have
shown potentially lower rates of gastrointestinal toxicity than traditional
NSAIDs (e.g., ibuprofen, sulindac, piroxicam), which inhibit both COX
isoforms (KULKARNI et al. 2000).

Interference with COX-2 expression is also a potential strategy for reducing carcinogenesis. The COX-2 gene is located in both the endoplasmic reticulum and nuclear membranes; gene expression is upregulated via signal
transduction pathways in response to growth factors, tumor promoters,
cytokines, and oncogenes (reviewed in HERSCHMAN 1999, SMITH et al. 2000;
FITZGERALD and PATRONO 2001, FUNK 2001). These include the oncogenes Ha-
ras, v-src, HER-2/neu, and wnt1, transforming growth factor-β1 (TGFβ1),
TGFα, tumor necrosis factor (TNF)-α, interferon and interleukins (ILs). The
effects of these stimuli may be upregulation of transcription, which
is mediated through multiple transcription factor binding sites within the

COX-2 gene promoter, such as those for cAMP, *myb*, nuclear factor-IL6 (NF-IL6), CCAAT/enhancer binding proteins (C/EBPs), NF-κB and Ets. COX-2 gene expression may also be modulated by effects on mRNA stability and protein synthesis and degradation (e.g., associated with regulatory elements in the 3' untranslated region of COX mRNA. Multiple regulatory elements have been identified in the COX-2 gene 3' untranslated region that control message stability and translational efficiency (SHENG et al. 2000; COK and MORRISON 2001; DIXON et al. 2001).

II. Leukotriene Synthetic Pathway

The burst of lipoxygenase (LOX) activity that is seen during inflammation is the first step in formation of LTs from AA. Available evidence suggests that the immediate products of LOX activity, hydroxyeicosatetrienoic acids (HETEs) and their hydroperoxy precursors (HPETEs), mediate cell proliferative aspects of carcinogenesis (STEELE et al. 1999). For example, compounds that suppress the formation of these free radicals and electrophiles (e.g., vitamin E, flavonoids, and tea polyphenols) inhibit tumor progression in mouse skin.

The LOXs are a family of nonheme iron-containing dioxygenases that catalyze the stereospecific oxygenation of the 5-, 12-, or 15-carbon atoms of AA to form the corresponding HETEs, which are metabolized to LTs or lipoxins through additional sequential cell-specific reactions (NEEDLEMAN et al. 1986; SAMUELSSON et al. 1987; STEELE et al. 1999; FUNK 2001). For example, in the presence of 5-LOX activating protein (FLAP), 5-LOX catalyzes the oxygenation of AA to 5-hydroperoxyeicosatetraenoic acid (HPETE); then 5-HPETE is dehydrated to form the epoxide LTA$_4$. LTA$_4$ is further metabolized to either LTB$_4$ via stereoselective hydration by LTA$_4$ hydrolase, or to LTC$_4$ through GSH conjugation catalyzed by LTC$_4$ synthase. Sequential metabolic reactions, catalyzed by γ-glutamyl transferase and a specific membrane-bound dipeptidase, convert LTC$_4$ into LTD$_4$ and LTE$_4$, respectively. These three sulfidopeptide LTs are commonly referred to as the slow-reacting substances of anaphylaxis. In the lung, sulfidopeptide LTs are known to act on a single high-affinity, smooth muscle receptor, the *cys*-LT$_1$ receptor, resulting in bronchoconstriction and alterations in vascular permeability and mucous secretion in this tissue. Important cellular sources of these LTs include eosinophils, mast cells, and basophils.

Acting via tissue and cell specific receptors, the LTs modulate the growth of several normal human cell types (T-lymphocytes, skin fibroblasts, epidermal keratinocytes, and glomerular epithelial cells). Both LTB$_4$ and LTC$_4$ increase growth of arterial smooth muscle cells, airway epithelial cells, and mitogen-stimulated lymphocytes in vitro. Besides these cells, LTs have a role in regulation of hematopoiesis. Specific factors that regulate LOX gene expression have been identified. Glucose, EGF, and angiotensin II stimulate 12-LOX mRNA expression, production of HETEs and hydroxyoctadecadienoic acids

(HODEs), and both IL-4 and IL-13 are positive regulators of monocyte 15-LOX gene expression.

LOX inhibition and blockade of LT receptors are the predominant methods for interfering with carcinogenesis-associated activities on this pathway. Inhibition of LOX may be the more effective cancer preventive activity because of the associated reduced production of oxygen radical intermediates.

The remainder of this chapter focuses primarily on the two molecular targets on the AA metabolic pathways that have thus far shown the greatest promise as targets for cancer preventive intervention – COX-2 on the PG pathway and 5-LOX on the LT pathway. Section B summarizes the research findings that qualify COX-2 and, to a lesser extent, 5-LOX as targets for cancer preventive intervention and progress in developing cancer prevention strategies involving modulation of these targets. Section C addresses possible lines of future research in this area.

B. COX-2 and 5-LOX as Molecular Targets for Cancer Prevention

The criteria describing a molecular target for cancer prevention are: (1) target is overexpressed in cancers and precancers compared with unaffected tissue, (2) blocking target does not interfere with normal cellular function, (3) mechanistic rationale(s) exist for participation of target in carcinogenesis, (4) modulation of target is measurable, (5) cancer preventive modulation of target is associated with low toxicity, and (6) modulation of target provides clinical benefit, directly or indirectly related to chemopreventive potential. The evidence that COX-2 and 5-LOX meet these criteria is summarized in the paragraphs following.

I. COX-2 as a Target for Cancer Prevention

1. COX-2 Expression in Carcinogenesis

In several respects, COX-2 is a near perfect molecular target for cancer prevention strategies (KELLOFF 2000; GUPTA and DUBOIS 2001; ANDERSON et al. 2002). First, it is expressed nearly ubiquitously in cancer and precancer tissues (see Table 1). It has been found in epithelial cancer cells, but a growing body of evidence suggests that its activity in the stroma (fibroblasts, immune cells, endothelial cells) may be more critical to carcinogenesis (KULKARNI et al. 2000; GUPTA and DUBOIS 2001; MASFERRER 2001). It is induced by cellular stress, such as during inflammation, and so is expected to be at very low or undetectable levels in unaffected cells. As summarized in Sect. A, mechanisms that control transcription and translation appear to contribute to and can be driven by the elevated expression of COX-2. Further, cellular and tissue functions in carcinogenesis are associated with COX-2 expression, including increased prolif-

Table 1. COX-2 and 5-LOX expression in human cancers

Target organ	COX-2 Precancer	COX-2 Cancer	5-LOX Cancer
Colon	√	√	√
Bladder	√	√	ND
Esophagus	√	√	ND
Skin	√	√	√
Head and neck	√	√	√
Leukemia	ND	ND	√
Lung	√	√	√
Breast	√	√	√
Prostate	√	√	√
Pancreas	ND	√	ND
CNS	ND	√	ND
Cervix	√	√	ND
Ovary	ND	√	ND
Liver	ND	√	ND
Stomach	√	√	ND

√, Expression observed in one or more published studies; ND, no data on expression were found (see Koki et al. 1999; Kelloff 2000; Soslow et al. 2000; Anderson et al. 2002).

eration, reduced apoptosis, angiogenesis, and cell migration and invasiveness (e.g., Herschman 1999; Gupta and Dubois 2001; Masferrer 2001).

a) Proliferation

Evidence shows that COX expression may modulate growth factor and growth factor receptor (e.g., EGFR) expression or by directly affecting downstream molecular targets on signal transduction pathways such as MAP kinase (Xie and Herschman 1996; Herschman et al. 1997; Subbaramaiah et al. 2002). Chronic inflammation is a known risk factor for epithelial carcinogenesis, as is suppressed immune response. Both processes are associated with elevated COX-2 expression (Weitzman and Gordon 1990; Kelloff 2000), which could lead to further stimulation of the signal transduction pathways involved in cell proliferation as stated in Sect. B.I.1. For example, in colorectal cancer, the production of PGs is associated with immune suppression and loss of HLA antigens (Balch et al. 1984; Mcdougall et al. 1990). PGE_2 produced by monocytes and macrophages suppresses factors required for immune surveillance, including lymphokines, T- and B-cell proliferation, and natural killer cell cytotoxic activity. COX-2 inhibitors suppress the inflammatory response and stimulate immune response. In UV-exposed skin, topical application of the COX-2 selective inhibitor celecoxib was shown to effectively decrease edema, dermal neutrophil infiltration and activation, PGE_2 levels, and the production of sunburn cells (Wilgus et al. 2000).

b) Apoptosis

Reduced apoptosis is prevalent in carcinogenesis (BEDI et al. 1995; TSUJII and DUBOIS 1995) and is associated with COX-2 expression, for example, by upregulation of *bcl*-2 (TSUJII and DUBOIS 1995). Induction of apoptosis is a potentially important cancer preventive mechanism of COX inhibitors, which have been found to induce apoptosis in cancer cells of the colon (HARA et al. 1997; SHENG et al. 1998; SMITH et al. 2000), bladder (MOHAMMED et al. 1999, 2002), stomach (SAWAOKA et al. 1998), prostate (LIU et al. 1998; HSU et al. 2000), pancreas (DING et al. 2000), esophagus (ZIMMERMANN et al. 1999), and lung (YAO et al. 2000), as well as in squamous cell carcinomas of the head and neck (NISHIMURA et al. 1999). Some molecular changes associated with the proapoptotic action of COX blocking agents are upregulation of prostate apoptosis response 4 gene, *fas*-L, and *bad*, and downregulation of *bcl*-2 and peroxisome proliferator activated receptor (PPAR)σ (although PPARσ appears to be more important to the inflammatory response) (LIU et al. 1998; SHENG et al. 1998; HE et al. 1999; YAO et al. 2000).

c) Angiogenesis

PGs stimulate tumor cell growth and neovascularization (TSUJII et al. 1998; TOMOZAWA et al. 2000; UEFUJI et al. 2000), and COX-2 is expressed in the angiogenic vasculature within tumors and preexisting vasculature adjacent to tumors in human breast, lung, pancreas, prostate, bladder, and colon cancers (reviewed in KOKI et al. 1999). COX inhibitors also decrease tumor blood vessel and capillary formation, inhibit expression of angiogenic growth factors such as vascular endothelial growth factor (VEGF) and basic fibroblast growth factor (bFGF), and are agonists of the antiangiogenic PPARγ (MASFERRER et al. 2000).

d) Invasiveness and Cell Migration

COX-2 expression has been directly associated with increased tumor cell adhesion, growth of endothelial cells and invasiveness (JONES et al. 1999; MASFERRER et al. 1999; SAWAOKA et al. 1999; SUH et al. 1999; MAJIMA et al. 2000; MEHTA et al. 2000; PETERS et al. 2000). For example, human colon cancer cells (CaCo-2) transfected with a COX-2 expression vector showed increased invasiveness, activation of matrix metalloproteinase-2 (MMP-2), and increased RNA levels for the membrane-type metalloproteinase (TSUJII et al. 1997); conversely, COX-2 inhibitors reversed invasiveness and MMP activation.

2. Epidemiological Evidence Associates Use of COX Inhibitors with Cancer Prevention

Chronic use of COX inhibitors has been associated with reduced cancer risk in many cancer target organs – colorectum, bladder, breast, esophagus, gynecological, lung, pancreas, prostate, skin, and stomach (ANDERSON et al. 2002;

THUN et al. 2002). The evidence is most striking for colorectal cancer. More than 20 studies have found a reduced incidence of colorectal cancers or precancerous adenomas associated with chronic use of aspirin or other NSAIDs. Since the use of COX-2 selective inhibitors is too recent for evaluation in such epidemiological studies, these observations are based on the use of aspirin and other nonselective COX inhibitors. However, it is very probable that the cancer preventive activity observed is due at least in part to COX-2 inhibition.

3. COX-2 Inhibitors Show Cancer Preventive Activity in Animal Models of Carcinogenesis

Table 2 summarizes published animal carcinogenesis studies in which COX-2 selective inhibitors have shown cancer preventive activity. This activity has

Table 2. COX-2 selective inhibitors demonstrate cancer preventive activity in animal models of carcinogenesis

Target organ/agents	Animal model	Reference(s)
Colon; Celecoxib	AOM-induced F344 rat; Min mouse	REDDY et al. 1996, 2000; KAWAMORI et al. 1998; JACOBY et al. 2000
MF Tricyclic	APC Δ^{716} mouse	OSHIMA et al. 1996
Tilmacoxib	APC Δ^{740} mouse	SASAI et al. 2000
Nimesulide	AOM-induced ICR mouse Min mouse	FUKUTAKE et al. 1998 NAKATSUGI et al. 1997
NS-398	AOM-induced F344 rat	YOSHIMI et al. 1999
Rofecoxib	APC Δ^{716} mouse	OSHIMA et al. 2001
Bladder; Celecoxib	OH-BBN-induced B6D2F1 mouse and F344 rat	GRUBBS et al. 2000
Nimesulide	OH-BBN-induced F344 rat	OKAJIMA et al. 1998
Lung NS-398	NNK-induced A/J mouse	RIOUX and CASTONGUAY 1998
Mammary; Celecoxib	DMBA-induced SD rat	HARRIS et al. 2000
Nabumetone	MNU-induced SD rat	MATSUNAGA et al. 1998
Oral cavity; Nimesulide	4-NQO-induced F344 rat	SHIOTANI et al. 2001
Skin; Celecoxib	UVB-induced Skh:HR-1 mice	FISCHER et al. 1999; PENTLAND et al. 1999
SC-51825	DMBA/TPA-induced NMRI mice	MULLER-DECKER et al. 1998

AOM, azoxymethane; DMBA, 7,12-dimethylbenz(a)anthracene; MNU, N-methyl-N-nitrosourea; NNK, 4-(methylnitrosamino)-1-(3-pyridyl)-1-butanone; NQO, 1-nitroquinoline-N-oxide; OH-BBN, N-butyl-N-(4-hydroxybutyl)nitrosamine; SD, Sprague-Dawley; TPA, 12-O-tetradecanoylphorbol-13-acetate.

been observed most consistently in studies of colon carcinogenesis, and activity has also been seen in bladder, skin, head and neck, lung, mammary gland and prostate. One interesting observation in these studies is that the COX-2 selective inhibitors are possibly more effective in reducing cancer progression than cancer incidence. This effect has been found in colon, skin, and bladder. For example, in rat bladder, the COX-2 selective inhibitor celecoxib reduced cancer incidence and multiplicity, but was most effective in preventing progression of dysplasia to cancers (GRUBBS et al. 2000). Similarly, in UV-induced mouse skin, the incidence of papillomas was reduced, but the most dramatic effects of 500 ppm celecoxib in the diet were the reductions in papilloma multiplicity (2/mouse in celecoxib treatment group vs. 18/mouse in UV control group) and size (1.3% >2 mm diameter in the celecoxib group vs. 12.5% >2 mm in UV control group) (FISCHER et al. 1999).

4. COX-2 Inhibitors Show High Promise of Cancer Preventive Activity in Clinical Intervention Studies – A Primary Target Is Regression and Prevention of the Obligate Precursor of Cancers, Intraepithelial Neoplasia

The rationales, evidence, and strategies supporting the use of intraepithelial neoplasia (IEN) endpoints for cancer prevention studies has been recently described (O'SHAUGHNESSY et al. 2002). Particularly strong evidence supports the use of colorectal adenomas. Several chemoprevention trials with colorectal adenoma recurrence and regression as endpoints have been undertaken with COX inhibitors in FAP patients. Sulindac has shown dramatic effects in causing the total or almost total regression of colorectal adenomatous polyps in patients with FAP (GIARDIELLO et al. 1993). A study completed in 1999 examined the effect of the COX-2 selective inhibitor celecoxib at two doses against colorectal polyps in subjects with FAP (STEINBACH et al. 2000).

In the randomized, double-blind, placebo-controlled study of 77 FAP patients, a 6-month intervention with 800 mg/day celecoxib significantly reduced polyp number by 28%, with 53% of treated subjects showing a >=25% reduction. A blinded physicians' assessment indicated a qualitative improvement in the colon and rectum, and to a lesser extent in the duodenum, of treated subjects. This trial led to accelerated FDA marketing approval of celecoxib as an adjunct to standard care for the regression and reduction of adenomatous polyps in FAP subjects. Although it can be inferred from data supporting the correlation of adenoma burden to colon cancer incidence, it remains to be demonstrated in a randomized, placebo-controlled clinical study that celecoxib will actually reduce cancer incidence. Nonetheless, this study was a landmark in chemoprevention research with precancer as an endpoint, demonstrating that adenomas can serve as an appropriate endpoint for quantitative and qualitative assessments of chemopreventive efficacy in FAP patients. Follow-up studies of celecoxib in patients with FAP as well as in subjects with sporadic adenomas are underway to assess the relative effect of celecoxib on polyp regression and prevention, and to determine whether greater efficacy can be engendered by combination therapy of celecoxib with other agents (such as eflornithine). Rofecoxib is also under evaluation for the prevention of sporadic adenomas (OSHIMA et al. 2001). Representative cancer prevention studies in progress with COX-2 inhibitors and using IEN as endpoints are summarized in Table 3. COX-2 inhibitors are under evaluation in prevention of superficial bladder cancers, regression and prevention of actinic keratosis, regression of Barrett's esophagus (a precursor of esophageal adenocarcinoma) and esophageal dysplasia (a precursor of squamous cell carcinoma of the esophagus), modulation of bronchial metaplasia/dysplasia, oral premalignant lesions (OPL) as well as modulation of biomarkers of prostate and breast carcinogenesis.

5. COX-2 Selective Inhibitors Show Low Toxicity and Have Promise of Providing Clinical Benefit in Several Chronic Diseases

COX inhibitors are already widely used to treat chronic inflammatory conditions, particularly osteo- and rheumatoid arthritis, and have additional indications in cardiovascular and, potentially, neurodegenerative (Alzheimer's) disease (KULKARNI et al. 2000). As described in Sect. A, there is significant toxicity associated with the use of nonselective COX inhibitors, primarily a result of inhibiting formation of the tissue protective PGs catalyzed by constitutive COX-1. For example, in 1997, there were approximately 16,000 deaths in the USA associated with NSAID use (WOLFE et al. 1999). In comparative studies of chronically administered COX-2 selective inhibitors with nonselective COX inhibitors, incidences of the most prevalent of these toxicities, gastrointestinal ulceration and bleeding, were reduced in patients using the COX-2 selective drugs (FITZGERALD and PATRONO 2001). Although the weight of evidence shows that COX-2 selective inhibitors are safe for chronic use, there is a very limited study suggesting that use of COX-2 selective NSAIDs may increase the risk of heart attack (MUKHERJEE et al. 2001), and there is the possibility that inhibition of COX-2 may affect kidney and reproductive function (WOLFE et al. 1999; KULKARNI et al. 2000; FITZGERALD and PATRONO 2001).

II. LOX as a Target for Cancer Prevention

1. LOX Expression in Carcinogenesis

There is a body of research suggesting that LOX and their products, LTs and HETEs, contribute to carcinogenesis (see Table 1). 12-LOX mRNA expression has been well-documented in many types of solid tumor cells, including those of prostate, colon, and epidermoid carcinoma (HONN et al. 1994a, TANG and HONN 1994). Additionally, the production of 12(S)-HETE by some tumor cells, including prostate cells, has been positively correlated to their metastatic potential (HONN et al. 1994a). Also, 12(S)-HETE is a critical intracellular

Table 3. Representative clinical cancer prevention studies of COX-2 selective inhibitors

Target organ/agent	Study cohort	Objective(s)
Colon		
Celecoxib	FAP patients >=18 years old	Regression/prevention of colorectal adenomas; modulation of duodenal dysplasia; modulation of biomarkers
Celecoxib ± eflornithine	"	"
Celecoxib	FAP genotype >=10 years old without FAP phenotype	Delay time to expression of FAP phenotype
Celecoxib	HNPCC	Modulation of biomarkers
Celecoxib	Previous colorectal adenoma	Prevention of colorectal adenomas; modulation of ACF and other biomarkers
Celecoxib	"	Prevention of colorectal adenomas
Bladder		
Celecoxib	Superficial TCC (Ta, T1/TIS) post-BCG	Increased time to recurrence of superficial TCC; modulation of biomarkers
Esophagus		
Celecoxib	Barrett's esophagus	Regression of Barrett's dysplasia
Celecoxib ± SeMet	Esophageal squamous dysplasia	Regression of dysplasia
Head and neck		
Celecoxib	OPL	Regression of OPL
Lung		
Celecoxib	Chronic smokers (mild COPD)	Modulation of biomarkers
Celecoxib	Previous stage I NSCLC	Prevention of lung cancers; modulation of precancerous changes
Prostate		
Celecoxib	Prostate cancer (scheduled for radical prostatectomy)	Modulation of biomarkers; pharmacodynamics
Skin		
Celecoxib	Fitzpatrick Skin Type I-IV photosensitivity	Decreased UV damage; modulation of biomarkers
Celecoxib	BCNS with previous BCC	Prevention of BCC
Celecoxib	AK (10–40 on upper extremities, neck and head)	Prevention and regression of AK; modulation of carcinogenesis biomarkers

ACF, aberrant crypt foci; AK, actinic keratosis; BCC, basal cell carcinoma; BCG, Bacillus Calmette-Guerin; BCNS, basal cell nevus syndrome; COPD, chronic obstructive pulmonary disease; FAP, familial adenomatous polyposis; HNPCC, hereditary non-polyposis colorectal cancer; NSCLC, non-small cell lung cancer; OPL, oral premalignant lesions; TCC, transitional cell carcinoma.
See www.cancertrials.nih.gov for more information on celecoxib studies.

signaling molecule that stimulates protein kinase C (PKC) and mediates the effects of growth factors (e.g., EGF, bFGF, PGDF) and cytokines (e.g., TNF, GM-CSF, IL-1, IL-3) on transcription factor activation and induction of oncogenes or other gene products needed for neoplastic cell growth (SCHADE et al. 1989; LIU et al. 1991, 1994a, 1997; DETHLEFSEN et al. 1994; TIMAR et al. 1996). Additionally, PKC activation by 12(S)-HETE mediates the release and secretion of cathepsin B, a cysteine protease involved in tumor metastasis and invasion, particularly in colon cancer cells (HONN et al. 1994b). Synthesis of 12(S)-HETE also stimulates adhesion by upregulating the surface expression of integrin receptors (CHOPRA et al. 1991; TANG et al. 1993). 5-LOX metabolites, particularly the 5-HETEs, have also specifically been implicated in cancer development. For example, recently published data have shown that 5-HETE directly stimulates prostate cancer cell growth (GHOSH and MYERS 1999; MYERS and GHOSH 1999). Like 12(S)-HETE, these molecules are capable of exerting pleiotropic effects on cells through autocrine- and paracrine-mediated mechanisms.

As inflammatory mediators, LTs elicit vessel wall adhesion, smooth muscle contraction, granulocyte degranulation, chemotaxis, and increased mucous secretion and vascular permeability (SAMUELSSON et al. 1987). A number of drugs which specifically inhibit the LOX metabolic pathway have been developed to treat inflammatory diseases such as asthma, ulcerative colitis, arthritis, and psoriasis (STEELE et al. 1999). Predominant among these are drugs affecting the 5-LOX pathway – 5-LOX inhibitors such as zileuton, FLAP inhibitors, and LTB$_4$ receptor antagonists such as zafirlukast, montelukast, and pranlukast.

2. Experimental Data Suggest that LOX Pathway Inhibition Has Cancer Preventive Potential, Although This Evidence Is Less Extensive and Conclusive than That for COX-2

The most compelling data are in lung (MOODY et al. 1998). A 5-LOX specific inhibitor (A 79175) (YAO et al. 2000) and a FLAP inhibitor (MK 966) have been shown to prevent lung adenomas induced by N-nitrosonornicotine (NNK) in Strain A/J mice (RIOUX and CASTONGUAY 1998). In human lung cancer cells, LOX inhibitors reduced 5-HETE-stimulated proliferation that was stimulated by 5-HETE (MOODY et al. 1998). Although no cancer preventive efficacy studies on LOX inhibitors in prostate have been reported, there are several studies showing that LOX products (particularly, 5-HETE) stimulate prostate cancer cell growth and that LOX-specific inhibitors reduce this growth (GHOSH and MYERS 1999; MYERS and GHOSH 1999). 5-HETE stimulates growth of human breast cancer cells; this growth is inhibited by 5-LOX and FLAP inhibitors (AVIS et al. 2001). Abundant data suggesting that fatty acid metabolites, including products of the LOX pathways, enhance tumorigenesis, and compounds which are nonspecific inhibitors of the LOX pathways, nordihydroguaiaretic acid (NDGA) and esculetin, prevent the development of N-methyl-N-nitrosourea (MNU)- and 7,12-dimethylbenz(a)anthracene (DMBA)-induced rat mammary gland tumors (MCCORMICK and SPICER 1987; KITAGAWA and NOGUCHI 1994; MATSUNAGA et al. 1998). The relevant studies in these three targets as well as data suggesting roles for LOX inhibition in cancer prevention of head and neck carcinogenesis, melanoma, and leukemia are described briefly in the following paragraphs.

a) Lung

In the lung cancer prevention study cited in Sect. B.II.2, the FLAP inhibitor MK 886 and the 5-LOX inhibitor, A 79175, reduced the multiplicity of NNK-induced tumors in strain A/J mice; A 79175 also reduced tumor incidence (RIOUX and CASTONGUAY 1998). Interestingly, in the same study, aspirin reduced tumor multiplicity and the combination of aspirin and A 79175 (i.e., inhibiting both the COX and LOX pathways) had synergistic activity in lowering tumor incidence and multiplicity. LOX metabolites have also been found to stimulate lung cancer cell growth. Studies in several human lung cancer cell lines found that 5-LOX stimulated by two autocrine growth factors, gastrin-releasing peptide (GRP) and IGF, both of which stimulate production of 5-HETE (AVIS et al. 1996). 5-HETE stimulated the growth of lung cancer cells, while the 5-LOX inhibitors NDGA, AA-861, and MK-886, decreased proliferation; the COX inhibitor aspirin had little effect. Expression of 5-LOX and FLAP mRNA by lung cancer cell lines was confirmed using RT-PCR, and the presence of 5-LOX mRNA was identified in samples of primary lung cancer tissue, including both small cell and non-small cell lung carcinomas. Also relevant to lung are studies demonstrating that LOXs mediate oxidation of potent carcinogens such as benzidine, o-dianisidine and benzo(a)pyrene; this activation can be blocked by the LOX inhibitors NDGA and esculetin (KULKARNI 2001).

b) Prostate

Initial studies found dramatically reduced levels of AA in prostate cancer; tenfold greater turnover in malignant vs. benign prostatic tissue suggested a possible increase in metabolism via the LOX and COX pathways in this tissue (CHAUDRY et al. 1991, 1994). In human prostate cancer cells, linoleic acid stimulated cell growth while COX inhibitors and a LOX inhibitor blocked it, suggesting the involvement of AA metabolism in prostate cancer cell proliferation (ROSE and CONNOLLY 1991). COX-specific inhibitors alone did not reduce human prostate PC3 cell DNA synthesis, while the AA antagonist eicosatetraynoic acid (ETYA) did reduce synthesis, suggesting that LOX products are essential to prostate cancer cell proliferation. A 5-LOX specific inhibitor (A63162) also reduced DNA synthesis and growth inhibition of prostate cancer cells (ANDERSON et al. 1994). Also, 5-HETE, particularly the 5-oxo-eicosatetraenoic form (5-oxo-ETE), stimulates PC-3 cell growth similarly to arachidonic acid; LTs had no effect. 5-HETEs also effectively reversed growth inhibition produced by the FLAP inhibitor MK-886. Both MK-886 and AA-861 effectively blocked prostate tumor proliferation induced by AA, while the COX inhibitor ibuprofen and 12-LOX inhibitors baicalein and N-benzyl-N-hydroxy-5-phenylpentanamide were ineffective (GHOSH and MYERS 1999).

c) Breast

5-LOX and FLAP inhibitors reduced growth, increased apoptosis and G_1 phase arrest in human breast cancer cells; PPARγ and PPARα were upregulated and may help mediate these effects (AVIS et al. 2001). Also, nonspecific and 12-LOX inhibition reduces growth and invasiveness of MDA-MB-435 breast cancer cells. For example, esculetin blocked linoleic acid- enhanced invasive capacity of these cells, while the COX-specific inhibitor piroxicam had no effect (LIU et al. 1996). The nonspecific LOX inhibitor NDGA inhibited adhesion to collagen IV induced by either A23187 or AA. In BT-20 breast cancer cells, NDGA inhibited LOX-mediated metabolism of linoleic acid to 13-HODE and blocked DNA synthesis induced by EGF and TGFα, suggesting a role for LOX in the EGFR signaling pathway (REDDY et al. 1997). NDGA administered postinitiation reduced mammary gland tumor multiplicity in rats induced with MNU (MCCORMICK and SPICER 1987). Esculetin significantly reduced DMBA-induced mammary gland tumor incidence and volume in rats fed high- and low-fat diets; piroxicam had no effect (KITAGAWA and NOGUCHI 1994). Both the COX-specific inhibitor nabumetone and esculetin reduced MNU-induced mammary gland tumor incidence in rats fed a standard diet (MATSUNAGA et al. 1998).

d) Other Cancers – Colon, Head and Neck, Melanoma, Leukemia

SC 41930, a competitive LTB$_4$ antagonist, inhibited LTB$_4$-induced growth stimulation in HT-29 colon cancer cells; similar inhibition was reported in mouse colon adenocarcinoma cell lines MAC16, MAC13, and MAC26 treated with other 5-LOX inhibitors, including BWA4C, BWB70C, and zileuton (DJURIC et al. 1989; TSAI et al. 1994). BWA4C was the most effective inhibitor in male NMRI mice transplanted with fragments of MAC26 or MAC16 colon tumors, decreasing both tumor volume and tumor growth rate after 8–13 days of treatment.

12- and 15-HETE are major AA metabolites in squamous epithelial carcinomas of the head and neck (EL ATTAR et al. 1985). Also, 12(S)-HETE is the predominant metabolic product of metastatic B16 melanoma cells (LIU et al. 1994b). Additionally, excess LT production, specifically LTC$_4$, has been documented in cells from patients with both acute and chronic leukemias (STENKE et al. 1990; ANDERSON et al. 1993, 1996). Adding 5-LOX-specific inhibitors SC41661A and A63162 to these cells reduced DNA labeling and decreased cell numbers within 72h (ANDERSON et al. 1996). Likewise, growth inhibition with other LOX inhibitors, including piriprost, NDGA, and BW755C, has been demonstrated in several malignant human hematopoietic cell lines; the COX inhibitor indomethacin lacked a suppressive effect in these cells (SNYDER and DESFORGES 1986; SNYDER et al. 1989).

3. Other Considerations in the Use of LOX Inhibitors for Cancer Prevention

In contrast to the extensive clinical development activity for COX-2 selective inhibitors in cancer prevention, there has been relatively little work on LOX inhibitors. Since oral 5-LOX pathway blocking agents are efficacious as anti-asthmatics, the lung has a high priority for future cancer prevention studies and applications of LOX inhibitors and LTA receptor antagonists. Cancer prevention testing of approved pharmaceuticals in this class such as zileuton, pranlukast, and zafirlukast, could be considered with oral formulations.

As suggested in Sect. A.II, LOX inhibition may be more fruitful for cancer prevention than LT receptor antagonism. However, the current 5-LOX inhibitors available as antiasthmatics have shown evidence of possibly significant liver toxicity. In a manufacturer-sponsored long-term safety study of zileuton, liver function was evaluated in 2,458 patients receiving zileuton plus normal asthma medications (LAZARUS et al. 1998). After 12 months of treatment, liver transaminase levels increased by 4.6% (three times the upper limit of normal) in the zileuton-treated group, compared with a 1.1% increase in patients receiving only the other asthma medications. Sixty-one percent of the liver enzyme elevations occurred within the first 2 months of zileuton treatment. Such toxicity could limit the use of these drugs for cancer prevention in asymptomatic populations.

Future studies may include the development of inhalant formulations, which may potentially reduce toxicity and allow for higher dose levels. Whether inhalant formulations of these agents would remain efficacious and exert cancer preventive activity remains to be determined. The prostate is also a cancer target of high interest based on the high rate of AA metabolism and antiproliferative activity of LOX inhibitors in prostate cancer cells. In this regard, inhibitors of the 12-LOX pathway may prove to be better candidates for cancer preventive intervention; however, this research will depend on the production and availability of such agents.

C. Promising Future Research Directions on AA Metabolic Pathways in Cancer Prevention

There is clearly overwhelming evidence that the AA metabolic pathways provide good targets for cancer preventive strategies, particularly the COX- and potentially the LOX-mediated arms. Future strategies will focus on optimizing the cancer preventive therapeutic index (TI) based on modulation of lead targets, particularly COX-2, as well as on identifying and developing strategies for other targets on these pathways.

One method of optimizing TIs is by combination therapy – pairing agents with complementary mechanisms of activity to enhance efficacy and/or reduce toxicity. Enhanced cancer preventive activity over either agent alone has been observed in combinations of a COX inhibitor with an anti-inflammatory inducible nitric oxide synthase inhibitor (RAO et al. 2002), EGFR inhibitor (TORRANCE et al. 2000), and a potent antiproliferative (eflornithine is an irreversible inhibitor of ornithine decarboxylase) (REDDY et al. 1990; RAO et al. 1991). In these examples, efficacy was seen at doses low enough to avoid or reduce toxicities associated with each of the agents. Particularly interesting for this review is the recent work with the dual COX/LOX inhibitor ML3000 (FIORUCCI et al. 2001). Although this drug has not been evaluated for cancer preventive activity, it shows potent anti-inflammatory activity in colon and no gastrointestinal toxicity.

Other molecular targets for cancer prevention have been associated with the COX and LOX pathways. For example, the drug R-flurbiprofen is an anti-inflammatory that inhibits COX-2 expression but not COX-2 activity that has shown cancer preventive activity in the Min mouse colon and TRAMP mouse prostate carcinogenesis models (WECHTER et al. 1997, 2000). Evidence suggests that the agent blocks COX-2 expression by inhibiting NF-κB mediated activation. Also, PPARγ agonists such as PGJ$_2$ and GW1929 inhibit COX-2 expression in a human neuroblastoma cell line; the inhibition is at least partially due to blocking the binding of the AP-1 transcription factor to the response site in the COX-2 gene promoter (HAN et al. 2001).

Independent of COX-2 expression, increased levels of PGE$_2$ are found in many cancers and precancers, including colorectal adenomas and adenocarcinomas. YOSHIMATSU et al. (2001) have reported an inducible PGE synthase which is overexpressed in these colorectal lesions. Interestingly, various molecular factors associated with carcinogenesis showed some differential effects on PGE synthase and COX-2 induction. Particularly, TNFα induced both COX-2 and PGE synthase, but PGE synthase was reduced earlier and at higher levels.

Like inhibitors of COX activity and expression, inhibitors of PG receptors have potential as cancer preventive agents. ONO-8711, a selective PGE receptor EP$_1$ antagonist, inhibited the formation of precancerous colorectal lesions in AOM-induced rats (aberrant crypt foci, ACF) and Min mice (intestinal adenomas) (WATANABE et al. 1999, 2000). This agent has also shown activity against carcinogen-induced rat mammary gland tumors (KAWAMORI et al. 2001). Elevated levels of COX-2 and PGE$_2$ in breast cancers compared with surrounding tissue coupled with evidence that PGE$_2$ stimulates transcription of the steroid aromatase gene (CYP19) via binding to the EP$_1$ and EP$_2$ receptors (ZHAO et al. 1996) suggest EP$_1$ antagonism as a potential target for decreasing estrogen biosynthesis and associated proliferative activity in breast carcinogenesis. Similarly, ONO-AE2-227 is an EP$_4$ antagonist that has been shown to inhibit AOM-induced ACF in C57BL/6Cr mice and polyp formation in Min mice (MUTOH et al. 2002).

In the LOX pathway, 15-LOX-1 and its product 13-*S*-HODE have been implicated as potential effectors of cancer preventive activity, and 15-LOX-1 has been suggested as a non-COX target for NSAID cancer preventive activity (Shureiqi and Lippman 2001; Shureiqi et al. 2000a,b, 2001). NSAIDs were found to induce apoptosis in colorectal cancer and esophageal cancer cells while upregulating 15-LOX-1.

Finally, effectors of PLA_2 activity show both the promise and complexity of modulating AA metabolism in cancer prevention. As stated in Sect. A, PLA_2 catalyzes release of AA from membrane phospholipids and is a potential target for cancer preventive intervention. Group IV cytosolic PLA_2 deficient Min mice showed reduced polyp burdens (Takaku et al. 2000; Hong et al. 2001). However, not all PLA_2 isoforms promote carcinogenesis. Min mice with Group IIA secretory PLA_2 isoform deficiency showed increased tumor burden (Cormier et al. 1997). As has also been observed in the LOX and COX pathways, these contradictory findings may be a result of the tissue and cell type specific control of PLA_2.

References

Anderson KM, Levin J, Jajeh A, Seed T, Harris JE (1993) Induction of apoptosis in blood cells from a patient with acute myelogenous leukemia by SC41661A, a selective inhibitor of 5-lipoxygenase. Prostaglandins Leukot Essent Fatty Acids 48:323–326

Anderson KM, Seed T, Ondrey F, Harris JE (1994) The selective 5-lipoxygenase inhibitor A63162 reduces PC3 proliferation and initiates morphologic changes consistent with secretion. Anticancer Res 14:1951–1960

Anderson KM, Seed T, Jajeh A, Dudeja P, Byun T, Meng J, Ou D, Bonomi P, Harris JE (1996) An in vivo inhibitor of 5-lipoxygenase, MK886, at micromolar concentration induces apoptosis in U937 and CML cells. Anticancer Res 16:2589–2599

Anderson WF, Umar A, Viner JL, Hawk ET (2002) The role of cyclooxygenase inhibitors in cancer prevention. Curr Pharm Des 8:1035–1062

Avis IM, Jett M, Boyle T, Vos MD, Moody T, Treston AM, Martinez A, Mulshine JL (1996) Growth control of lung cancer by interruption of 5-lipoxygenase- mediated growth factor signaling. J Clin Invest 97:806–813

Avis I, Hong SH, Martinez A, Moody T, Choi YH, Trepel J, Das R, Jett M, Mulshine JL (2001) 5-Lipoxygenase inhibitors can mediate apoptosis in human breast cancer cell lines through complex eicosanoid interactions. FASEB J 15:2007–2009

Balch CM, Dougherty PA, Cloud GA, Tilden AB (1984) Prostaglandin E2-mediated suppression of cellular immunity in colon cancer patients. Surgery 95:71–77

Bedi A, Pasricha PJ, Akhtar AJ, Barber JP, Bedi GC, Giardiello FM, Zehnbauer BA, Hamilton SR, Jones RJ (1995) Inhibition of apoptosis during development of colorectal cancer. Cancer Res 55:1811–1816

Chaudry A, McClinton S, Moffat LE, Wahle KW (1991) Essential fatty acid distribution in the plasma and tissue phospholipids of patients with benign and malignant prostatic disease. Br J Cancer 64:1157–1160

Chaudry AA, Wahle KW, McClinton S, Moffat LE (1994) Arachidonic acid metabolism in benign and malignant prostatic tissue in vitro: effects of fatty acids and cyclooxygenase inhibitors. Int J Cancer 57:176–180

Chopra H, Timar J, Chen YQ, Rong XH, Grossi IM, Fitzgerald LA, Taylor JD, Honn KV (1991) The lipoxygenase metabolite 12(*S*)-HETE induces a cytoskeleton-dependent increase in surface expression of integrin alpha IIb beta 3 on melanoma cells. Int J Cancer 49:774–786

Clark MA, Ozgur LE, Conway TM, Dispoto J, Crooke ST, Bomalaski JS (1991) Cloning of a phospholipase A_2-activating protein. Proc Natl Acad Sci U S A 88:5418–5422

Cok SJ, Morrison AR (2001) The 3'-untranslated region of murine cyclooxygenase-2 contains multiple regulatory elements that alter message stability and translational efficiency. J Biol Chem 276:23179–23185

Cormier RT, Hong KH, Halberg RB, Hawkins TL, Richardson P, Mulherkar R, Dove WF, Lander ES (1997) Secretory phospholipase Pla2g2a confers resistance to intestinal tumorigenesis. Nat Genet 17:88–91

Dannenberg AJ, Altorki NK, Boyle JO, Dang C, Howe LR, Weksler BB, Subbaramaiah K (2001) Cyclo-oxygenase 2:a pharmacological target for the prevention of cancer. Lancet Oncol 2:544–551

Dethlefsen SM, Shepro D, D'Amore PA (1994) Arachidonic acid metabolites in bFGF, PDGF-, and serum-stimulated vascular cell growth. Exp Cell Res 212:262–273

Ding XZ, Tong WG, Adrian TE (2000) Blockade of cyclooxygenase-2 inhibits proliferation and induces apoptosis in human pancreatic cancer cells. Anticancer Res 20:2625–2631

Dixon DA, Tolley ND, King PH, Nabors LB, McIntyre TM, Zimmerman GA, Prescott SM (2001) Altered expression of the mRNA stability factor HuR promotes cyclooxygenase-2 expression in colon cancer cells. J Clin Invest 108:1657–1665

Djuric SW, Collins PW, Jones PH, Shone RL, Tsai BS, Fretland DJ, Butchko GM, Villani-Price D, Keith RH, Zemaitis JM (1989) 7-[3-(4-acetyl-3-methoxy-2-propylphenoxy)propoxy]-3,4-dihydro-8-propyl-$2H$-1-benzopyran-2-carboxylic acid: an orally active selective leukotriene B_4 receptor antagonist. J Med Chem 32:1145–1147

El Attar TM, Lin HS, Vanderhoek JY (1985) Biosynthesis of prostaglandins and hydroxy fatty acids in primary squamous carcinomas of head and neck in humans. Cancer Lett 27:255–259

Fiorucci S, Meli R, Bucci M, Cirino G (2001) Dual inhibitors of cyclooxygenase and 5-lipoxygenase. A new avenue in anti-inflammatory therapy? Biochem. Pharmacol 62:1433–1438

Fischer SM, Lo HH, Gordon GB, Seibert K, Kelloff G, Lubet RA, Conti CJ (1999) Chemopreventive activity of celecoxib, a specific cyclooxygenase-2 inhibitor, and indomethacin against ultraviolet light-induced skin carcinogenesis. Mol. Carcinog 25:231–240

FitzGerald GA, Patrono C (2001) The Coxibs, selective inhibitors of cyclooxygenase-2. N Engl J Med 345:433–442

Fukutake M, Nakatsugi S, Isoi T, Takahashi M, Ohta T, Mamiya S, Taniguchi Y, Sato H, Fukuda K, Sugimura T, Wakabayashi K. 1998. Suppressive effects of nimesulide, a selective inhibitor of cyclooxygenase-2, on azoxymethane-induced colon carcinogenesis in mice. Carcinogenesis 19:1939–1942

Funk CD (2001) Prostaglandins and leukotrienes: advances in eicosanoid biology. Science 294:1871–185

Ghosh J, Myers CE (1999) Central role of arachidonate 5-lipoxygenase in the regulation of cell growth and apoptosis in human prostate cancer cells. Adv Exp Med Biol 469:577–582

Giardiello FM, Hamilton SR, Krush AJ, Piantadosi S, Hylind LM, Celano P, Booker SV, Robinson CR, Offerhaus GJ (1993) Treatment of colonic and rectal adenomas with sulindac in familial adenomatous polyposis. N Engl J Med 328: 1313–1316

Grubbs CJ, Lubet RA, Koki AT, Leahy KM, Masferrer JL, Steele VE, Kelloff GJ, Hill DL, Seibert K (2000) Celecoxib inhibits N-butyl-N-(4-hydroxybutyl)-nitrosamine-induced urinary bladder cancers in male B6D2F1 mice and female Fischer-344 rats. Cancer Res 60:5599–5602

204 G.J. KELLOFF and C.C. SIGMAN

Gupta RA, DuBois RN (2001) Colorectal cancer prevention and treatment by inhibition of cyclooxygenase-2. Nat Rev Cancer 1:11–21
Han S, Wada RK, Sidell N (2001) Differentiation of human neuroblastoma by phenylacetate is mediated by peroxisome proliferator-activated receptor γ. Cancer Res 61:3998–4002
Hara A, Yoshimi N, Niwa M, Ino N, Mori H (1997) Apoptosis induced by NS-398, a selective cyclooxygenase-2 inhibitor, in human colorectal cancer cell lines. Jpn J Cancer Res 88:600–604
Harris RE, Alshafie GA, Abou-Issa H, Seibert K (2000). Chemoprevention of breast cancer in rats by celecoxib, a cyclooxygenase 2 inhibitor. Cancer Res 60:2101–2103
He TC, Chan TA, Vogelstein B, Kinzler KW (1999) PPARσ is an APC-regulated target of nonsteroidal anti-inflammatory drugs. Cell 99:335–345
Herschman HR (1999) Function and regulation of prostaglandin synthase 2. Adv Exp Med Biol 469:3–8
Herschman HR, Reddy ST, Xie W (1997) Function and regulation of prostaglandin synthase-2. Adv Exp Med Biol 407:61–66
Hong KH, Bonventre JC, O'Leary E, Bonventre JV, Lander ES (2001) Deletion of cytosolic phospholipase A(2) suppresses Apc(Min)-induced tumorigenesis. Proc Natl Acad Sci U S A 98:3935–3939
Honn KV, Tang DG, Gao X, Butovich IA, Liu B, Timar J, Hagmann W (1994a) 12-lipoxygenases and 12(S)-HETE: role in cancer metastasis. Cancer Metastasis Rev 13:365–396
Honn KV, Timar J, Rozhin J, Bazaz R, Sameni M, Ziegler G, Sloane BF (1994b) A lipoxygenase metabolite, 12-(S)-HETE, stimulates protein kinase C- mediated release of cathepsin B from malignant cells. Exp Cell Res 214:120–130
Hsu AL, Ching TT, Wang DS, song X, Rangnekar VM, Chen CS (2000) The cyclooxygenase-2 inhibitor celecoxib induces apoptosis by blocking Akt activation in human prostate cancer cells independently of Bcl-2. J Biol Chem 275:11397–11403
Jacoby RF, Seibert K, Cole CE, Kelloff G, Lubet RA (2000) The cyclooxygenase-2 inhibitor celecoxib is a potent preventive and therapeutic agent in the min mouse model of adenomatous polyposis. Cancer Res 60:5040–5044
Jones MK, Wang H, Peskar BM, Levin E, Itani RM, Sarfeh IJ, Tarnawski AS (1999) Inhibition of angiogenesis by nonsteroidal anti-inflammatory drugs: insight into mechanisms and implications for cancer growth and ulcer healing. Nat Med 5:1418–423
Kawamori T, Rao CV, Seibert K, Reddy BS (1998) Chemopreventive activity of celecoxib, a specific cyclooxygenase-2 inhibitor, against colon carcinogenesis. Cancer Res. 58:409–412
Kawamori T, Uchiya N, Nakatsugi S, Watanabe K, Ohuchida S, Yamamoto H, Maruyama T, Kondo K, Sugimura T, Wakabayashi K (2001) Chemopreventive effects of ONO-8711, a selective prostaglandin E receptor EP(1) antagonist, on breast cancer development. Carcinogenesis 22:2001–2004
Kelloff GJ (2000) Perspectives on cancer chemoprevention research and drug development. Adv Cancer Res 78:199–334
Kelloff GJ, Boone CW, Steele VE, Fay JR, Lubet RA, Crowell JA, Sigman CC (1994) Mechanistic considerations in chemopreventive drug development. J Cell Biochem Suppl 20:1–24
Kitagawa H, Noguchi M (1994) Comparative effects of piroxicam and esculetin on incidence, proliferation, and cell kinetics of mammary carcinomas induced by 7,12- dimethylbenz[a]anthracene in rats on high- and low-fat diets. Oncology 51:401–410
Koki AT, Leahy KM, Masferrer JL (1999) Potential utility of COX-2 inhibitors in chemoprevention and chemotherapy. Expert Opin Investig Drugs 8:1623–1638
Kulkarni AP (2001) Lipoxygenase–a versatile biocatalyst for biotransformation of endobiotics and xenobiotics. Cell Mol Life Sci 58:1805–1825

Kulkarni SK, Jain NK, Singh A (2000) Cyclooxygenase isoenzymes and newer therapeutic potential for selective COX-2 inhibitors. Methods Find Exp Clin Pharmacol 22:291–298

Lazarus SC, Lee T, Kemp JP, Wenzel S, Dube LM, Ochs RF, Carpentier PJ, Lancaster JF (1998) Safety and clinical efficacy of zileuton in patients with chronic asthma. Am J Manag Care 4:841–848

Lippman SM, Lee JJ, Sabichi AL (1998) Cancer chemoprevention: progress and promise. J Natl Cancer Inst 90:1514–1528

Liu B, Maher RJ, Hannun YA, Porter AT, Honn KV (1994a) 12(S)-HETE enhancement of prostate tumor cell invasion: selective role of PKC alpha. J Natl Cancer Inst 86:1145–1151

Liu B, Marnett LJ, Chaudhary A, Ji C, Blair IA, Johnson CR, Diglio CA, Honn KV (1994b) Biosynthesis of 12(S)-hydroxyeicosatetraenoic acid by B16 amelanotic melanoma cells is a determinant of their metastatic potential. Lab Invest 70:314–323

Liu B, Timar J, Howlett J, Diglio CA, Honn KV (1991) Lipoxygenase metabolites of arachidonic and linoleic acids modulate the adhesion of tumor cells to endothelium via regulation of protein kinase C. Cell Regul 2:1045–1055

Liu XH, Connolly JM, Rose DP (1996) Eicosanoids as mediators of linoleic acid-stimulated invasion and type IV collagenase production by a metastatic human breast cancer cell line. Clin Exp Metastasis 14:145–152

Liu XH, Yao S, Kirschenbaum A, Levine AC (1998) NS398, a selective cyclooxygenase-2 inhibitor, induces apoptosis and down-regulates bcl-2 expression in LNCaP cells. Cancer Res 58:4245–4249

Liu YW, Chen BK, Chen CJ, Arakawa T, Yoshimoto T, Yamamoto S, Chang WC (1997) Epidermal growth factor enhances transcription of human arachidonate 12-lipoxygenase in A431 cells. Biochim Biophys Acta 1344:38–46

Majima M, Hayashi I, Muramatsu M, Katada J, Yamashina S, Katori M (2000) Cyclooxygenase-2 enhances basic fibroblast growth factor-induced angiogenesis through induction of vascular endothelial growth factor in rat sponge implants. Br J Pharmacol 130:641–649

Marnett LJ (1992) Aspirin and the potential role of prostaglandins in colon cancer. Cancer Res 52:5575–5589

Marnett LJ (1995) Aspirin and related nonsteroidal anti-inflammatory drugs as chemopreventive agents against colon cancer. Prev Med 24:103–106

Masferrer J (2001) Approach to angiogenesis inhibition based on cyclooxygenase-2. Cancer J 7 Suppl 3:S144–S150

Masferrer JL, Koki A, Seibert K (1999) COX-2 inhibitors. A new class of antiangiogenic agents. Ann N Y Acad Sci 889:84–86

Masferrer JL, Leahy KM, Koki AT, Zweifel BS, Settle SL, Woerner BM, Edwards DA, Flickinger AG, Moore RJ, Seibert K (2000) Antiangiogenic and antitumor activities of cyclooxygenase-2 inhibitors. Cancer Res 60:1306–1311

Matsunaga K, Yoshimi N, Yamada Y, Shimizu M, Kawabata K, Ozawa Y, Hara A, Mori H (1998) Inhibitory effects of nabumetone, a cyclooxygenase-2 inhibitor, and esculetin, a lipoxygenase inhibitor, on N-methyl-N-nitrosourea-induced mammary carcinogenesis in rats. Jpn J Cancer Res 89:496–501

McCormick DL, Spicer AM (1987) Nordihydroguaiaretic acid suppression of rat mammary carcinogenesis induced by N-methyl-N-nitrosourea. Cancer Lett 37:139–146

McDougall CJ, Ngoi SS, Goldman IS, Godwin T, Felix J, DeCosse JJ, Rigas B (1990) Reduced expression of HLA class I and II antigens in colon cancer. Cancer Res 50:8023–8027

Mehta RG, Williamson E, Patel MK, Koeffler HP (2000) A ligand of peroxisome proliferator-activated receptor γ, retinoids, and prevention of preneoplastic mammary lesions. J Natl Cancer Inst 92:418–423

Mohammed SI, Bennett PF, Craig BA, Glickman NW, Mutsaers AJ, Snyder PW, Widmer WR, DeGortari AE, Bonney PL, Knapp DW (2002) Effects of the cyclooxygenase inhibitor, piroxicam, on tumor response, apoptosis, and angiogenesis in a canine model of human invasive urinary bladder cancer. Cancer Res 62:356–358

Mohammed SI, Knapp DW, Bostwick DG, Foster RS, Khan KN, Masferrer JL, Woerner BM, Snyder PW, Koki AT (1999) Expression of cyclooxygenase-2 (COX-2) in human invasive transitional cell carcinoma (TCC) of the urinary bladder. Cancer Res 59:5647–5650

Moody TW, Leyton J, Martinez A, Hong S, Malkinson A, Mulshine JL (1998) Lipoxygenase inhibitors prevent lung carcinogenesis and inhibit non small cell lung cancer growth. Exp Lung Res 24:617–628

Mukherjee D, Nissen SE, Topol EJ (2001) Risk of cardiovascular events associated with selective COX-2 inhibitors. JAMA 286:954–959

Muller-Decker K, Kopp-Schneider A, Marks F, Seibert K, Furstenberger G (1998) Localization of prostaglandin H synthase isoenzymes in murine epidermal tumors: suppression of skin tumor promotion by inhibition of prostaglandin H synthase-2. Mo. Carcinog 23:36–44

Mutoh M, Watanabe K, Kitamura T, Shoji Y, Takahashi M, Kawamori T, Tani K, Kobayashi M, Maruyama T, Kobayashi K, Ohuchida S, Sugimoto Y, Narumiya S, Sugimura T, Wakabayashi K (2002) Involvement of prostaglandin E receptor subtype EP(4) in colon carcinogenesis. Cancer Res 62:28–32

Myers CE, Ghosh J (1999) Lipoxygenase inhibition in prostate cancer. Eur Urol 35:395–398

Nakatsugi S, Fukutake M, Takahashi M, Fukuda K, Isoi T, Taniguchi Y, Sugimura T, Wakabayashi K (1997) Suppression of intestinal polyp development by nimesulide, a selective cyclooxygenase-2 inhibitor, in Min mice. Jpn J Cancer Res 88:1117–1120

Needleman P, Turk J, Jakschik BA, Morrison AR, Lefkowith JB (1986) Arachidonic acid metabolism. Annu Rev Biochem 55:69–102

Nishimura G, Yanoma S, Mizuno H, Kawakami K, Tsukuda M (1999) A selective cyclooxygenase-2 inhibitor suppresses tumor growth in nude mouse xenografted with human head and neck squamous carcinoma cells. Jpn J Cancer Res 90:1152–1162

Okajima E, Denda A, Ozono S, Takahama M, Akai H, Sasaki Y, Kitayama W, Wakabayashi K, Konishi Y (1998) Chemopreventive effects of nimesulide, a selective cyclooxygenase-2 inhibitor, on the development of rat urinary bladder carcinomas initiated by N-butyl-N-(4-hydroxybutyl)nitrosamine. Cancer Res 58:3028–3031

O'Shaughnessy JA, Kelloff GJ, Gordon GB, Dannenberg AJ, Hong WK, Fabian CJ, Sigman CC, Bertagnolli MM, Stratton SP, Lam S, Nelson WG, Meyskens FL, Alberts DS, Follen M, Rustgi AK, Papadimitrakopoulou V, Scardino PT, Gazdar AF, Wattenberg LW, Sporn MB, Sakr WA, Lippman SM, Von Hoff DD (2002) Treatment and prevention of intraepithelial neoplasia: an important target for accelerated new agent development. Clin Cancer Res 8:314–346

Oshima M, Dinchuk JE, Kargman SL, Oshima H, Hancock B, Kwong E, Trzaskos JM, Evans JF, Taketo MM (1996) Suppression of intestinal polyposis in Apc delta716 knockout mice by inhibition of cyclooxygenase 2 (COX-2). Cell 87:803–809

Oshima M, Murai N, Kargman S, Arguello M, Luk P, Kwong E, Taketo MM, Evans JF (2001) Chemoprevention of intestinal polyposis in the ApcΔ^{716} mouse by rofecoxib, a specific cyclooxygenase-2 inhibitor. Cancer Res 61:1733–1740

Pai R, Szabo IL, Giap AQ, Kawanaka H, Tarnawski AS (2001) Nonsteroidal anti-inflammatory drugs inhibit re-epithelialization of wounded gastric monolayers by interfering with actin, Src, FAK, and tensin signaling. Life Sci 69:3055–3071

Pentland AP, Schoggins JW, Scott GA, Khan KN, Han R. 1999. Reduction of UV-induced skin tumors in hairless mice by selective COX-2 inhibition. Carcinogenesis 20:1939–1944

Peters JM, Lee SS, Li W, Ward JM, Gavrilova O, Everett C, Reitman ML, Hudson LD, Gonzalez FJ (2000) Growth, adipose, brain, and skin alterations resulting from targeted disruption of the mouse peroxisome proliferator-activated receptor $\beta(\delta)$. Mol Cell Biol 20:5119–5280

Rao CV, Tokumo K, Rigotty J, Zang E, Kelloff G, Reddy BS (1991) Chemoprevention of colon carcinogenesis by dietary administration of piroxicam, alpha-difluoromethylornithine, 16 alpha-fluoro-5-androsten- 17-one, and ellagic acid individually and in combination. Cancer Res 51:4528–4534

Rao CV, Indranie C, Simi B, Manning PT, Connor JR, Reddy BS (2002) Chemopreventive properties of a selective inducible nitric oxide synthase inhibitor in colon carcinogenesis, administered alone or in combination with celecoxib, a selective cyclooxygenase-2 inhibitor. Cancer Res 62:165–170

Reddy BS, Nayini J, Tokumo K, Rigotty J, Zang E, Kelloff G (1990) Chemoprevention of colon carcinogenesis by concurrent administration of piroxicam, a nonsteroidal anti-inflammatory drug with D,L-alpha- difluoromethylornithine, an ornithine decarboxylase inhibitor, in diet. Cancer Res 50:2562–2568

Reddy BS, Rao CV, Seibert K (1996) Evaluation of cyclooxygenase-2 inhibitor for potential chemopreventive properties in colon carcinogenesis. Cancer Res 56:4566–4569

Reddy BS, Hirose Y, Lubet R, Steele V, Kelloff G, Paulson S, Seibert K, Rao CV (2000) Chemoprevention of colon cancer by specific cyclooxygenase-2 inhibitor, celecoxib, administered during different stages of carcinogenesis. Cancer Res 60:293–297

Reddy N, Everhart A, Eling T, Glasgow W (1997) Characterization of a 15-lipoxygenase in human breast carcinoma BT-20 cells: stimulation of 13-HODE formation by TGF"/EGF. Biochem Biophys Res Commun 231:111–116

Rioux N, Castonguay A (1998) Inhibitors of lipoxygenase: a new class of cancer chemopreventive agents. Carcinogenesis 19:1393–1400

Rose P, Connolly JM (1991) Effects of fatty acids and eicosanoid synthesis inhibitors on the growth of two human prostate cancer cell lines. Prostate 18:243–254

Samuelsson B, Dahlen SE, Lindgren JA, Rouzer CA, Serhan CN (1987) Leukotrienes and lipoxins: structures, biosynthesis, and biological effects. Science 237:1171–1176

Sasai H, Masaki M, Wakitani K (2000) Suppression of polypogenesis in a new mouse strain with a truncated Apc(Delta474) by a novel COX-2 inhibitor, JTE-522. Carcinogenesis 21:953–958

Sawaoka H, Kawano S, Tsuji S, Tsujii M, Gunawan ES, Takei Y, Nagano K, Hori M (1998) Cyclooxygenase-2 inhibitors suppress the growth of gastric cancer xenografts via induction of apoptosis in nude mice. Am J Physiol 274: G1061–G1067

Sawaoka H, Tsuji S, Tsujii M, Gunawan ES, Sasaki Y, Kawano S, Hori M (1999) Cyclooxygenase inhibitors suppress angiogenesis and reduce tumor growth in vivo. Lab Invest 79:1469–1477

Schade UF, Ernst M, Reinke M, Wolter DT (1989) Lipoxygenase inhibitors suppress formation of tumor necrosis factor in vitro and in vivo. Biochem Biophys Res Commun 159:748–754

Sheng H, Shao J, Morrow JD, Beauchamp RD, DuBois RN (1998) Modulation of apoptosis and Bcl-2 expression by prostaglandin E2 in human colon cancer cells. Cancer Res 58:362–366

Sheng H, Shao J, Dixon DA, Williams CS, Prescott SM, DuBois RN, Beauchamp RD (2000) Transforming growth factor-beta1 enhances Ha-*ras*-induced expression of cyclooxygenase-2 in intestinal epithelial cells via stabilization of mRNA. J Biol Chem 275:6628–6635

Shiotani H, Denda A, Yamamoto K, Kitayama W, Endoh T, Sasaki Y, Tsutsumi N, Sugimura M, Konishi Y (2001) Increased expression of cyclooxygenase-2 protein in 4-nitroquinoline-1- oxide-induced rat tongue carcinomas and chemopreventive efficacy of a specific inhibitor, nimesulide. Cancer Res 61:1451–1456

Shureiqi I, Lippman SM (2001) Lipoxygenase modulation to reverse carcinogenesis. Cancer Res 61:6307–6312

Shureiqi I, Chen D, Lee JJ, Yang P, Newman RA, Brenner DE, Lotan R, Fischer SM, Lippman SM (2000a) 15-LOX-1:a novel molecular target of nonsteroidal anti-inflammatory drug-induced apoptosis in colorectal cancer cells. J Natl Cancer Inst 92:1136–1142

Shureiqi I, Chen D, Lotan R, Yang P, Newman RA, Fischer SM, Lippman SM (2000b) 15-Lipoxygenase-1 mediates nonsteroidal anti-inflammatory drug-induced apoptosis independently of cyclooxygenase-2 in colon cancer cells. Cancer Res 60:6846–6850

Shureiqi I, Xu X, Chen D, Lotan R, Morris JS, Fischer SM, Lippman SM (2001) Nonsteroidal anti-inflammatory drugs induce apoptosis in esophageal cancer cells by restoring 15-lipoxygenase-1 expression. Cancer Res 61:4879–4884

Smith ML, Hawcroft G, Hull MA (2000) The effect of nonsteroidal anti-inflammatory drugs on human colorectal cancer cells: evidence of different mechanisms of action. Eur J Cancer 36:664–674

Smith WL, Marnett LJ, DeWitt DL (1991) Prostaglandin and thromboxane biosynthesis. Pharmacol Ther 49:153–179

Smith WL, DeWitt DL, Garavito RM (2000) Cyclooxygenases: structural, cellular, and molecular biology. Annu Rev Biochem 69:145–182

Snyder DS, Castro R, Desforges JF (1989) Antiproliferative effects of lipoxygenase inhibitors on malignant human hematopoietic cell lines. Exp Hematol 17:6–9

Snyder DS, Desforges JF (1986) Lipoxygenase metabolites of arachidonic acid modulate hematopoiesis. Blood 67:1675–1679

Soslow RA, Dannenberg AJ, Rush D, Woerner BM, Khan KN, Masferrer J, Koki AT (2000) COX-2 is expressed in human pulmonary, colonic, and mammary tumors. Cancer 89:2637–645

Steele VE, Holmes CA, Hawk ET, Kopelovich L, Lubet RA, Crowell JA, Sigman CC, Kelloff GJ (1999) Lipoxygenase inhibitors as potential cancer chemopreventives. Cancer Epidemiol Biomarkers Prev 8:467–483

Steinbach G, Lynch PM, Phillips RK, Wallace MH, Hawk E, Gordon GB, Wakabayashi N, Saunders B, Shen Y, Fujimura T, Su LK, Levin B (2000) The effect of celecoxib, a cyclooxygenase-2 inhibitor, in familial adenomatous polyposis. N Engl J Med 342:1946–1952

Stenke L, Samuelsson J, Palmblad J, Dabrowski L, Reizenstein P, Lindgren JA (1990) Elevated white blood cell synthesis of leukotriene C4 in chronic myelogenous leukemia but not in polycythaemia vera. Br J Haematol 74:257–263

Subbaramaiah K, Norton L, Gerald W, Dannenberg AJ (2002) Cyclooxygenase-2 is overexpressed in HER-2/neu-positive breast cancer. Evidence for involvement of AP-1 and PEA3. J Biol Chem 277:18649–18657

Suh N, Wang Y, Williams CR, Risingsong R, Gilmer T, Willson TM, Sporn MB (1999) A new ligand for the peroxisome proliferator-activated receptor-((PPAR-(), GW7845, inhibits rat mammary carcinogenesis. Cancer Res 59:5671–5673

Takaku K, Sonoshita M, Sasaki N, Uozumi N, Doi Y, Shimizu T, Taketo MM (2000) Suppression of intestinal polyposis in Apc() 716) knockout mice by an additional mutation in the cytosolic phospholipase A(2) gene. J Biol Chem 275:34013–34016

Taketo MM (1998a) Cyclooxygenase-2 inhibitors in tumorigenesis (Part I). J Natl Cancer Inst 90:1529–1536

Taketo MM (1998b) Cyclooxygenase-2 inhibitors in tumorigenesis (Part II). J Natl Cancer Inst 90:1609–1620

Tang DG, Grossi IM, Chen YQ, Diglio CA, Honn KV (1993) 12(S)-HETE promotes tumor-cell adhesion by increasing surface expression of alpha V beta 3 integrins on endothelial cells. Int J Cancer 54:102–111

Tang DG, Honn KV (1994) 12-Lipoxygenase, 12(S)-HETE, and cancer metastasis. Ann NY Acad Sci 744:199–215

Thun MJ, Henley SJ, Patrono C (2002) Nonsteroidal anti-inflammatory drugs as anti-cancer agents: mechanistic, pharmacologic, and clinical issues. J Natl Cancer Inst 94:252–266

Timar J, Raso E, Fazakas ZS, Silletti S, Raz A, Honn KV (1996) Multiple use of a signal transduction pathway in tumor cell invasion. Anticancer Res 16:3299–3306

Tomozawa S, Tsuno NH, Sunami E, Hatano K, Kitayama J, Osada T, Saito S, Tsuruo T, Shibata Y, Nagawa H (2000) Cyclooxygenase-2 overexpression correlates with tumour recurrence, especially haematogenous metastasis, of colorectal cancer. Br J Cancer 83:324–328

Torrance CJ, Jackson PE, Montgomery E, Kinzler KW, Vogelstein B, Wissner A, Nunes M, Frost P, Discafani CM (2000) Combinatorial chemoprevention of intestinal neoplasia. Nat Med 6:1024–1028

Tsai BS, Keith RH, Villani-Price D, Kachur JF, Yang DC, Djuric SW, Yu S (1994) The in vitro pharmacology of SC-51146:a potent antagonist of leukotriene B4 receptors. J Pharmacol Exp Ther 268:1499–1505

Tsujii M, DuBois RN (1995) Alterations in cellular adhesion and apoptosis in epithelial cells overexpressing prostaglandin endoperoxide synthase 2. Cell 83:493–501

Tsujii M, Kawano S, DuBois RN (1997) Cyclooxygenase-2 expression in human colon cancer cells increases metastatic potential. Proc Natl Acad Sci U S A 94:3336–3340

Tsujii M, Kawano S, Tsuji S, Sawaoka H, Hori M, DuBois RN (1998) Cyclooxygenase regulates angiogenesis induced by colon cancer cells. Cell 93:705–716

Uefuji K, Ichikura T, Mochizuki H (2000) Cyclooxygenase-2 expression is related to prostaglandin biosynthesis and angiogenesis in human gastric cancer. Clin Cancer Res 6:135–138

Watanabe K, Kawamori T, Nakatsugi S, Ohta T, Ohuchida S, Yamamoto H, Maruyama T, Kondo K, Ushikubi F, Narumiya S, Sugimura T, Wakabayashi K (1999) Role of the prostaglandin E receptor subtype EP1 in colon carcinogenesis. Cancer Res 59:5093–5096

Watanabe K, Kawamori T, Nakatsugi S, Ohta T, Ohuchida S, Yamamoto H, Maruyama T, Kondo K, Narumiya S, Sugimura T, Wakabayashi K (2000) Inhibitory effect of a prostaglandin E receptor subtype EP(1) selective antagonist, ONO-8713, on development of azoxymethane-induced aberrant crypt foci in mice. Cancer Lett 156:57–61

Wechter WJ, Kantoci D, Murray ED, Jr., Quiggle DD, Leipold DD, Gibson KM, McCracken JD (1997) R-flurbiprofen chemoprevention and treatment of intestinal adenomas in the APC(Min)/+ mouse model: implications for prophylaxis and treatment of colon cancer. Cancer Res 57:4316–4324

Wechter WJ, Leipold DD, Murray ED, Jr., Quiggle D, McCracken JD, Barrios RS, Greenberg NM (2000) E-7869 (R-flurbiprofen) inhibits progression of prostate cancer in the TRAMP mouse. Cancer Res 60:2203–2208

Weitzman SA, Gordon LI (1990) Inflammation and cancer: role of phagocyte-generated oxidants in carcinogenesis. Blood 76:655–663

Wilgus TA, Ross MS, Parrett ML, Oberyszyn TM (2000) Topical application of a selective cyclooxygenase inhibitor suppresses UVB mediated cutaneous inflammation. Prostaglandins Other Lipid Mediat 62:367–384

Wolfe MM, Lichtenstein DR, Singh G (1999) Gastrointestinal toxicity of nonsteroidal anti-inflammatory drugs. N Engl J Med 340:1888–1899

Xie W, Herschman HR (1996) Transcriptional regulation of prostaglandin synthase 2 gene expression by platelet-derived growth factor and serum. J Bio. Chem 271:31742–31748

Yao R, Rioux N, Castonguay A, You M (2000) Inhibition of COX-2 and induction of apoptosis: two determinants of nonsteroidal anti-inflammatory drugs' chemopreventive efficacies in mouse lung tumorigenesis. Exp. Lung Res 26:731–742

Yoshimatsu K, Golijanin D, Paty PB, Soslow RA, Jakobsson PJ, DeLellis RA, Subbaramaiah K, Dannenberg AJ (2001) Inducible microsomal prostaglandin E

    synthase is overexpressed in colorectal adenomas and cancer. Clin Cancer Res
        7:3971–3976
Yoshimi N, Shimizu M, Matsunaga K, Yamada Y, Fujii K, Hara A, Mori H. 1999. Chemo-
        preventive effect of N-(2-cyclohexyloxy-4-nitrophenyl)methane sulfonamide (NS-
        398), a selective cyclooxygenase-2 inhibitor, in rat colon carcinogenesis induced by
        azoxymethane. Jpn J Cancer Res 90:406–412
Zhao Y, Agarwal VR, Mendelson CR, Simpson ER (1996) Estrogen biosynthesis prox-
        imal to a breast tumor is stimulated by PGE2 via cyclic AMP, leading to activa-
        tion of promoter II of the CYP19 (aromatase) gene. Endocrinology 137:5739–5742
Zimmermann KC, Sarbia M, Weber AA, Borchard F, Gabbert HE, Schror K (1999)
        Cyclooxygenase-2 expression in human esophageal carcinoma. Cancer Res
        59:198–204

Infections, Inflammation and Cancer: Roles of Reactive Oxygen and Nitrogen Species

H. Ohshima and M. Tatemichi

A. Introduction

It has been estimated that about 16% (1,450,000 cases) of the worldwide incidence of cancer in 1990 can be attributed to infection with either the hepatitis B and C viruses, the human papilloma viruses, Epstein-Barr virus, human T-cell lymphotropic virus I, human immunodeficiency virus (HIV), the bacterium *Helicobacter pylori*, schistosomes or liver flukes (Pisani et al. 1997). This estimate was made following the evaluations of the IARC monographs program, which has evaluated several infectious agents as carcinogenic to humans (IARC Working Group on the Evaluation of Carcinogenic Risks to Humans 1994a,b, 1995, 1996, 1997). Table 1 summarizes some human cancers for which infection and inflammation have been associated with increased risk. Chronic infection by a variety of viruses, bacteria, or parasites and tissue inflammation such as gastritis and hepatitis, which are often caused by chronic infection, are recognized risk factors for human cancers at various sites. Moreover, the chronic inflammation induced by chemical and physical agents such as cigarette smoke and asbestos and autoimmune and inflammatory reactions of uncertain etiology (e.g., pernicious anemia, ulcerative colitis, pancreatitis, etc.) are also associated with an increased risk of cancer. Thus a significant fraction of the global cancer burden is attributable to chronic infection and inflammation. It is estimated that there would be 21% fewer cases of cancer in developing countries (1,000,000 fewer cases per year) and 9% fewer cases in developed countries (375,000 fewer cases per year) if these known infectious diseases were prevented (Pisani et al. 1997).

B. Infection and Cancer-Possible Mechanisms

Three main mechanisms have been proposed for infection-associated carcinogenesis [see, for example, review (Parsonnet 2001)]:

1. *Direct action of infectious agent on host cells or tissues.*
   Integration of viral DNA into the human genome often results in alterations of host DNA (insertion, deletion, translocation, and amplification). Products of integrated viral DNA (e.g., the X-protein of hepatitis B virus, the E6 and E7 proteins of human papilloma virus) also interact with tumor-

Table 1. Infections and inflammatory conditions at risk factors in human cancers

Cancer site	Infection/inflammation
Breast	Inflammatory breast cancer
Cervix	Human papilloma viruses, Herpes simplex virus
Esophagus	Barrett's esophagitis
Gall bladder and extrahepatic biliary ducts	Stone/cholecystitis, *Salmonella typhimurium*
Kaposi's sarcoma	Human immunodeficiency viruses and human T-cell lymphotropic viruses
Large intestine (colon/rectum)	Inflammatory bowel diseases, *Schistosomiasis japonicum*
Leukemia/lymphoma	Human T cell leukemia virus, Epstein-Barr virus, malaria
Liver and intrahepatic biliary ducts	Hepatitis viruses B and C, cirrhosis, *Opisthorchis viverrini, Clonorchis sinensis, S. japonicum*
Lung	Cigarette smoke, particles (asbestos, silica dust, etc.)
Nasopharynx	Epstein-Barr virus
Oral cavity	Leukoplakia
Pancreas	Pancreatitis
Pleura (mesothelioma)	Asbestos
Stomach	*Helicobacter pylori*, chronic atrophic gastritis, Epstein-Barr virus
Urinary bladder	Stones, bacterial infection, *S. haematobium*

suppressor gene products such as pRB, p53, and Bax, inactivating them in host cells. Viral products may also immortalize infected cells (e.g., the E6 and E7 proteins of human papilloma virus in human genital keratinocytes) and interact with transcription factors of host genes (e.g., activation of *c-myc* by the X-protein of hepatitis B virus), deregulating the cell cycle or cell growth and death.

2. *Immunosuppression.*
   Viral infection (e.g., with human immunodeficiency virus) may induce immunosuppression, which can enhance some types of malignancy (e.g., Kaposi's sarcoma).

3. *Production of reactive oxygen species (ROS) and reactive nitrogen species (RNS).*
   Chronic inflammation induced by infection (e.g., *H. pylori* infection, liver flukes) results in prolonged activation of inflammatory cells, which gener-

ate ROS and RNS that can damage host DNA and tissues and contribute to carcinogenesis.

At many sites, however, mechanisms for cancers associated with infection have not been fully elucidated. It is probable that both direct (integration of virus DNA into host genome) and indirect (activation of inflammatory cells, and involvement of genetic or other host factors) mechanisms cooperate in many cases. This is evident because (a) many infectious agents associated with human cancer are ubiquitous and widely distributed, but only a small portion of infected subjects develop cancer, (b) there is a long latency period between initial infection and cancer development and (c) other lifestyle factors (e.g., smoking habits, diet etc.) are known to modify cancer risks associated with infection.

C. The Inflammatory Process

Inflammation is the normal physiological response to tissue injury. The cellular and tissue responses to injury include an increased supply of blood, enhanced vascular permeability, and migration of white blood cells to damaged sites. Thus granulocytes, monocytes, and lymphocytes are recruited in the affected area with concomitant production of soluble mediators such as acute-phase proteins, eicosanoids, interleukins, and cytokines. Granulocytes include neutrophils [also called polymorphonuclear leukocytes (PMNs)], basophils, and eosinophils. Monocytes mature into macrophages, which are also the main phagocytes in the body, like neutrophils. During inflammation, these inflammatory cells are activated to produce potent oxidants primarily to attack and destroy invading microorganisms and foreign bodies. However, if infection is not resolved rapidly, or the control of the immune response is not well regulated, inflammation becomes chronic, which often causes extensive tissue damage, due to continuous production of excess active proteolytic enzymes and potent oxidants.

D. The Respiratory Burst

Phagocytic cells (PMNs, eosinophils, and mononuclear phagocytes) consume significantly increased amounts of oxygen during phagocytosis. This process is termed the respiratory burst (DAHLGREN and KARLSSON 1999). Phagocytic cells possess the NADPH oxidase system, which is a membrane-associated enzyme complex that transfers electrons from NADPH to oxygen to generate superoxide (O_2^-). The respiratory burst is triggered by many factors, including phagocytosed insoluble particles, immune complexes, viruses such as influenza and Sendai viruses, a variety of proinflammatory chemotactic agents such as bacterial formylpeptides, complement fragment C5a, platelet-activating factor, leukotriene B_4, and chemicals such as the tumor promoter phorbol 12-

myristate 13-acetate (PMA) [see, for example, review (Christen et al. 1999)]. In addition, many proinflammatory cytokines including tumor necrosis factor (TNF)-α, interleukin-1β, 6 and others, and interferon-γ can contribute to activation of phagocytic cells. Polymorphism of genes encoding cytokines has been associated with increased risk of certain cancer. Examples include TNF-α polymorphism and non-Hodgkin's lymphoma (Warzocha et al. 1998) and prostate cancer (Oh et al. 2000), and interleukin-1β polymorphism and *H. pylori*-associated gastric cancer (El Omar et al. 2000). Enhanced production of such cytokines may increase cancer risks by inducing or activating enzymes involving in the respiratory burst.

E. Production of ROS and RNS

As shown in Fig. 1, various oxidant-generating enzymes are induced and activated under pathophysiological conditions, including NADPH oxidase and xanthine oxidase, which produce superoxide anion ($O_2^{\cdot-}$) in phagolysosomes or in the extracellular fluid. $O_2^{\cdot-}$ itself is a weak oxidant, but two molecules of $O_2^{\cdot-}$ can interact spontaneously to generate one molecule of hydrogen peroxide (H_2O_2), which is a more potent oxidant than $O_2^{\cdot-}$. H_2O_2 is also produced from $O_2^{\cdot-}$ by superoxide dismutases (SODs). H_2O_2 reacts with reduced transition metals (either free or bound to macromolecules such as DNA) to generate the highly toxic hydroxyl radical (HO$^{\cdot}$) or a metal-peroxide complex (Me-OOH). $O_2^{\cdot-}$ also reacts with nitric oxide (NO$^{\cdot}$) rapidly (reaction rate, 6.7×10^9 M^{-1} s^{-1}) to form peroxynitrite anion (ONOO$^-$), which is a highly reactive nitrating and oxidizing species (Beckman and Koppenol 1996; Ducrocq et al. 1999).

Myeloperoxidase (MPO), present in PMNs and monocytes, uses H_2O_2 to generate hypochlorous acid (HOCl) in the presence of chloride ion (Cl$^-$). In the case of parasitic infections and allergic inflammatory disorders such as asthma, eosinophil peroxidase (EPO) is activated in eosinophils, generating hypobromous acid (HOBr) from H_2O_2 and bromide ion (Br$^-$) (Wu et al. 1999a). These hypohalous acids (HOCl and HOBr) are much more potent oxidants than $O_2^{\cdot-}$ and H_2O_2.

Another enzyme that contributes to cytotoxicity of phagocytes is inducible nitric oxide synthase (iNOS). This enzyme can be induced in a variety of human cells and tissues upon stimulation with lipopolysaccharide, cytokines and interferon-γ (Alderton et al. 2001; Bogdan 2001). The enzyme utilizes L-arginine, NADPH and O_2 as substrates, producing nitrogen oxide, NADP$^+$ and citrulline. It remains, however, a matter of debate as to whether NOS synthesizes NO$^{\cdot}$ or not. Recent studies suggest that NOS does not produce NO$^{\cdot}$, but produces NO$^-$ especially in the absence of tetrahydrobiopterin (BH$_4$) (Adak et al. 2000; Rusche et al. 1998); NO$^-$ is then converted to NO$^{\cdot}$ by SOD or other electron acceptors (Hobbs et al. 1994; Schmidt et al. 1996). In the presence of BH$_4$ NO$^{\cdot}$ formation seems favored, with arginine as substrate (Rusche et al. 1998). This issue is important because BH$_4$ has antioxidant

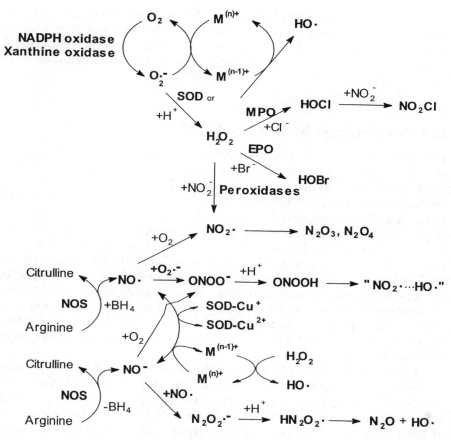

Fig. 1. Production of a variety of ROS and RNS by various oxidant-generating enzymes. New potent oxidants are also formed by interactions of NO·, O_2^-, H_2O_2 and HOCl. These oxidants damage DNA, RNA, lipids and proteins by nitration, oxidation and chlorination (bromination). *SOD*, superoxide dismutase; *MPO*, myeloperoxidase; *EPO*, eosinophil peroxidase

activity and its level is reduced during oxidative stress (NAKAMURA et al. 2001). In addition, NO· and NO⁻ have significantly different reactivity towards many biological molecules (MA et al. 1999). Several studies show that NO· generated from NO· donors is anti-inflammatory and cytoprotective, because NO· can form complexes with transitional metals, inhibiting the Fenton-type reaction (YOSHIE and OHSHIMA 1997) and also terminate radical chain-propagation reactions of lipid peroxidation by radical–radical reactions between NO· and lipid hydroperoxy radicals (LOO·) and alkoxyl radicals (LO·) (RUBBO et al. 1995). On the other hand, NO⁻ generated from an NO⁻ donor (Angeli's salt) exerts strong cytotoxic effects (Wink et al. 1998a), possibly producing HO· or generating peroxynitrite (Ohshima et al. 1999b). Inhibition of NOS leads to anti-inflammatory and cytoprotective effects in many experimental systems (Hobbs et al. 1999). This can be explained if NOS synthesizes cytotoxic NO⁻, but not protective NO·.

F. DNA Damage by ROS and RNS

ROS in the presence of free or DNA-bound transition metals can cause oxidative damage to nucleobases and sugar moieties of DNA and RNA. More than 30 different products have been identified (Dizdaroglu 1994). The best studied include 8-oxo-7,8-dihydro-2′-deoxyguanosine (8-oxo-dG), thymidine glycol and 5-hydroxymethyl-2′-deoxyuridine. Oxidative damage can lead to single- or double-strand breaks, to point and frameshift mutations, and to chromosome abnormalities [see, for example, review (Christen et al. 1999)]. 8-Oxo-dG has been measured as a marker of oxidative DNA damage (Kasai 1997). However, this compound may be easily formed during extraction of DNA and analysis (Helbock et al. 1998). It is also easily converted to further oxidized products such as spiroiminodihydantoin nucleoside by various oxidants including peroxynitrite and HOCl (Niles et al. 2001; Suzuki et al. 2001). Therefore, care is needed if this modified base is measured as a biomarker of oxidative damage.

The reaction of HOCl with various nucleosides yields chlorinated nucleosides, including 8-chloro-2′-deoxyguanosine, 8-chloro-2′-deoxyadenosine and 5-chloro-2′-deoxycytidine. These products are also formed by human MPO or activated human neutrophils in the presence of H_2O_2 and Cl⁻ (Henderson et al. 1999; Masuda et al. 2001). Using electrospray ionization tandem mass spectrometry, it has been shown that several chlorinated nucleosides are also formed following exposure of isolated DNA or RNA to HOCl. Micromolar concentrations of tertiary amines such as nicotine and trimethylamine dramatically enhance the chlorination of free (2′-deoxy)nucleosides and nucleosides in RNA by HOCl. As the G–463A polymorphism of the *MPO* gene, which strongly reduces expression of MPO mRNA, is associated with reduced risk of lung cancer, chlorination damage of DNA or RNA and nucleosides by MPO and its enhancement by nicotine may be important in the pathophysiology of human diseases associated with tobacco habits (Masuda et al. 2001). Similarly, HOBr produced by EPO in the presence of H_2O_2 and Br⁻ can brominate nucleosides to generate 8-bromo-2′-deoxyguanosine, 8-bromo-2′-deoxyadenosine and 5-bromo-2′-deoxycytidine (Shen et al. 2001). These halogenated nucleosides may be measurable as specific biomarkers of DNA damage mediated by MPO/EPO during inflammation.

NO· can be converted, in the presence of oxygen, into the strong nitrosating agent N_2O_3, which can deaminate various DNA bases (e.g., guanine to xanthine and oxanosine, adenine to hypoxanthine, cytosine to uracil, 5-

methylcytosine to thymine). N_2O_3 reacts with secondary amines to form carcinogenic N-nitrosamines, which can damage DNA by alkylation. Increased formation of nitrosamines has been reported to occur in vivo in experimental animals with acute and chronic inflammation as well as in human subjects with infection and inflammation (OHSHIMA and BARTSCH 1999).

The diffusion-controlled coupling of NO· with $O_2^{·-}$ forms a highly reactive nitrating and oxidizing species, peroxynitrite anion ($ONOO^-$) (BECKMAN and KOPPENOL 1996; DUCROCQ et al. 1999). DNA damage induced by peroxynitrite has been reviewed recently (SZABO and OHSHIMA 1997). Treatment of isolated DNA and RNA with authentic peroxynitrite led to dose-dependent formation of 8-nitroguanine (YERMILOV et al. 1995) (MASUDA et al. 2002). The MPO-H_2O_2-NO_2^- system and activated human neutrophils can also nitrate the C-8 position of 2'-deoxyguanosine to form 8-nitroguanine (BYUN et al. 1999) and can nitrate RNA to form 8-nitroguanosine (MASUDA et al. 2002).

On the other hand, peroxynitrite induced only small increases in levels of some oxidized bases, including highly cytotoxic base-propenals (base-CH=CH–CHO) and 8-oxoguanine (DOUKI and CADET 1996; YERMILOV et al. 1995). One possible explanation is that oxidized bases such as 8-oxoguanine are further oxidized by peroxynitrite to ring-cleavage products (NILES et al. 1999). Peroxynitrite and HO· can also induce DNA single strand breakage, which activates the nuclear enzyme poly-ADP ribosylase. Rapid activation of this enzyme results in depletion of its substrate, NAD^+, leading to loss of ATP synthesis and to acute cell dysfunction and cell death (SZABO and OHSHIMA 1997).

NO^- can generate oxidants, possibly highly toxic hydroxyl radicals (HO·), which may be generated by the rapid reaction between NO^- and NO· (reaction rate, $1.7 \times 10^9\ M^{-1}\,s^{-1}$) (OHSHIMA et al. 1999b). More recently, it has been shown that strong oxidants are generated from the NO^--generating agent, Angeli's salt, especially in the presence of H_2O_2 plus Fe(III)-EDTA or Cu(II) (CHAZOTTE-AUBERT et al. 1999). NO· released from diethylamine-NONOate had no such effect. The distinct effects of HO· scavengers and patterns of site-specific DNA cleavage caused by Angeli's salt alone or by Angeli's salt with H_2O_2 plus metal ion suggest that NO^- acts as a reductant to mediate formation of HO· from H_2O_2 plus Fe(III) and formation of Cu(I)-peroxide complexes, that have reactivity similar to that of HO·, from H_2O_2 and Cu(II). NO^- may be formed in vivo under a variety of physiological conditions, including by NO· synthase (see Sect. E.). As stimulated immune cells including neutrophils and macrophages can produce H_2O_2, one may expect that, during an inflammatory process, the formation of both NO^- and H_2O_2 could dramatically enhance the antimicrobial and tumoricidal activity.

In addition to DNA base modifications caused directly by ROS and RNS, base modifications can be induced by lipid peroxidation products (malondialdehyde, 4-hydroxynonenal etc.) to form cyclic adducts including malondialdehyde-guanine and etheno-DNA adducts (SINGER and BARTSCH 1999).

G. Mutations Caused by ROS and RNS

Most ROS and RNS are genotoxic [see, for example, review (Christen et al. 1999)]. The types of mutation depend on the experimental system, especially on the host cells (bacteria or mammalian) in which the DNA was replicated, possibly due to the different DNA repair systems within the host. The most common point mutations induced by H_2O_2/Fe^{3+}-EDTA-altered DNA (*supF*) replicated in monkey kidney cells (CV-1) are G:C to A:T transitions, followed by G:C to T:A and G:C to C:G transversions (Moraes et al. 1989). The mutation spectrum is similar to those found in spontaneous mutants. The same plasmid treated with Fe^{2+}-EDTA alone and replicated in *E. coli* contained predominantly G:C to C:G and G:C to T:A transversions predominantly (Akasaka and Yamamoto 1995). Jeong et al. (1998) reported that base substitutions are the major form of mutation induced in a plasmid replicated in human (AD293) cells by peroxynitrite (84%) and singlet ($^1O_2^*$) (71%), whereas HO· (generated by γ-radiation) induced a lower proportion (49%). G:C to T:A transversions were the most common form of base substitution in each case. These mutations are clustered in hot spots of certain DNA sequences. 8-Oxo-dG in DNA causes mainly G:C to T:A transversions (Shibutani et al. 1991). This type of mutation can be induced by other base modifications (e.g., apurinic sites). 8-Chloro-2'-deoxyguanosine or 8-bromo-2'-deoxyguanosine formed in DNA by HOCl or HOBr may also induce the same G:C to T:A transversions. 5-Chloro- or 5-bromo-2'-deoxyuridine may induce G:C to A:T transitions. The NOx-mediated deamination of DNA bases leads to a variety of mutations (Tannenbaum et al. 1994), the majority of point mutations being G:C to A:T transitions. Deamination of 5-methylcytosine at CpG by NOx results in formation of thymine, inducing G:C to A:T transitions at CpG, one of the most frequently detected mutations in the *TP53* gene and the *Hprt* locus. However, it has been reported that 5-methylcytosine in codon 248 of the *TP53* gene, which is one of the hot spots for G:C to A:T mutations at CpG sites, is not deaminated when human bronchial epithelial cells are exposed to an NO·-releasing compound (Felley Bosco et al. 1995). Recently, the G:C to A:T mutation at codon 248 of the *TP53* gene was observed after cells were exposed to both an NO·-releasing compound and an $O_2^{\cdot-}$-generating hypoxanthine/xanthine oxidase system (Souici et al. 2000).

In addition to various in vitro studies showing that ROS and RNS are genotoxic, several in vivo systems also clearly show mutagenic effects of activated PMNs and macrophages. Human phagocytes stimulated by either bacteria or PMA induced a variety of cytogenetic changes in cocultured cells (Weitzman and Gordon 1990). Addition of SOD, catalase and antioxidants inhibited these genotoxic effects. RNS formed by activated macrophages were also responsible for increased mutation frequency (in the *lacZ* gene of the pUR288 plasmid) in the spleen of transgenic SJL mice (Gal and Wogan 1996). This increase was prevented by administration of *N*-methylarginine, an inhibitor of NOS. Recent studies have shown that iNOS of PMNs infiltrating into tumors induced mutation in the *Hprt* locus of tumor cells (SANDHU et al. 2000). The authors proposed that genotoxic ROS or RNS produced by tumor-infiltrating immune cells contribute to the burden of genetic abnormalities associated with tumor progression. Finally, PMA-activated human PMNs can also cause malignant transformation in C3H 10T1/2 mouse fibroblasts (WEITZMAN et al. 1985).

H. Protein Damage Induced by ROS and RNS

ROS and RNS react with proteins to modify amino acid residues by oxidation, nitrosation, nitration, and halogenation. Modified forms of proteins accumulate during aging, oxidative stress and some pathological conditions, resulting in alterations of the protein structure and function (BERLETT and STADTMAN 1997; DAVIS et al. 2001; ISCHIROPOULOS 1998). Tyrosine residues in protein react with various RNS to form 3-nitrotyrosine (NTYR) (ISCHIROPOULOS 1998; OHSHIMA et al. 1990; 1999a). MPO and EPO can also nitrate tyrosine to form NTYR using H_2O_2 and nitrite (NO_2^-) as substrates (EISERICH et al. 1998; WU et al. 1999b). Tyrosine residues in protein are also chlorinated by HOCl, human MPO and activated human neutrophils in the presence of H_2O_2 and Cl^- to form 3-chlorotyrosine (HAZEN et al. 1996; HAZEN and HEINECKE 1997). Similarly, EPO brominates tyrosine to form 3-bromotyrosine with HOBr generated from H_2O_2 and Br^- (WU et al. 1999a). In addition, dityrosine, carbonyl groups (as measured by reaction with 2,4-dinitrophenylhydrazine) and lipid peroxidation product-protein adducts (e.g., malondialdehyde and 4-hydroxynonenal-protein adducts) have been measured as markers of oxidative damage in proteins (BERLETT and STADTMAN 1997; HEINECKE et al. 1993; UCHIDA and STADTMAN 1992). Other types of protein modification include interactions of ROS and RNS with thiols, metals, and radical residues (DAVIS et al. 2001).

I. Protein Damage as an Epigenetic Effect of ROS and RNS in Carcinogenesis

Alterations of protein structure and function induced by ROS and RNS may contribute to carcinogenesis. Using antibodies against NTYR-containing proteins, many studies have shown that the levels of nitrated proteins are elevated in inflamed tissues, such as gastric mucosa of patients with *H. pylori*-induced gastritis (LI et al. 2001; PIGNATELLI et al. 2001a) and plasma of lung cancer patients and cigarette smokers (PIGNATELLI et al. 2001b). Various proteins or enzymes have been reported to be nitrated, and this modification often results in loss of enzyme activity [see, for example, (AULAK et al. 2001; DAVIS et al. 2001; ISCHIROPOULOS 1998)]. Table 2 summarizes the effects of NO· on enzymes and other proteins especially associated with carcinogenesis. Mammalian cells

Table 2. NO· and other RNS mediated modulations of enzymes/proteins in carcinogenesis

Activation	Inhibition
Ras p21 protein	p53 protein
Metalloproteinases	Caspases
Cycloxygenase-2	Fas (APO-1, CD95)
Soluble guanylate cyclase	Antioxidant enzymes (glutathione reductase/superoxide dismutase)
DNA methyltransferase	Glutathione S-transferases
Telomerase	Ribonucleotide reductase
Src kinase	DNA repair enzymes (OGG1, O^6-methylguanine transferase, etc)
VEGF/bFGF	NF-κB
Heme oxygenase-I	c-fos
	Cytochrome P450s

incubated with excess NO· accumulate the p53 tumor-suppressor protein but concomitantly this p53 loses its capacity for binding to its DNA consensus sequence (Calmels et al. 1997; Cobbs et al. 2001). This alteration could be due to modification(s) of p53 protein by NO·, including formation of disulfide bonds through S-nitrosylation (Calmels et al. 1997) and/or nitration of tyrosine residues (Chazotte-Aubert et al. 2000). Conversely, NO· is capable of activating the protooncogene c-Ha-ras product, p21 protein via S-nitrosation (Lander et al. 1995). These posttranslational modifications of p53 and ras p21 proteins may occur through over-production of NO· in inflamed tissues. Interestingly, over-expression of iNOS has been observed in a variety of premalignant and malignant tissues. Inactivation of p53 through mutations occurs in one-half of human cancers. The ras gene mutations are also found only in some tumors. In view of these observations, one can hypothesize that in some of the tumors carrying wild-type p53 and ras genes, epigenetic events, such as inactivation of p53 protein and activation of ras p21 protein by overproduction of NO·, may play an important role in carcinogenesis. The tumor-suppressor activity of p53 has been reported to be inhibited by a proinflammatory cytokine, macrophage migration inhibitory factor (MIF) (Hudson et al. 1999), although it is not clear whether this inactivation is mediated by NO· or other reactive species.

Other roles of NO· and/or other reactive species in carcinogenesis include inhibition of important enzymes including various DNA repair enzymes (Jaiswal et al. 2001; Wink et al. 1998b) and caspases and other proapoptotic enzymes, which prevent apoptotic cell death (Kim et al. 1997; Mannick et al. 1994). NO· and/or other reactive species, however, can also activate various

Table 3. Roles of ROS and RNS in various stages of carcinogenesis

DNA damage/mutation	
Inhibition of antioxidant enzymes	
Inhibition of DNA repair enzymes	
Inhibition of apoptosis	(Evading apoptosis)
Functional inactivation of tumor-suppressor gene products (e.g., p53 protein)	(Insensitivity to antigrowth signals)
Functional activation of oncogene products (e.g., *ras* p21)	(Self-sufficiency in growth signals)
Telomerase activation	(Limitless replicative potential)
Increased vascular permeability	
Induction of angiogenesis factor production	(Sustained angiogenesis)
Activation of metalloproteinase	(Tissue invasion)
Subversion of host immune system	

Six hallmark capabilities necessary for tumorigenesis, proposed by HANAHAN and WEINBERG (2000), are shown in parentheses.

enzymes such as telomerase, by the action of which cells acquire replicative potential (VASA et al. 2000), DNA methyltransferase, which suppresses gene expression (e.g., tumor-suppressor genes) (HMADCHA et al. 1999), and metalloproteases, which facilitate invasion by cancer cells into surrounding tissues (OKAMOTO et al. 2001). NO· can also activate the enzyme cyclooxygenase-2 which plays pivotal roles in the progression of a variety of cancers through its role in prostaglandin synthesis (GOODWIN et al. 1999; MEI et al. 2000). In addition, stimulation of angiogenesis (GARCIA-CARDENA and FOLKMAN 1998) and subversion of immunity by inhibition of lymphocyte proliferation (HEGARDT et al. 2000; LEJEUNE et al. 1994) are also mediated by ROS and RNS. Thus NO· and/or other reactive species can play important roles in various stages of carcinogenesis (Table 3).

J. Chemoprevention by Anti-inflammatory Agents and Antioxidants

Cancer prevention by antioxidants, anti-inflammatory agents, antagonists against TNF, interleukin, and other cytokines and nonsteroidal anti-inflammatory drugs (NSAIDs) has been studied extensively (BALKWILL and MANTOVANI 2001; WEISBURGER 2001). IARC WORKING GROUP ON THE EVALUATION OF CANCER-PREVENTIVE AGENTS (1997) recently reviewed the cancer-preventive activity of four NSAIDs: aspirin, indomethacin, sulindac, and piroxicam. There is limited evidence in humans that aspirin reduces the risk for colorectal cancer and that sulindac has cancer-preventive activity in patients with familial adenomatous polyposis. Recently, more specific inhibitors against cyclooxygenase-2 (e.g., celecoxib) have been shown to prevent colon and other cancers successfully, although the mechanism by which they inhibit cancer growth is a matter of debate (Marx 2001).

K. Conclusion

Hanahan and Weinberg (2000) recently proposed six hallmark capabilities of cells and tissues necessary for tumorigenesis. These include (a) *self-sufficiency in growth signals*, (b) *insensitivity to antigrowth signals*, (c) *evading apoptosis*, (d) *limitless replicative potential*, (e) *sustained angiogenesis* and (f) *tissue invasion and metastasis*. ROS and RNS can not only damage DNA and induce mutations, but also participate in most of these events by activating and/or inactivating enzymes and proteins involved in these process (Tables 2, 3). Thus, inflammation facilitates the initiation of normal cells and their growth and progression to malignancy. Appropriate treatment of inflammation should be further explored for chemoprevention of human cancers, especially those known to be associated with chronic inflammation.

Acknowledgments. The authors thank Dr. J. Cheney for editing the manuscript, Ms. P. Collard for secretarial assistance.

References

Adak S, Wang Q, Stuehr DJ (2000) Arginine conversion to nitroxide by tetrahydrobiopterin-free neuronal nitric-oxide synthase: Implications for mechanism. J Biol Chem 275:33554–33561

Akasaka S, Yamamoto K (1995) Mutational specificity of the ferrous ion in a supF gene of Escherichia coli. Biochem Biophys Res Commun 213:74–80

Alderton WK, Cooper CE, Knowles RG (2001) Nitric oxide synthases: structure, function and inhibition. Biochem J 357:593–615

Aulak KS, Miyagi M, Yan L, West KA, Massillon D, Crabb JW, Stuehr DJ (2001) Proteomic method identifies proteins nitrated in vivo during inflammatory challenge. Proc Natl Acad Sci USA 98:12056–12061

Balkwill F, Mantovani A (2001) Inflammation and cancer: back to Virchow? Lancet 357:539–545

Beckman JS, Koppenol WH (1996) Nitric oxide, superoxide, and peroxynitrite: the good, the bad, and ugly. Am J Physiol 271:C1424–37

Berlett BS, Stadtman ER (1997) Protein oxidation in aging, disease, and oxidative stress. J Biol Chem 272:20313–20316

Bogdan C (2001) Nitric oxide and the immune response. Nat Immunol 2:907–916

Byun J, Mueller DM, Heinecke JW (1999) 8-Nitro-2'-deoxyguanosine, a specific marker of oxidation by reactive nitrogen species, is generated by the myeloperoxidase-hydrogen peroxide-nitrite system of activated human phagocytes. Biochemistry 38:2590–2600

Calmels S, Hainaut P, Ohshima H (1997) Nitric oxide induces conformational and functional modifications of wild-type p53 tumor suppressor protein. Cancer Res 57:3365–3369

Chazotte-Aubert L, Hainaut P, Ohshima H (2000) Nitric oxide nitrates tyrosine residues of tumor-suppressor p53 protein in MCF-7 cells. Biochem Biophys Res Commun 267:609–613

Chazotte-Aubert L, Oikawa S, Gilibert I, Bianchini F, Kawanishi S, Ohshima H (1999) Cytotoxicity and site-specific DNA damage induced by nitroxyl anion (NO$^-$) in the presence of hydrogen peroxide. Implications for various pathophysiological conditions. J Biol Chem 274:20909–20915

Christen S, Hagen TM, Shigenaga MK, Ames BN (1999) Chronic Inflammation, Mutation, and Cancer. In: Parsonnet J (ed) Microbes and Malignancy. Infection as a cause of human cancers. Oxford University Press, New York, Oxford, p 35

Cobbs CS, Samanta M, Harkins LE, Gillespie GY, Merrick BA, MacMillan-Crow LA (2001) Evidence for Peroxynitrite-Mediated Modifications to p53 in Human Gliomas: Possible Functional Consequences. Arch Biochem Biophys 394:167–172

Dahlgren C, Karlsson A (1999) Respiratory burst in human neutrophils. J Immunol Methods 232:3–14

Davis KL, Martin E, Turko IV, Murad F (2001) Novel effects of nitric oxide. Annu Rev Pharmacol Toxicol 41:203–36

Dizdaroglu M (1994) Chemical determination of oxidative DNA damage by gas chromatography-mass spectrometry. Methods Enzymol 234:3–16

Douki T, Cadet J (1996) Peroxynitrite mediated oxidation of purine bases of nucleosides and isolated DNA. Free Radic Res 24:369–380

Ducrocq C, Blanchard B, Pignatelli B, Ohshima H (1999) Peroxynitrite: an endogenous oxidizing and nitrating agent. Cell Mol Life Sci 55:1068–1077

Eiserich JP, Hristova M, Cross CE, Jones AD, Freeman BA, Halliwell B, van der Vliet A (1998) Formation of nitric oxide-derived inflammatory oxidants by myeloperoxidase in neutrophils. Nature 391:393–397

El Omar EM, Carrington M, Chow WH, McColl KE, Bream JH, Young HA, Herrera J, Lissowska J, Yuan CC, Rothman N, Lanyon G, Martin M, Fraumeni JF, Jr., Rabkin CS (2000) Interleukin-1 polymorphisms associated with increased risk of gastric cancer. Nature 404:398–402

Felley Bosco E, Mirkovitch J, Ambs S, Mace K, Pfeifer A, Keefer LK, Harris CC (1995) Nitric oxide and ethylnitrosourea: relative mutagenicity in the p53 tumor suppressor and hypoxanthine-phosphoribosyltransferase genes. Carcinogenesis 16:2069–2074

Gal A, Wogan GN (1996) Mutagenesis associated with nitric oxide production in transgenic SJL mice. Proc Natl Acad Sci USA 93:15102–15107

Garcia-Cardena G, Folkman J (1998) Is there a role for nitric oxide in tumor angiogenesis? J Natl Cancer Inst 90:560–561

Goodwin DC, Landino LM, Marnett LJ (1999) Effects of nitric oxide and nitric oxide-derived species on prostaglandin endoperoxide synthase and prostaglandin biosynthesis. FASEB J 13:1121–1136

Hanahan D, Weinberg RA (2000) The hallmarks of cancer. Cell 100:57–70

Hazen SL, Heinecke JW (1997) 3-Chlorotyrosine, a specific marker of myeloperoxidase-catalyzed oxidation, is markedly elevated in low density lipoprotein isolated from human atherosclerotic intima. J Clin Invest 99:2075–2081

Hazen SL, Hsu FF, Mueller DM, Crowley JR, Heinecke JW (1996) Human neutrophils employ chlorine gas as an oxidant during phagocytosis. J Clin Invest 98:1283–1289

Hegardt P, Widegren B, Sjogren HO (2000) Nitric-oxide-dependent systemic immunosuppression in animals with progressively growing malignant gliomas. Cell Immunol 200:116–127

Heinecke JW, Li W, Daehnke HL, Goldstein JA (1993) Dityrosine, a specific marker of oxidation, is synthesized by the myeloperoxidase-hydrogen peroxide system of human neutrophils and macrophages. J Biol Chem 268:4069–4077

Helbock HJ, Beckman KB, Shigenaga MK, Walter PB, Woodall AA, Yeo HC, Ames BN (1998) DNA oxidation matters: the HPLC-electrochemical detection assay of 8-oxo-deoxyguanosine and 8-oxo-guanine. Proc Natl Acad Sci USA 95:288–293

Henderson J P, Byun J, Heinecke JW (1999) Molecular chlorine generated by the myeloperoxidase-hydrogen peroxide-chloride system of phagocytes produces 5-chlorocytosine in bacterial RNA. J Biol Chem 274:33440–33448

Hmadcha A, Bedoya FJ, Sobrino F, Pintado E (1999) Methylation-dependent gene silencing induced by interleukin 1beta via nitric oxide production. J Exp Med 190:1595–1604

Hobbs AJ, Fukuto JM, Ignarro LJ (1994) Formation of free nitric oxide from l-arginine by nitric oxide synthase: direct enhancement of generation by superoxide dismutase. Proc Natl Acad Sci USA 91:10992–10996

Hobbs AJ, Higgs A, Moncada S (1999) Inhibition of nitric oxide synthase as a potential therapeutic target. Annu Rev Pharmacol Toxicol 39:191–220

Hudson JD, Shoaibi MA, Maestro R, Carnero A, Hannon GJ, Beach DH (1999) A proinflammatory cytokine inhibits p53 tumor suppressor activity. J Exp Med 190: 1375–1382

IARC Working Group on the Evaluation of Cancer Preventive Agents (1997) IARC Handbooks of Cancer Prevention Nonsteroidal Anti-Inflammatory Drugs. 1, International Agency for Research on Cancer, Lyon, France

IARC Working Group on the Evaluation of Carcinogenic Risks to Humans (1994a) IARC Monographs on the Evaluation of Carcinogenic Risks to Humans: vol. 59: Hepatitis Viruses. International Agency for Research on Cancer, Lyon, France

IARC Working Group on the Evaluation of Carcinogenic Risks to Humans (1994b) IARC Monographs on the Evaluation of Carcinogenic Risks to Humans: vol. 61: Schistosomes, Liver Flukes and Helicobacter pylori. International Agency for Research on Cancer, Lyon, France

IARC Working Group on the Evaluation of Carcinogenic Risks to Humans (1995) IARC Monographs on the Evaluation of Carcinogenic Risks to Humans: vol. 64: Human Papilloma viruses. International Agency for Research on Cancer, Lyon, France

IARC Working Group on the Evaluation of Carcinogenic Risks to Humans (1996) IARC Monographs on the Evaluation of Carcinogenic Risks to Humans: vol. 67: Human Immunodeficiency Viruses and Human T-cell Lymphotropic Viruses. International Agency for Research on Cancer, Lyon, France

IARC Working Group on the Evaluation of Carcinogenic Risks to Humans (1997) IARC Monographs on the Evaluation of Carcinogenic Risks to Humans: vol. 70: Epstein-Barr Viruses and Kaposi's Sarcoma Herpesviruses/Human Herpesvirus. International Agency for Research on Cancer, Lyon, France

Ischiropoulos H (1998) Biological tyrosine nitration: a pathophysiological function of nitric oxide and reactive oxygen species. Arch Biochem Biophys 356:1–11

Jaiswal M, LaRusso NF, Nishioka N, Nakabeppu Y, Gores GJ (2001) Human Ogg1, a protein involved in the repair of 8-oxoguanine, is inhibited by nitric oxide. Cancer Res 61:6388–6393

Jeong JK, Juedes MJ, Wogan GN (1998) Mutations induced in the supF gene of pSP189 by hydroxyl radical and singlet oxygen: relevance to peroxynitrite mutagenesis. Chem Res Toxicol 11:550–556

Kasai H (1997) Analysis of a form of oxidative DNA damage, 8-hydroxy-2'-deoxyguanosine, as a marker of cellular oxidative stress during carcinogenesis. Mutat Res 387:147–163

Kim YM, Talanian RV, Billiar TR (1997) Nitric oxide inhibits apoptosis by preventing increases in caspase-3-like activity via two distinct mechanisms. J Biol Chem 272: 31138–31148

Lander HM, Ogiste JS, Pearce SF, Levi R, Novogrodsky A (1995) Nitric oxide-stimulated guanine nucleotide exchange on p21ras. J Biol Chem 270:7017–7020

Lejeune P, Lagadec P, Onier N, Pinard D, Ohshima H, Jeannin JF (1994) Nitric oxide involvement in tumor-induced immunosuppression. J Immunol 152:5077–5083

Li CQ, Pignatelli B, Ohshima H (2001) Increased oxidative and nitrative stress in human stomach associated with cagA+ Helicobacter pylori infection and inflammation. Dig Dis Sci 46:836–844

Ma XL, Gao F, Liu GL, Lopez BL, Christopher TA, Fukuto JM, Wink DA, Feelisch M (1999) Opposite effects of nitric oxide and nitroxyl on postischemic myocardial injury. Proc Natl Acad Sci USA 96:14617–14622

Mannick JB, Asano K, Izumi K, Kieff E, Stamler JS (1994) Nitric oxide produced by human B lymphocytes inhibits apoptosis and Epstein-Barr virus reactivation. Cell 79:1137–1146

Marx J (2001) Anti-inflammatories inhibit cancer growth-but how? Science 291: 581–582

Masuda M, Suzuki T, Friesen MD, Ravanat JL, Cadet J, Pignatelli B, Nishino H, Ohshima H (2001) Chlorination of guanosine and other nucleosides by hypochlorous acid and myeloperoxidase of activated human neutrophils. Catalysis by nicotine and trimethylamine. J Biol Chem 276:40486–40496

Masuda M, Nishino H, Ohshima H (2002) Formation of 8-nitroguanosine in cellular RNA as a biomarker of exposure to reactive nitrogen species. Chem Biol Interact 139:187–197

Mei JM, Hord NG, Winterstein DF, Donald SP, Phang JM (2000) Expression of prostaglandin endoperoxide H synthase-2 induced by nitric oxide in conditionally immortalized murine colonic epithelial cells. FASEB J 14:1188–1201

Moraes EC, Keyse SM, Pidoux M, Tyrrell RM (1989) The spectrum of mutations generated by passage of a hydrogen peroxide damaged shuttle vector plasmid through a mammalian host. Nucleic Acids Res 17:8301–8312

Nakamura K, Bindokas VP, Kowlessur D, Elas M, Milstien S, Marks JD, Halpern HJ, Kang UJ (2001) Tetrahydrobiopterin scavenges superoxide in dopaminergic neurons. J Biol Chem 276:34402–34407

Niles JC, Burney S, Singh SP, Wishnok JS, Tannenbaum SR (1999) Peroxynitrite reaction products of 3′,5′-di-O-acetyl-8-oxo-7, 8-dihydro-2′-deoxyguanosine. Proc Natl Acad Sci USA 96:11729–11734

Niles JC, Wishnok JS, Tannenbaum SR (2001) Spiroiminodihydantoin is the major product of the 8-oxo-7,8-dihydroguanosine reaction with peroxynitrite in the presence of thiols and guanosine photooxidation by methylene blue. Org Lett 3:963–966

Oh BR, Sasaki M, Perinchery G, Ryu SB, Park YI, Carroll P, Dahiya R (2000) Frequent genotype changes at – 308, and 488 regions of the tumor necrosis factor-alpha (TNF-alpha) gene in patients with prostate cancer. J Urol 163:1584–1587

Ohshima H, Bartsch H (1999) Quantitative estimation of endogenous N-nitrosation in humans by monitoring N-nitrosoproline in urine. Methods Enzymol 301:40–49

Ohshima H, Celan I, Chazotte L, Pignatelli B, Mower HF (1999a) Analysis of 3-nitrotyrosine in biological fluids and protein hydrolyzates by high-performance liquid chromatography using a postseparation, on-line reduction column and electrochemical detection: results with various nitrating agents. Nitric Oxide 3:132–141

Ohshima H, Friesen M, Brouet I, Bartsch H (1990) Nitrotyrosine as a new marker for endogenous nitrosation and nitration of proteins. Food Chem Toxicol 28: 647–652

Ohshima H, Gilibert I, Bianchini F (1999b) Induction of DNA strand breakage and base oxidation by nitroxyl anion (NO⁻) through hydroxyl radical production. Free Radic Biol Med 26:1305–1313

Okamoto T, Akaike T, Sawa T, Miyamoto Y, van der Vliet A, Maeda H (2001) Activation of matrix metalloproteinases by peroxynitrite-induced protein S-glutathiolation via disulfide S-oxide formation. J Biol Chem 276:29596–29602

Parsonnet J (2001) Microbes and malignancy. Infection as a cause of human cancers. Oxford University Press, New York; Oxford

Pignatelli B, Bancel B, Plummer M, Toyokuni S, Patricot L-M, Ohshima H (2001a) Helicobacter pylori eradication attenuates oxidative stress in human gastric mucosa. Am J Gastroenterol 96:1758–1766

Pignatelli B, Li CQ, Boffetta P, Chen Q, Ahrens W, Nyberg F, Mukeria A, Bruske-Hohlfeld I, Fortes C, Constantinescu V, Ischiropoulos H, Ohshima H (2001b) Nitrated and oxidized plasma proteins in smokers and lung cancer patients. Cancer Res 61:778–784

Pisani P, Parkin DM, Munoz N, Ferlay J (1997) Cancer and infection: estimates of the attributable fraction in 1990. Cancer Epidemiol Biomarkers Prev 6:387–400

Rubbo H, Parthasarathy S, Barnes S, Kirk M, Kalyanaraman B, Freeman BA (1995) Nitric oxide inhibition of lipoxygenase-dependent liposome and low-density lipoprotein oxidation: termination of radical chain propagation reactions and formation of nitrogen-containing oxidized lipid derivatives. Arch Biochem Biophys 324:15–25

Rusche KM, Spiering MM, Marletta MA (1998) Reactions catalyzed by tetrahydrobiopterin-free nitric oxide synthase. Biochemistry 37:15503–15512

Sandhu JK, Privora HF, Wenckebach G, Birnboim HC (2000) Neutrophils, nitric oxide synthase, and mutations in the mutatect murine tumor model. Am J Pathol 156: 509–518

Schmidt HH, Hofmann H, Schindler U, Shutenko ZS, Cunningham DD, Feelisch M (1996) No .NO from NO synthase. Proc Natl Acad Sci USA 93:14492–14497

Shen Z, Mitra SN, Wu W, Chen Y, Yang Y, Qin J, Hazen SL (2001) Eosinophil peroxidase catalyzes bromination of free nucleosides and double-stranded DNA. Biochemistry 40:2041–2051

Shibutani S, Takeshita M, Grollman AP (1991) Insertion of specific bases during DNA synthesis past the oxidation-damaged base 8-oxodG. Nature 349:431–434

Singer B and Bartsch H (1999) Exocyclic DNA Adducts in Mutagenesis and Carcinogenesis. IARC Sci. Publ. 150, International Agency for Research on Cancer, Lyon, France

Souici AC, Mirkovitch J, Hausel P, Keefer K, Felley-Bosco E (2000) Transition mutation in codon 248 of the p53 tumor suppressor gene induced by reactive oxygen species and a nitric oxide-releasing compound. Carcinogenesis 21:281–287

Suzuki T, Masuda M, Friesen MD, Ohshima H (2001) Formation of spiroiminodihydantoin nucleoside by reaction of 8-oxo-7,8-dihydro-2′-deoxyguanosine with hypochlorous acid or a myeloperoxidase-H2O2-Cl- system. Chem Res Toxicol 14:1163–1169

Szabo C, Ohshima H (1997) DNA damage induced by peroxynitrite: subsequent biological effects. Nitric Oxide Biol Chem 1:373–385

Tannenbaum SR, Tamir S, Rojas-Walker TD, Wishnok JS (1994) DNA damage and cytotoxicity caused by nitric oxide. ACS Symp Ser 553:120–135

Uchida K, Stadtman ER (1992) Modification of histidine residues in proteins by reaction with 4-hydroxynonenal. Proc Natl Acad Sci USA 89:4544–4548

Vasa M, Breitschopf K, Zeiher AM, Dimmeler S (2000) Nitric oxide activates telomerase and delays endothelial cell senescence. Circ Res 87:540–542

Warzocha K, Ribeiro P, Bienvenu J, Roy P, Charlot C, Rigal D, Coiffier B, Salles G (1998) Genetic polymorphisms in the tumor necrosis factor locus influence non-Hodgkin's lymphoma outcome. Blood 91:3574–3581

Weisburger JH (2001) Antimutagenesis and anticarcinogenesis, from the past to the future. Mutat Res 480–481:23–35

Weitzman SA, Gordon LI (1990) Inflammation and cancer: role of phagocyte-generated oxidants in carcinogenesis. Blood 76:655–663

Weitzman SA, Weitberg AB, Clark EP, Stossel TP (1985) Phagocytes as carcinogens: malignant transformation produced by human neutrophils. Science 227:1231–1233

Wink DA, Feelisch M, Fukuto J, Chistodoulou D, Jourd'heuil D, Grisham MB, Vodovotz Y, Cook JA, Krishna M, DeGraff WG, Kim S, Gamson J, Mitchell JB (1998a) The cytotoxicity of nitroxyl: possible implications for the pathophysiological role of NO. Arch Biochem Biophys 351:66–74

Wink DA, Vodovotz Y, Laval J, Laval F, Dewhirst MW, Mitchell JB (1998b) The multifaceted roles of nitric oxide in cancer. Carcinogenesis 19:711–721

Wu W, Chen Y, d'Avignon A, Hazen SL (1999a) 3-Bromotyrosine and 3,5-dibromotyrosine are major products of protein oxidation by eosinophil peroxidase: potential markers for eosinophil- dependent tissue injury in vivo. Biochemistry 38:3538–3548

Wu W, Chen Y, Hazen SL (1999b) Eosinophil peroxidase nitrates protein tyrosyl residues. Implications for oxidative damage by nitrating intermediates in eosinophilic inflammatory disorders. J Biol Chem 274:25933–25944

Yermilov V, Rubio J, Ohshima H (1995) Formation of 8-nitroguanine in DNA treated with peroxynitrite in vitro and its rapid removal from DNA by depurination. FEBS Lett 376:207–210

Yoshie Y, Ohshima H (1997) Nitric oxide synergistically enhances DNA strand breakage induced by polyhydroxyaromatic compounds, but inhibits that induced by the Fenton-reaction. Arch Biochem Biophys 342:13–21

CHAPTER 13

Infections and the Etiology of Human Cancer: Epidemiological Evidence and Opportunities for Prevention

F.X. Bosch, S. de Sanjosé, J. Ribes, and C.A. González

A. Cancer Burden Related to Infections

Recent estimates of the cancer burden in the world indicate that as of the year 2000 10.1 million new cases arise annually. Mortality from cancer accounts for 6.2 million cases. The 5-year prevalence, which estimates the burden of disease that requires care and close surveillance, is estimated at 22.4 million cases worldwide. Incidence reflects, on a broad scale, the impact of the disease as well as the burden of diagnostic and first treatment requirements. Mortality reflects the number of potential years of life lost to cancer and its relation to cancer incidence (i.e., incidence to mortality ratio) and is used as a global index of the diagnostic and therapeutic efficiency of the health system. Currently, the most common cancers in the world are lung cancer (1.2 million new cases), and breast cancer (1 million new cases) followed by colon and rectum combined and stomach cancer (875,000 to 1 million new cases). Cancers of the liver, prostate, and cervix uteri contribute 400–600,000 new cases each. In terms of prevalence, the cancer sites that account for most of the disease burden include the locations with high incidence rates (such as lung cancer) and the relatively less frequent locations for which effective treatments are available, to a substantial fraction of the cases (such as cervix uteri). In these instances, survival of at least 5 years is reasonably good. The most prevalent cancers worldwide are breast (3.8 million cases) and colon and rectum (2.4 million), followed by stomach, cervix uteri, prostate and lung (between 1.3 and 1.5 million each). More developed countries have age-adjusted incidence rates about twice the rates in the developing parts of the world (301 per 100,000 vs. 154 per 100,000 among males and 218 per 100,000 vs. 128 per 100,000 among females). However, over half of the new cancer cases in the world are currently arising from less developed countries, a growing concern for health planners (PARKIN et al. 2001). The differential pattern of cancer incidence by level of development reproduces to some extent within developed countries (i.e., across Europe and across social groups within a given country) and for each cancer location.

Approximately 18% of all human cancers have been linked to persistent infections from viruses, bacteria, or parasites. For some specific sites, infections are responsible for the large majority of the cases, offering challenging options for cancer prevention. These proportions vary considerably according to the

level of development. In the most developed parts of western countries, infections account for 9%–10% of the total number of cancer cases, whereas in
developing regions infections account for 20% of the common cancers. This
percentage is consistently more important among women, largely due to the
association between human papillomavirus (HPV) and cervical cancer.

Table 1 shows in numerical terms the impact of infections as a cause of
cancer. The table identifies the agent, the estimated number of cases associated with the infections, the cancer sites involved with the corresponding estimates of the number of cases, and the proportion of the total burden of cancer
in the world that each infection-induced cancer represents.

Figures 1 and 2 show for males and females and for developed and developing countries the number of cancer cases linked to infections and the per-

Table 1. Infection and the estimated burden of cancer worldwide in 2000 (Parkin, M.
personal communication)

Infectious agents	No. of cases related to the infection	Cancer site[a] (no. of cases)	% Of the total cancer incidence[b] attributable to the infection
Human papillomavirus (HPV)	536 000	Cervix, anogenital area	5.3
Hepatitis B and C viruses (HBV, HCV)	508 000	Liver	5.0
Helicobacter pylori (HP)	453 000	Stomach (442 000) Lymphoma (11 000)	4.5
Human immunodeficiency virus (HIV)	193 000	KS (134 000) NHL (55 000) Hodgkin's (4 400)	1.9
Epstein-Barr Virus (EBV)	99 000	NPC (63 000) Hodgkin's (29 000) Burkitt's lymphoma (6 500)	1.0
Schistosoma	10 000	Urinary bladder	0.1
Human T-cell leukemia virus type 1 (HTI-V 1)	3 000	ATLL	0.03
Liver flukes	1 000	Liver	0.01
Total	1 801 000		17.9

[a] KS, Kaposi's sarcoma; NHL, non-Hodgkin's lymphoma; NPC, nasopharyngeal carcinoma; ATLL, acute T-cell leukemia-lymphoma.
[b] 10 055 544 new cases worldwide. ( ): number of cases.

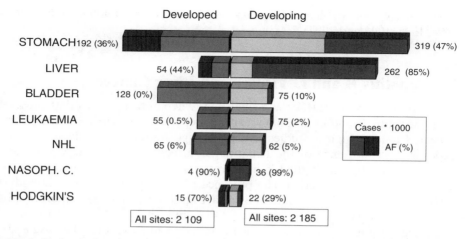

Fig. 1. Estimated number of new cases of cancer caused by infectious agents – males

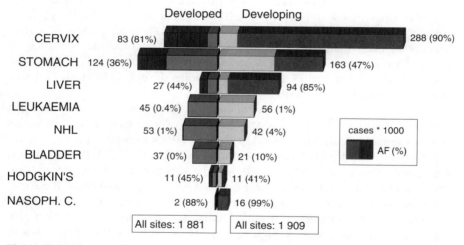

Fig. 2. Estimated number of new cases of cancer caused by infectious agents – females

centage of each cancer location that is attributable to the infection. The most remarkable examples are gastric cancer, 40%–50% of which has been linked to *Helicobacter pylori* infections; liver cancer, 80% of which is related to Hepatitis B (HBV) or C (HCV) infections in developing countries; and cervical cancer, a major human cancer, which is currently believed to be attributable to Human Papillomavirus (HPV) infections in above 90% of the cases worldwide.

The study of infections and cancer has made substantial progress with regard to the developments of molecular biomarkers and excellent reviews are regularly being published (Goedert 2000; Newton et al. 1999; IARC 1992 1994, 1995, 1996 and 1997).

B. Hepatitis B and C Viruses and Liver Cancer

The hepatitis B virus (HBV) is a small DNA hepatotropic virus that causes acute hepatitis B and occasionally chronic hepatitis, liver cirrhosis, and liver cancer. Epidemiological studies use the antigen/antibody profile to assess exposure. The presence of the hepatitis B surface antigen (HBsAg) in the serum of a healthy individual is interpreted as a marker of persistent (frequently subclinical) infection. The presence of the hepatitis B core antibody (HBcAb) with or without hepatitis B surface antibody (HBsAg) is interpreted as a marker of past (solved) exposure. Other biomarkers of interest for epidemiological studies are the hepatitis Be antigen and antibodies (HBeAg and HBeAb) and HBV DNA, measured with amplification methods in either serum or tissue.

The hepatitis C virus (HCV) is a positive-strand RNA virus distantly related to pestiviruses and flaviviruses. It is a human virus that can infect chimpanzees, but no natural equivalent of animal HCVs have been identified. Biomarkers to investigate the epidemiology of HCV include the detection in serum of antibodies to HCV (HCVAb) and viral nucleic acid (HCV RNA) by reverse transcription and PCR. HCV antibodies do not distinguish between current and past HCV infections.

Current estimates of the prevalence of hepatitis B surface Antigen (HBsAg) of anti-HCVAb and of the incidence of liver cancer (LC) in males show a significant correlation worldwide (for HBsAg correlation coefficient: $0.67, p < 0.001$ and for HCVAb correlation coefficient: $0.37, p < 0.001$) (Bosch et al. 1999). The areas at highest risk are the sub-Saharan African countries, China and South East Asia and some isolated populations in Alaska, the Amazonian basin and New Zealand. Prevalence of HCV infection is perhaps less well known but available information indicates that the areas at high risk largely overlap the areas at high risk of HBV. The Mediterranean basin, notably Southern Italy and Greece, are areas of high prevalence of both HBV and HCV, as well as of liver cancer in males.

Some dramatic examples of iatrogenically induced HCV infections and of liver cancer have been reported in Japan and in Egypt. In Japan, increasing LC incidence and mortality trends since the early 1970s have been partially attributed to exposure of the population to HCV through blood transfusion or contaminated needles (Okuda 1991). In Egypt, the reported HCV prevalence in the population has been estimated to be of the order of 6%–9% in the urban areas and 27%–30% in the rural parts of the Nile delta, one of the highest ever found. A carefully documented epidemiological study traced the source of the infection to the massive treatment campaigns against schistosomal infestation conducted in the interval 1920–1970. The treatment typically included several courses of intramuscular or intravenous drugs against schistosoma that were delivered under nonsterile conditions (FRANK et al. 2000).

Table 2 summarizes current estimates of the risk factors for liver cancer in areas of high (Africa and Asia) and low (western Europe and northern America) incidence. Japan has a peculiar pattern of liver cancer incidence in what is a fairly developed country and yet has a very high incidence rate of HBV- and HCV-related liver cancer.

Overall 75%–80% of the LC cases can be related to persistent viral infections with either HBV (50%–55%) or HCV (25%–30%).

The epidemiology of liver cancer and HBV has been largely conducted using the viral antigen/antibody profiles in cases and controls. Updated technology, however, is showing that current data may underestimate the attributable fractions (BRÉCHOT et al. 1998). A meta-analysis on viral factors and LC reported summary odds ratios (OR) for HBsAg positivity without HCV Ab or HCV/RNA of 22.5 (95% CI: 19.5–26.0). The OR for HCV Ab/ HCV RNA positivity and HBsAg negativity was 17.3 (95% CI: 13.9–21.6), and the OR for positivity to both markers was 165 (95% CI: 81.2–374), suggesting a synergism of the two viral infection in the causation of LC (DONATO et al. 1998). The IARC's MONOGRAPH program evaluated HBV and HCV viruses in relation to liver cancer as human carcinogens (Class 1; IARC 1994).

I. Opportunities for Prevention of Liver Cancer

Screening of blood and blood products has successfully reduced HBV transmission, and vaccination against hepatitis B has already shown that prevention of liver cancer is feasible and likely to be of public health relevance in the years to come.

One major intervention trial in a highly endemic area in Africa is underway to demonstrate that infant immunization against HB prevents liver cancer in adulthood. Short-term results from The GAMBIA HEPATITIS INTERVENTION STUDY (GHIS) estimated that protection against HB infection using three doses of HBV vaccine is high (84%; 95% CI = 78%–89%) and against the HBsAg carrier state is also high (94%; 95% CI = 84%–98%) (FORTUIN et al. 1993). With longer follow-up, a reduction in incidence of liver cancer of 70% or greater is expected. These results are consistent with the findings of several follow-up studies in different populations using different vaccination products.

In 1996, the NATIONAL HB IMMUNIZATION PROGRAM and the LIVER CANCER STUDY GROUP in Taiwan reported that a program of immunization of newborns against HBV that was initiated in 1984 achieved national coverage in 1986. Among the cohorts of HB vaccinated infants, followed to 1993, no cases of liver cancer were identified in children 6–8 years old in contrast to an expected yearly average of 6–7 hepatocellular carcinoma cases per year in the preceding 6 years. If the observation is confirmed over time, this will be the first proof

F.X. Bosch et al.

Table 2. Risk factors of liver cancer and estimates of the attributable fractions (adapted from Bosch et al. 1999)

Risk factors	Europe and the US		Japan		Africa and Asia	
	Estimate	Range	Estimate	Range	Estimate	Range
Hepatitis B virus	22%	4%–58%	20%	18%–44%	60%	40%–90%
Hepatitis C virus[a]	60%	12%–72%	63%	48%–94%	20%	9%–56%
Alcohol	45%	8%–57%	20%	15%–33%	–	11%–41%
Tobacco	12%	0%–14%	40%	9%–51%	22%[b]	–
Oral contraceptives	–	10%–50%[c]	NE	–	8%[d]	–
Aflatoxin	Limited exposure	–	Limited exposure[e]	–	Important exposure[e]	–
Other	<5%	–	–	–	<5%	–

NE, not evaluated (limited exposure).
[a] Not including double infections with HBV and HCV.
[b] Estimates for HBsAg-negative, black men.
[c] Restricted to liver cancer in women.
[d] Restricted to liver cancer in black women.
[e] Attributable risk not quantified.
Note: attributable fractions do not necessarily add to 100% because of multiple exposures and possible interactions between risk factors.

of the success of HB vaccination in the prevention of a major cancer in South East Asia (CHANG et al. 1998). Similar examples have been reported in Korea and other high-risk populations (LEE et al. 1998). In 1991 and 1992, the WORLD HEALTH ASSEMBLY recommended integrating the HB vaccination of infants into their EPI delivery services. In 1994, 72 countries had national HB immunization programs and in 1997, the number reached 90. These countries represent roughly 40% of the world's newborns and almost 60% of the world's 350 million carriers (VAN DAMME 1997). Some countries in Europe (i.e., UK) decided, however, not to introduce HBV vaccination into their standardized vaccination protocols. Availability of the HBV vaccine to the most deprived populations at risk is now the greatest challenge.

At present, there is no vaccine available against HCV. Prevention of HCV infection should be based on screening blood products and on the implementation of education programs among potential and high-risk populations. HBV and HCV screening of blood products can effectively reduce the incidence of posttransfusion hepatitis (TABOR 1999; GONZÁLEZ et al. 1995). However, there is yet no direct evidence of the effect of this screening in the reduction of LC incidence. It has been postulated that syringe exchange programs among drug addict populations could reduce transmission of HBV, HCV, and HIV. However, the results to date are inconsistent (HAGAN et al. 1995, 1999).

C. Human Papillomavirus and Cancer of the Anogenital Tract

The human papillomavirus (HPV) is a family of small DNA viruses that infect the skin and the mucosae. Some HPV types induce verrucae and condylomas (genital warts) and other types, also called high-risk types are strongly related to carcinomas in the genital tract, the skin, and in some locations in the oral cavity.

The evidence relating HPV infections to cervical cancer includes a large and consistent body of studies indicating a strong and specific role of the viral infection in all countries where investigations have taken place. The association has been recognized as causal in nature by a number of international review parties since the early 1990s (IARC 1992, IARC 1995, NATIONAL INSTITUTES OF HEALTH 1996). Nucleic acid amplification techniques regularly identify HPV DNA in 90%–95% of the cervical cancer specimens both squamous cell and adenocarcinomas. Detailed investigations of the few cervical cancer specimens that appear as HPV DNA negatives in every series has been conducted and the results strongly suggest that these are largely false negatives. The reasons for nondetection are attributable to: (a) poor quality of the specimen, poor preservation or absence of cancer tissue (b) HPV DNA integration into cellular DNA with increased target fragmentation (more often seen with HPV 18), and (c) length and target sequences of the βglobin probes and of the HPV-type-specific probes (BOSCH et al. 1995; WALBOOMERS et al. 1999).

I. HPV Type Distribution in Cervical Cancer Cases

Of the more than 35 HPV types found in the genital tract, approximately ten (HPV types 16, 18, 31, 33, 35, 45, 51, 52, 58, and 59) have been adequately evaluated as high risk types in relation to invasive cervical cancer. HPV 16 accounts for approximately 50%–60% of the types found in cervical cancer cases in most countries, followed by HPV 18 (10%–12%) and HPV 31 and 45 (4%–5% each). Cervical adenocarcinomas showed a slightly different distribution and the most common types are HPV 16 (approximately 45%), HPV 18 (approximately 40%), and HPV 45 and 59 (4%–5% each). In series of women without cervical lesions, (corresponding to controls in most case-control studies or ad-hoc HPV prevalence surveys from the general population) the HPV-type-specific distribution embraces a much larger series of viral types. HPV 16 remains again the most common type (approximately 20%), followed by HPV 18 (approximately 10%), HPV 45 (approximately 8%), HPV 59 (approximately 2%), and smaller proportions of approximately 30 additional HPV types. Many of these rare types are occasionally found in controls and still convey a high risk for cervical cancer (Bosch et al. 2001).

It is of interest to notice that the geographical variation in type distribution has not been fully documented. For example, high rates of HPV 35 and 58 in the general population in Mozambique are now being reported (Castellsagué et al. 2001). New technical developments are also describing high frequencies of multiple HPV infections that were most probably undetected by previous testing systems.

II. Risk Estimates from Case-Control Studies

The IARC research program on HPV organized a series of case-control studies in different countries, mostly in areas at high risk for invasive cervical cancer. To date, this represents the largest data set on invasive cancer in high-risk countries and a major source of reference data. Preliminary results on the pooled analyses of studies in nine countries included approximately 2,288 invasive squamous cell carcinomas, 141 adenocarcinomas, and 2,513 matched controls (Bosch et al. 2001). The adjusted ORs (the factor by which the risk of cervical cancer of a given woman is multiplied if HPV DNA is detected) for HPV DNA detection was OR = 83.3 (95% CI: 54.9–105.3). Type-specific risk estimates were as follows: HPV 16: OR = 182; HPV 18: 231; HPV 45 OR = 148; HPV 31 OR = 71.5; HPV 33 OR = 77.6; HPV 35 OR = 34.8; HPV 51, OR = 42.7; HPV 52 OR = 145.7; HPV 58 OR = 78.9; HPV 59 OR = 347.3. The risk for any given high-risk type was not statistically different from the risk reported for HPV 16. Multiple infections did not increase significantly the risk of single infections. The estimates of the attributable fraction AF%, (the proportion of disease that is related to HPV DNA) in most studies range from 90% to 98%. Studies on HPV variants (variation within HPV types affecting down to one nucleotide of the viral genome) are beginning to reveal that the risk of some HPV 16 variants may differ. According to these results, non-European variants would convey higher risk than the HPV 16 European prototype (HILDESHEIM et al. 2001).

III. New Options for Screening and Triage in Cervical Cancer Prevention

Several studies in both developed and developing countries have shown that HPV- and HPV-type distribution is related to cervical cancer precursor lesions with the same strength than the more advanced invasive cancers (MORENO et al. 1995; LIAW et al. 1995; KJAER et al. 1996; HERRERO et al. 2000). Testing for the presence of viral DNA is currently being evaluated as adjuvant in cytology-based screening programs and as a stand-alone screening test in primary screening programs. As the HPV detection methods developed, the prevalence of HPV DNA in LGSIL/HGSIL increased steadily to levels of 80%–90%. In fact, the very high prevalence observed in recent studies of LGSIL promoted the notion that HPV testing would not be suitable for triage of LGSIL (ALTS STUDY GROUP 2000). In contrast, HPV testing has been shown to enhance the sensitivity of screening programs whenever used in conjunction with cytology in cases of ambiguous results. As a discriminant in cases of a cytological diagnosis of abnormality of uncertain nature (ASCUS/AGUS), HPV tests have a better sensitivity than a repeated Pap smear. A substantial part of the variability in the HPV prevalence in LSIL observed across studies is related to variability in the definition of the preneoplastic lesions rather than variability in HPV testing. As a stand-alone screening test, HPV testing is being evaluated in low-equipped areas where cytology-based screening has proven to be difficult to sustain and yet there is a medium level of technological sophistication.

IV. Immune Response to HPV Infection and Implications for Vaccine Development

Prevention of HPV infections is becoming the newly defined target for cervical cancer prevention in developing countries. Serologically based follow-up studies strongly suggest that antibody responses are dependent on the duration of the detection of HPV DNA in the cervical tissue. However, HPV antibodies are largely type-specific and infection with one high-risk HPV type does not offer protection against a second infection with other HPV types (THOMAS et al. 2000). HPV vaccines should, then, consider at least two viral types (HPV 16 and 18). The prospects for developing HPV vaccines are advanced. Animal studies have shown the ability of pseudo viral particles (VLP) based upon the L1 major capsid protein to induce virion-neutralizing antibodies that protect animals from challenge with species-specific viruses. Therapeutic vaccines seek to generate cell-mediated immune response to non-virion HPV proteins in established lesions. Phase I studies in humans are under active research and have shown safety and immunogenicity. Phase II–III trials involving large numbers of participants from the general population should be initiated in the years 2000–2001. The aim of these studies is the demonstration of a reduction in mortality from cervical cancer in the vaccinated group. The completion of this work may offer realistic preventive options to third world countries in the future.

D. *Helicobacter pylori* and Gastric Cancer

Helicobacter pylori (HP) is a Gram-negative spiral-shaped bacteria, with two to six unipolar flagella, and remarkable motility in viscous solution. It was isolated by accidental extended incubation in 1982 and today HP is recognized as one of the commonest bacterial pathogens in humans, associated with gastritis, peptic ulcer disease, and gastric cancer. HP is uniquely adapted to grow in an acidic environment through its urease activity and, in the stomach, bacterial colonization usually occurs initially in the antrum. HP does not colonize gastric mucosa that has undergone intestinal metaplasia thereby reducing the gastric acid secretion. Several HP strains have been identified. Factors related to bacterial virulence [cytotoxin CagA, vacuolating cytotoxin (VacA) and neutrophil activating factor (NAF)] may influence HP putative carcinogenic potential. Strain-specific genetic diversity is thought to be involved in the organism's ability to cause different diseases, although subjects may be infected with multiple strains and no clustering of disease-specific strains have been shown so far.

Colonization of the gastric mucosa with HP is widespread. Very high infection rates (80%–90%) have been found in many populations in developing countries. In developed populations the prevalence is lower (30%–50%), notably among children. The annual incidence has been estimated to be 0.3%–0.7% in developed countries and 6%–14% in developing countries, including primary acquisition of infection or reinfection after successful eradication. However, HP acquisition and transmission pathways are not fully elucidated (GOODMAN and COCKBURN 2001). Direct person-to-person is possible, but the relative importance of fecal–oral, oral–oral or gastric–oral (through vomiting) routes are not well established. Transmission by gastroenterologic medical procedures has been documented. Waterborne transmission has been suggested, while vectorborne transmission is unlikely. Host factors that facilitate acquisition and transmission of infection are not well identified. (BROWN 2000). The prevalence of the infection is inversely related to socioeconomic level and hygiene practices, and directly related to age. On the contrary, the HP prevalence seems not to be related to gender, ethnicity, or geography. Inconsistent associations have been found with smoking, alcohol consumption, dietary habits, and occupational exposures. The prevalence of HP exposure increases with age, translating the cumulative risk of acquisition, and tends to decrease with birth cohort, probably in relation to the increasing socioeconomic level. Children are particularly vulnerable to exposure, notably whenever poor socioeconomic conditions occur (crowding, sharing beds, institutionalized children).

The relationship between HP infections and gastric cancer in humans was reviewed in 1994 by the Monograph program at IARC, which considered HP to be a human carcinogen (Class 1; IARC 1994).

The prevalence of HP in gastric cancer, as determined by histology, ranged from 40% to 80% in most populations similar for the incidence of intestinal and diffuse types of gastric carcinomas. Case-control studies of gastric cancer have provided risk estimates ranging from nonsignificant OR of 1.5 to significant ORs of five- to sixfold increase in risk for HP carriers. Part of the variability in results is attributable to the different sensibility and specificity of methods of detection of HP (LOGAN and WALKER 2001). These included methods based on gastric biopsies (histological examination, culture and rapid urease test), methods based on breath samples (urea breath test), methods based on serological assays (usually used in large epidemiological studies), and methods based on stool and saliva specimens, which are still in development.

A recent combined analysis of case-control studies nested within cohorts including over 1,200 cases of gastric cancer concluded that the association of HP is largely restricted to gastric cancers arising in nongastric cardia and that the best estimate of the association for this anatomic site is an OR of sixfold. HP was not related to an increased risk of gastric cardia. The study indicated also that several HP markers of exposure are lost during the carcinogenic process. As a consequence, case-control studies that evaluated HP close to the time of cancer diagnosis may substantially decrease the prevalence estimates in the cases and the magnitude of the risk (HELICOBACTER AND CANCER COLLABORATIVE GROUP 2001). The conclusions are consistent with the results of follow-up studies in high risk countries (UEMURA et al. 2001).

A specific relationship has been established between HP infections and the relatively rare gastric lymphoma, a clinical entity that seems to originate in the lymphocytes infiltrating the gastric mucosa following HP infestation. The OR for gastric lymphoma related to HP seropositivity was estimated to be a sixfold increase in a nested case-control study in Norway and the United States. (PARSONNET et al. 1994). Antibiotic treatment has been shown to achieve eradication of *H. pylori* and histological regression of localized low-grade MALT gastric lymphoma in over 60% of patients (ZUCCA and ROGGERO 1996).

I. Opportunities for Prevention of Gastric Cancer

Links between *Helicobacter pylori* and gastric cancer have prompted intervention trials using active antimicrobial therapy with the aim of reducing the burden of infection and hopefully of HP-related cancers.

Treatment of HP infections with combinations of antibiotics and acid inhibitors successfully limits the infection and eventually eradicates the bacteria from the stomach. However, at the population level, eradication has proven to be a difficult task. Reinfections occur often and sensitivity of the bacteria to antibiotics is less obvious in vivo that it is in vitro. Better success has been achieved in the treatment of other HP-related conditions such as duodenal ulcer and gastric lymphoma. Prevention of gastric cancer following interventions to eradicate HP infections at the population level has not been achieved even in limited size controlled studies.

HP vaccination is being investigated actively following the characterization of the natural immune response that follows HP infections. However, as it is currently known, immune response does not eradicate current infections and it is thus uncertain what the mechanisms of prevention should target. Some animal experiments in mice (a species that has species-specific *Helicobacter* infection) Mongolian gerbils, and beagle dogs have provided encouraging results. Meanwhile, the best approach for the prevention of gastric cancer risk is to encourage the consumption of vegetables and fruits, to decrease the intake of preserved foods (salted and smoked) and to avoid smoking.

E. Epstein-Barr Virus, Other Infections and Malignant Lymphomas

The role of infectious agents in lymphomas has been suspected for a long time, following repeated observations of apparent clusters of cases in certain geographical and familial settings and the variation in the age-specific incidence rates in different populations. However, the confirmation of the cluster observation over and above the spontaneous occurrence of random clusters and the identification of a biological agent responsible for a sensible fraction of the cases has remained elusive. More recently, two observations triggered a wealth of epidemiological research. The first observation was the confirmation of a significant increase in the cases of lymphomas over time in many populations, as reported by cancer registries (Cartwright et al. 1999; Hartge et al. 1994). The second observation was that immune suppressed subjects (either because of therapeutic suppression following transplants or because of HIV infections) were at an increased risk of cancer, notably of lymphomas (Swinnen 2000). The results to date seem to point at a certain number of different biological agents involved in the pathogenesis of lymphomas. These are the Epstein-Barr virus (EBV), the human immunodeficiency virus (HIV), the human herpes virus type 8 (HHV-8), and the human T-cell leukemia and lymphoma virus (HTLV-1). The bacteria *Helicobacter pylori* (HP) has also been related to MALT gastric lymphoma. Other agents that may also play a role are HCV, *Borrelia vincentii*, *Vibrio cholerae*, *Strongyloides stercolaris* and *Plasmodium falciparum*.

EBV is a γ herpes virus endemic in the human population that infects B-cells. By the third decade of life, more than 80% of the adult population have been infected with EBV through breastfeeding and saliva. In developing countries primary infection generally takes place in the first years of life, while in developed societies, primary infection is often delayed until adolescence. About half of these cases will be diagnosed with infectious mononucleosis. EBV will persist lifelong in its host in a latent form in the resting memory B cells. In immune competent subjects, EBV persists in the host through periodic reactivation of the latently infected memory B-cell. Healthy carriers of EBV will have detectable antibodies to the capside proteins of the virus (VCA, gp350 and EBNA-1). The latent viral gene products of EBV are the EBV nuclear antigens (EBNA-1, -2 and -3), latent membrane protein (LMP-1 and -2) and EBV-encoded RNA (EBER-1 and 2). These proteins will be expressed in the tumor cells with specific latency patterns in different EBV-related diseases. Disrupture of the immune system is a key factor to trigger viral replication and establishment of cell transformation. The EBV-related lymphoid malignancies can be diagnosed as Hodgkin's lymphoma (HL), B-cell lymphoma, and T-cell lymphoma and they are common among immuno-suppressed patients (PALLESEN et al. 1993).

Expression of latent viral proteins EBER and LMP is observed in about half of the cases with Hodgkin's lymphoma. However, HL cases negative for EBV in the tumoral tissue have EBV-specific CTL in the blood (DOLCETTI et al. 1995) suggesting that no detection of EBV in the tumor does not exclude EBV as a cause of the cellular damage. Other interesting aspects that strongly supports the association of EBV and HL is the repeated observation that recent history of infectious mononucleosis increases about threefold the risk for HL and that in some reports, antibody titers against the EBV capside increase before the onset of disease (MUELLER et al. 1989, IARC 1997).

Within B-cell lymphomas, EBV is consistently associated to Burkitt's lymphoma (BL) occurring in endemic areas of Plasmodium Falciparum. The EBV expression in tumor cells of BL is characteristically restricted to EBERs and EBNA-1 but not LMP. EBV will be detected in only 10%–20% of sporadic BL cases, in about 40% of HIV associated B-cell lymphomas, and in the majority of B-cell lymphomas arising in iatrogenic immune suppressed patients (JAFFE et al. 2001). The contribution of EBV in other B-cell lymphomas in immune competent subjects is still under research.

Within lymphomas of T-cell origin, sinonasal T-cell lymphomas has been consistently associated to EBV. Other extranodal T-cell lymphomas have a wide range of EBV positivity (18%–70%) depending on the histological type. Angioimmunoblastic lymphomas generally are EBV positive, while mycosis fungoides is rarely associated to EBV.

Patients with a severe impairment of the cell-mediated immunity like organ-transplanted recipients or AIDS patients undergo an inhibition of the cytotoxic T-lymphocytes which leads to an outgrowth of EBV-infected B-lymphocytes. This may derive into AIDS-related lymphomas (ARL) and posttransplant lymphoproliferative disorders (PTLD). HIV-1 is generally the immunosuppression viral type involved (IARC 1996). About 3%–5% of the patients with HIV will develop a LN as a first AIDS-defining disease which represents a 60- to 200-fold increased risk for developing a lymphoma compared to the general population (Jaffe et al. 2001). The ARL are not clinically different from those occurring in immune competent patients, although they tend to be aggressive B-cell lymphomas and more than 40% occur in uncommon sites such as the brain or the heart (Levine et al. 1992). In countries where highly active antiretroviral therapy is being used, a decrease of incidence of LN in these locations has been reported. The mechanisms of action of HIV in the pathogenesis of lymphoma is suggested to be a multistep one. HIV patients seem to have chronic antigen stimulation, multiple genetic abnormalities, increased release of cytokines IL6 and IL10, and a high prevalence of EBV or HHV-8. EBV biomarkers are found in more than 60% of HIV-related lymphomas, but particularly in central nervous system lymphomas, primary effusion lymphomas and immunoblastic diffuse large B-cell lymphomas. Almost all HL cases occurring in HIV patients are also EBV positive. HHV-8 related lymphoma are almost always seen in the context of HIV infected patients.

PTLD and posttransplant lymphomas (PTL) are generally associated with EBV infection and are due to the proliferation of B-cell due to the immunosuppressive therapy. PTLD tend to regress with reduction of the immune suppression. In contrast, PTL have a poor prognosis and occur in 0.7%–6% of the organ-transplant recipients. The majority of the PTL originate in the host and are likely to be diagnosed within the first years after the allograft. Early monitoring for EBV reactivation has been reported to be a marker of future lymphoma development. The fact that the risk of lymphoma is allograft-site-dependent has been related to the intensity of the immunosuppression. Heart transplant patients receive a very aggressive immunosuppressive therapy and have a risk for lymphoma that is around six times higher than the risk observed among patients receiving a liver or kidney transplant. This risk is 35-fold higher when heart-allografted patients are compared to the general population (Domingo-Domenech et al. 2001).

Kaposi's sarcoma-associated herpes virus, also known as human herpes virus 8 (HHV-8) has been shown to be causally associated with Kaposi's sarcoma, primary effusion lymphoma and multicentric Castleman's disease. Like EBV, HHV-8 is a γ herpes virus that contains some genes similar to other well known viral and cellular oncogenes and growth controlling factors (interleukin 6, bcl2, D-type cyclin and a chemokine receptor). These genes are believed to affect cell proliferation, cell transformation, and have also antiapoptotic properties. HHV-8 is found in B-cells, macrophages and dendritic cells and like EBV, will establish latency in the host cells (IARC 1997).

Kaposi's sarcoma in its classic form is a tumor arising in the skin, generally of the lower limbs and has an indolent evolution. KS in immunosuppressed subjects is more aggressive, tends to spread to internal organs, and has a short survival time. However, if the immune suppression is restored soon after diagnosis of KS, the tumor can regress. In geographical regions where HHV-8 is endemic, e.g., Italy, Israel, and sub-Saharan Africa, KS is also a common tumor in its classical form. Since the epidemic of HIV, the incidence of KS around the world parallels the incidence of AIDS (WHITBY et al. 1998). HHV-8 DNA is generally detected in all the cells of Kaposi's lesions and the serological response to HHV-8 consistently shows higher response in affected patients as compared to controls. The infection seems also to precede the development of the disease.

All cancer cells of primary effusion lymphoma (PEL) harbor HHV-8 and in many occasions also EBV. This is a rare condition that develops in severely affected HIV patients in HHV-8 endemic areas and in allografted patients. Multiple myeloma has been associated in some cases to the detection of HHV-8 in tumor cells; however, results are inconsistent. Multicentric Castleman's disease is a lymphoproliferative disorder described in HIV patients who also tend to develop HHV-8 related KS.

The monograph program has classified HHV-8 as a probable carcinogen (Group 2A) owing to the scarcity of studies in humans (IARC 1997).

Hepatitis C virus (HCV) has been related to lymphoplasmacytic lymphomas associated with type II cryoglobulinemia and with some lymphomas of the liver and salivary glands. In one study, the risk of B-cell lymphoma was three times higher among individuals with anti-HCV and the prevalence of anti-HCV among the subgroup of lymphoplasmacytic lymphomas was as high as 30% (SILVESTRI et al. 1996). Another study reported a higher prevalence of HCV among patients with low grade lymphoma as compared to those with intermediate grade or high grade (MAZZARO et al. 1996). It has been hypothesized that HCV could act as H pylori or EBV in inducing benign lymphoproliferative disorders. The persistence of the infection could in the long run generate genetic instability leading to malignant proliferation (PERSING and PRENDERGAST 1999). *Borrelia burgdorferi* has been implicated in the pathogenesis of cutaneous MALT lymphomas and mixed bacterial infections in intestinal MALT lymphoma associated with immunoproliferative small intestinal diseases (PRICE 1990).

Finally, HTLV-1 infections are associated with T-cell leukemia and lymphomas particularly in Japan, Africa and in the Caribbean. This association is very rare in other world's regions.

F. Epstein-Barr Virus, Nasopharyngeal Carcinoma and Other Cancers

Nasopharyngeal carcinoma (NPC) is a rare cancer arising in the lymphoid rich tissue of the Rosenmuller fossa or the roof of the nasopharynx.

High incidence rates correspond to regions in Southern China, the Inuit populations in Alaska and Greenland, other countries in South East Asia, and a belt in Northern Africa and the Middle East countries. (Parkin et al. 1997). Migrant studies tend to confirm that first generation migrants retain the risk levels of their populations of origin. NPC incidence increases with age in most populations; however, as is the case with HD, a peak in incidence has been observed in adolescents in several populations at low/moderate risk. Additional established risk factors for NPC are the Chinese-style salted fish, other preserved foods, and smoking. Genetic factors may operate in some populations, although definite biomarkers of risk have not been identified.

Epidemiological studies on EBV and NPC are difficult to conduct due to the relatively rarity of the tumor in most populations, the diversity of the biomarkers that have been used, and the widespread exposure of the human population to the virus. A limited number of case-control studies have been reported from high-risk populations in China, most of which were based on the presence of antibodies to the viral capsid antigen (VCA). Most of the studies found high relative risks (i.e., >10) and, in some, dose response relationships were observed with antibody titers. Serological surveys have reported a high incidence of NPC among anti-VCA carriers. Molecular studies showed that EBV DNA is regularly found in NPC cells, and in virtually all the undifferentiated carcinomas, but not in the normal epithelium of the nasopharynx. Tumors are monoclonal, and all cancerous cells retain EBV DNA.

An increasing number of reports have suggested the association of EBV with gastric cancer. The proportion of gastric carcinoma that show EBV markers range from 16.8% in Chile (Corvalan et al. 2001) to 6.9% in Japan (Tokunaga et al. 1993a). However, the geographic variation of gastric cancer rates within nine Japanese cities does not correlate with EBV prevalence (Tokunaga et al. 1993b). Associations with histological type and anatomical subsite are inconsistent. It is possible that EBV infection is involved in some gastric carcinoma mainly with lymphoid stroma (termed lymphoepithelioma-like carcinoma). An etiological role of EBV in lymphoepithelial and adenocarcinomas has not been conclusively established yet (IARC 1997).

The IARC monograph reviewed the carcinogenicity of EBV and classified it as a human carcinogen (class 1) related to BL, HL, lymphoma in the immunosuppressed, NPC and sinonasal angiocentric T-cell-lymphoma (IARC 1997).

G. Cancer Incidence in HIV-Infected Persons

In the year 2000, approximately 36 million adults worldwide were HIV-positive and rising incidence rates were reported in India, Africa, and Latin America. Since 1993, three cancer sites were recognized as AIDS-defining conditions among HIV-positive subjects. These were Kaposi's sarcoma, non-Hodgkin's lymphoma, and invasive cervical cancer. However, HIV-infected patients have been consistently associated with an increased risk of other

Table 3. Cancer and HIV: linkage studies in the United States (SELIK and RABKIN 1998)

Cancer site	RR
Kaposi	1 322
NHL	136
HD	11
Rectal	6.8
Lung	2.8
Oral	2.0
Leukemia	1.7
Males	**RR**
Testicular	4.1
M. Myeloma	3.0
Bone/sarcoma	2.1
Liver	1.9
Females	**RR**
Larynx	28
Cervical	5.5
Uterine	4.5
Kidney/bladder	2.7

cancer sites, most of which are related to coinfections with oncogenic viruses. Table 3 summarizes the results of a very large linkage study in the US in which mortality registries in young adults were linked to AIDS registries. The excess mortality related to cancer was computed by comparisons to expected numbers from a reference population. Patients with HIV or AIDS were found to be at increased risk of Kaposi's sarcoma, non-Hodgkin's lymphoma, Hodgkin's lymphoma, and cervical cancer. These patients were also found to be at moderately increased risk of rectal cancer, lung and oral cancers, and leukemias. HIV-positive men showed, in addition, an increased risk of testicular cancer, multiple myeloma, bone cancer, a range of sarcomas, and liver cancer. HIV-positive women showed an increased risk of uterine and cervical cancer, bladder cancers, and cancer of the larynx. These population-based observations found confirmation and additional support in a substantial number of case-control and cohort studies that have increased the list of associated cancers to include childhood leiomyosarcomas and conjunctival cancer. Occasional moderate excess in incidence has been reported for skin, breast, brain, and thyroid cancers (LI et al. 2002; BERAL and NEWTON 1998).

Liver cancer is not commonly found in excess in HIV-positive cohorts, or in case-control studies. The negative finding is consistent in the United States cohorts and in South Africa, a country with high rates of HIV and early exposure to HBV (SITAS et al. 2000). The singularity of liver cancer model suggests that an intact immune response is of importance in the mechanisms of HBV or HCV carcinogenesis. It also underlines the complexity of the viral/host interactions in the carcinogenic process.

I. Anogenital Cancer in HIV-Positive and AIDS Patients

Cervical cancer was included among the AIDS-defining conditions in January 1993. Although some studies failed to observe an increased risk, there is growing evidence of an interaction between the two infections in causing cervical and other anogenital cancers (PALEFSKY 1994).

Among women with AIDS reported to the Italian AIDS-Registry between 1993 and 1995, the frequency of cervical cancer as one of the AIDS-defining conditions was nearly three times higher among intravenous drug users than those infected by heterosexual contact. In Italy, the linkage of the National AIDS Registry and the populations cancer registries showed a 15-fold increased risk for cervical cancer for women with AIDS (FRANCESCHI et al. 1998). The joint Italian–French follow-up study of HIV-positive women also showed a 13-fold increased rate of cervical cancer for HIV-positive women (SERRAINO et al. 1999). In Spain, the Catalonian AIDS surveillance system detected 58 cases of invasive cervical cancer among 823 HIV-positive women, an 18-fold increased risk as compared to the general population (VALL MAYANS and DE SANJOSÉ 2000). FRUCHTER reported that HIV-positive women in New York had a threefold increase in invasive cervical cancer as compared to HIV-negative women. Independent predictors of cervical cancer were the duration of symptoms and lack of screening (FRUCHTER et al. 1998). Similarly, CHIN in the United States reported an increased risk of cervical cancer among black and Hispanic women in the Sentinel Hospital Surveillance System (CHIN et al. 1999). SITAS in South Africa reported an increased risk of cervical (OR: 1.6) and vulvar (OR: 4.8) cancer among HIV-1 infected patients as compared to hospital controls (SITAS et al. 2000).

Anal cancer is a tumor that is more common in women than in men. Homosexual men and HIV-positive homosexual men have considerably higher rates of anal cancer than any other sexually active group (PALEFSKY 2000). Rates of anal cancer have been reported to increase in homosexual population groups and communities long before the AIDS epidemic (PALEFSKY, 1994).

With the AIDS epidemic, anal cytology became a recommended screening procedure in high-risk groups. Anal preneoplastic lesions are often seen in HIV-infected people, in those with high HIV load, and in women with an abnormal cervical cytology (HOLLY et al. 2001). The AIDS-CANCER MATCH REGISTRY in the United States has been collecting data since 1978 and indicates that in the anogenital region, anal cancer is the site most commonly seen in HIV infected people (FRISCH and GOODMAN 2000). A large proportion of cases with anal preneoplastic lesions or invasive cancer will have an HPV-associated infection (MELBYE et al. 1990). The mechanisms of HIV and HPV interaction are under research.

II. Opportunities for Prevention of HIV-Associated Cancers

Awareness of the most common cancers in developing HIV-positive persons and AIDS patients calls for organ specific surveillance protocols. Screening for anogenital neoplasm by clinical inspection, and cytology with or without HPV testing may prevent some invasive cancers in long-term AIDS survivors. More research is warranted among long term HIV carriers to investigate the occurrence of other cancers and in exploring the presence of viral markers in cancers that at present are not suspected of having a viral origin and yet occur with increased frequency among HIV carriers.

H. Conclusion

The recognition that 15%–20% of human cancers are related to infectious agents represented a major progress in the understanding of cancer etiology and is opening challenging new perspectives in cancer prevention.

Acknowledgments. The authors acknowledge with gratitude the contributions of Mireia Diaz in elaborating incidence and mortality data and of Cristina Rajo in the preparation of the manuscript. Partial support has been granted by the Fondo de Investigaciones Sanitarias of the Spanish government FIS 01/1237.

References

ALTS Study Group (The Atypical Squamous Cell of Undetermined Significance/Low-grade squamous Intraepithelial Lesions Triage Study Group) (2000) Human Papillomavirus Testing for Triage of Women With Cytologic Evidence of Low-Grade Squamous Intraepithelial Lesions: Baseline Data From a Randomized Trial. J Natl Cancer Inst 92(5): 397–402

Beral V, Newton R (1998) Overview of the Epidemiology of Immunodeficiency-Associated Cancers. J Natl Cancer Inst Monogr 23:1–6

Bosch FX, Manos MM, Muñoz N, Sherman M, Jansen AM, Peto J, Schiffman MH, Moreno V, Kurman R, Shah KV, International biological Study on Cervical Cancer (IBSCC) Study Group (1995) Prevalence of Human Papillomavirus Cervical Cancer: a Worldwide Perspective. J Natl Cancer Inst 87(11): 796–802

Bosch FX, Ribes J, Borras J (1999) Epidemiology of Primary Liver Cancer. Semin Liver Dis, 19:271–285

Bosch FX, Rohan T, Schneider A, Frazer I, Pfister H, Castellsagué X, de Sanjosé S, Moreno V, Puig-Tintoré LM, Smith PG, Muñoz N, Zur Hausen H (2001) Papillomavirus research update: highlights of the Barcelona HPV 2000 International Papillomavirus Conference. J Clin Pathol 54(1): 163–175

Bréchot C, Jaffredo F, Lagorce D, Gerken G, Büschenfelde KM, Papakonstontinou A, Hadziyannis S, Romeo R, Colombo M, Rodes J, Bruix J, Williams R, Naoumov N (1998) Impact of HBV, HCV and GBV-C/HGV on hepatocellular carcinomas in Europe: results of a European concerted action. J Hepatol 29:173–183.

Brown ML (2000) *Helicobacter pylori*: Epidemiology and routes of transmission. Epidemiologic Reviews 22:293–297

Cartwright R, Brincker H, Carli PM, Clayden D, Coebergh JW, Jack AD, McNally R, Morgan G, de Sanjosé S, Tumino R, Vornanen M (1999) The rise in incidence of lymphomas in Europe 1985–1992. Eur J Cancer 35:627–633

Castellsagué X, Menéndez C, Loscertales M-P, Kornegay R, dos Santos F, Gómez-Olivé FX, Lloveras B, Abarca N, Vaz N, Barreto A, Bosch FX, Alonso P (2001) Human papillomavirus genotypes in rural Mozambique. Lancet 358:1429

Chang MH, Chen ChJ, Lai MS, Hsu HM, Wu TC, Kong MS, Liang DC, Shau WY, Chen DS (1998) Universal Hepatitis B Vaccination in Taiwan and The Incidence of Hepatocellular Carcioma in Children. New Engl J Med 336(26): 1855–1907

Chin PL, Chu DZ, Clarke KG, Odom-Maryon T, Yen Y, Wagman LD (1999) Ethnic differences in the behavior of hepatocellular carcinoma. Cancer 85:1931–1936.

Corvalan A, Koriyama C, Akiba S, Eizuru Y, Backhouse C, Palma M, Argandona J, Tokunaga M (2001) Epstein-Barr virus in gastric carcinoma is associated with location in the cardia and with a diffuse histology: a study in one area of Chile. Int J Cancer 94(4): 527–530

Dolcetti R, Gloghini A, de Vita S, Vaccher E, de Re V, Tirelli U, Carbone A, Boiocchi M (1995) Characteristics of EBV-infected cells in HIV-related lymphadenopathy: implications for the pathogenesis of EBV-associated and EBV-unrelated lymphomas of HIV-seropositive individuals. Int J Cancer 63:652–659

Domingo-Domenech, E, de Sanjosé S, González Barca E, Romagosa V, Domingo-Clarós A, il-Vernet S, Figueras J, Manito N, Otón B, Petit J, Grañena A, Fernández de Sevilla A (2001) Post-transplant lymphomas: a 20-year epidemiologic, clinical and pathologic study in a single center. Haematologica 86:715–721

Donato F, Boffetta P, Puoti M (1998) A meta-analysis of epidemiological studies on the combined effect of hepatitis B and C virus infections in causing hepatocellular carcinoma. Int J Cancer 75:347–354

Fortuin M, Chotard J, Jack AD, Maine NP, Mendy M, Hall AJ, Inskip HM, Ceorge MO, Whittle HC (1993) Efficacy of hepatitis B vaccine in the Gambian expanded programme on immunisation. Lancet 341:1129–31

Franceschi S, Dal Maso L, Arniani S, Crosignani P, Vercelli M, Simonato L, Falcini F, Zanetti R, Barchielli A, Serraino D, Rezza G for the Cancer and AIDS Registry Linkage Study (1998) Br J Cancer 78(7): 966–970

Frank C, Mohamed MK, Strickland GT, Lavanchy D, Arthur RR, Magder LS, El-Khoby T, Abdel Wahab Y, Aly Ohn ES, Anwar W, Sallam I (2000) The role of parenteral antischistosomal therapy in the spread of hepatitis C virus in Egypt. Lancet 355: 887–891

Frisch M, Goodman MT (2000) Human Papilllomavirus-associated carcinomas in Hawaii and the Mainland U.S. Cancer 88:1464–1469

Fruchter RG, Maiman M, Arrastia CD, Matthews R, Gates EJ, Holcomb K (1998) Is HIV infection a risk factor for advanced cervical cancer? J Acquir Immune Defic Syndr Hum Retrovirol 18(3):241–5

Goedert JJ ed. (2000) Infectious Causes of Cancer. Targets for Intervention. Humana Press, New Jersey

Gonzalez A, Esteban JI, Madoz P, Viladomiu L, Genesca J, Muniz E, Enriquez J, Torras X, Hernandez JM, Quer J, et al. (1995) Efficacy of screening donors for antibodies to the hepatitis C virus to prevent transfusion-associated hepatitis: final report of a prospective trial. Hepaology 22:439–445

Goodman KJ, Cockburn M (2001) The role of epidemiology in understanding the health effects of *Helicobacter pylori*. Epidemiology 12:266–271

Hagan H, Jarlais DC, Friedman SR, Purchase D, Alter MJ (1995) Reduced risk of hepatitis B and hepatitis C among injection drug users in the Tacoma syringe exchange program. Am J Public Health 85:1531–1537

Hagan H, McGough JP, Thiede H, Weiss NS, Hopkins S, Alexander ER (1999) Syringe exchange and risk of infection with hepatitis B and C viruses. Am J Epidemiol 149(3):203–313.

Hartge P, Devesa SS, Fraumeni Jr. J F (1994) Hodgkin's and Non-Hodgkin's Lymphomas. Cancer Surv 19/20:423–453

Helicobacter and Cancer Collaborative Group (2001) Gastric cancer and *Helicobacter pylori*: a combined analysis of 12 case control studies nested within prospective cohorts. Gut 49:347–353

Herrero R, Hildesheim A, Bratti C, Sherman ME, Hutchinson M, Morales J, Balmaceda I, Greenberg MD, Alfaro M, Burk RD, Wacholder S, Plummer M, Schiffman M (2000) Population-Based Study of Human Papillomavirus Infection and Cervical Neoplasia in Rural Costa Rica. J Natl Cancer Inst 92(6): 464–474

Hildesheim A, Schiffman M, Bromley C, Wacholder S, Herrero R, Rodriguez AC, Bratti MC, Sherman ME, Scarpidis U, Lin QQ, Terai M, Bromley RL, Buetow K, Apple RJ, Burk RD (2001) Human Papillomavirus Type 16 Variants and Risk of Cervical Cancer. J Natl Cancer Inst 93(4): 315–318

Holly EA, Ralston ML, Darragh TM, Greenblatt RM, Jay N, Palefsky JM (2001) Prevalence and Risk Factors for Anal Squamous Intraepithelial Lesions in Women. J Natl Cancer Inst 93(11): 843–849

IARC (1992) The Epidemiology of Cervical Cancer and Human Papillomavirus. Muñoz N, Bosch FX, Shah KV, Meheus A eds. Vol. 119. IARC Scientific Publications, International Agency for Research on Cancer, Lyon

IARC (1994) Hepatitis Viruses. IARC Monographs on the evaluation of carcinogenic risks to humans. Vol. 59. IARC Scientific Publications, International Agency for Research on Cancer, Lyon

IARC (1995) Human Papillomaviruses. Vol. 64. IARC monographs on the evaluation of carcinogenic risks to humans, IARC Scientific Publications, International Agency for Research on Cancer, Lyon

IARC (1996) Human Immunodeficiency Viruses and Human T-cell Lymphotropic Viruses. Vol. 67. IARC monographs on the evaluation of carcinogenic risks to humans, International Agency for Research on Cancer, Lyon

IARC (1997) Epstein-Barr virus and Kaposi's sarcoma Herpesvirus/Human Herpesvirus 8 Vol. 70. IARC monographs on the evaluation of carcinogenic risks to humans, International Agency for Research on Cancer, Lyon

Jaffe E, Lee Harris N, Stein H, Vardiman JW (2001) Pathology & Genetics. Tumours of Haematopoietic and Lymphoid Tissues. IARC Press, Lyon

Kjaer SK, Van der Brule AJC, Boch JE, Poll PA, Poll PA, Sherman ME, Walboomers JMM, Meijer CJLM (1996) Human papillomavirus–the most significant risk determinant of cervical intraepithelial neoplasia. Int J Cancer 65, 601–606

Lee MS, Kim DH, Kim H, Lee HS, Kim CY, Park TS, Yoo KY, Park BJ, Ahn YO (1998) Hepatitis B vaccination and reduced risk of primary liver cancer among male adults: a cohort study in Korea. Int J Epidemiol 27(2):316–319

Levine AM, Shibata D, Sullivan-Halley J, Nathwani B, Brynes R, Slovak,ML, Mahterian S, Lynn Riley C, Weiss L, Levine PH, Rasheed S, Bernstein L (1992) Epidemiological and biological study of acquired immunodeficiency syndrome-related lymphoma in the country of Los Angeles: preliminary results. Cancer Research 52:5482–5484

Li Y, Law M, McDonald A, Correll P, Kaldor JM, Grulich AE (2002) Estimation of Risk of Cancers before Occurrence of Acquired Immunodeficiency Syndrome in Persons Infected with Human Immunodeficiency Virus. Am J Epidemiol 155(2): 153–158

Liaw KL, Hsing AW, Chen C-J, Schiffman MH, Zhang TY, Hsieh CY, Greer CE, You SL, Huang TW, Wu TC, O'Leary TJ, Seidman JD, Blot WJ, Meinert CL and Manos MM (1995) Human papillomavirus and cervical neoplasia: a case-control study in Taiwan Int J Cancer 62:565–571

Logan RP, Walker MM (2001) ABC of the upper gastrointestinal tract: Epidemiology and diagnosis of *Helicobacter pylori* infection. BMJ 323(7318): 920–922

Mazzaro C, Zagonel V, Monfardini S, Tulissi P, Pussini E, Fanni M, Sorio R, Bortolus R, Crovatto M, Santini G, Tiribelli C, Sasso F, Masutti R, Pozzato G (1996) Hepatitis C virus and non-Hodgkin's lymphomas. Br J Haematol 77(12):2604–2613

Melbye M, Palefsky JM, Gonzales J, Ryder LP, Nielsen H, Bergmann O, Pindborg J, Biggar RJ. (1990) Immune status as a determinant of human papillomavirus detection and its association with anal epithelial abnormalities. Int J Cancer 46:203–206

Moreno V, Muñoz N, Bosch FX, De Sanjosé S, Gonzalez LC, Tafur L, Gili M, Izarzugaza I, Navarro C, Vergara A, Viladiu P, Ascunce N and Shah K (1995) Risk factors for progression of cervical intraepithelial neoplasm grade III to invasive cervical cancer. Cancer Epidemiol Biomark Prev 4:459–467

Mueller N, Evans A, Harris NL, Comstock GW, Jellum E, Magnus K, Orentreich N, Polk BF, Vogelman J (1989) Hodgkin's disease and Epstein Barr virus. Altered antibody pattern before diagnosis. N Engl J Med 320:689–695
NIH Consensus Development Panel (1996) National Institutes of Health Consensus Development Conference Statement: Cervical Cancer, April 1–3, 1996 J Natl Cancer Inst Monographs 21:7–13
Newton R, Beral V, Weiss RA, Tooze J ed. (1999) Infections and Human Cancer. Vol. 33 Cancer Surveys. Cold Spring Harbor Laboratory Press, USA
Okuda K (1991) Hepatitis C Virus and Hepatocellular Carcinoma. In: Tabor E, di Bisceglie AM, Purcell RH (Eds.) Etiology, pathology, and treatment of hepatocellular carcinoma in North America. Chapter 9. PPC – Gulf Publishing Company, Houston, pp. 119–126.
Palefsky J (1994) Anal human papillomavirus infection and cancer in HIV-positive individuals. An emerging problem. AIDS 8:295
Palefsky M (2000) Anal squamous intraepithelial lesions in human immunodeficiency virus-positive men and women. Semin Oncol 27, 471–479
Pallesen G, Hamilton-Dutoit SJ, Zhou B (1993) The association of Epstein-Barr virus (EBV) with T-cell lymphoproliferations and Hosdgkin's disease: two new developments in the EBV field. Advances in Cancer Research Vol. 62 Academia Press Inc., pp. 179–239
Parkin DM, Whelan SL, Ferlay J, Raymond L, Young J (1997) Cancer Incidence in Five Continents. Vol. VII, No: 143. IARC Scientific Publications, Lyon
Parkin DM, Bray F, Ferlay J, Pisani P (2001) Estimating the world cancer burden: Globocan 2000. Int J Cancer 94:153–156
Parsonnet J., Hansen S, Rodriguez L, Gelb AB, Warnke RA, Jellum E, Orentreich N, Vogelman JH, Friedman GD (1994) Helicobacter pylori infection and gastric lymphoma. New Engl J Med 330:1267–1271
Persing DH, Prendergast FG (1999) Infection, Immunity and Cancer. Arch Pathol Lab Med 123:1015–1022
Price (1990) Immunoproliferative small intestinal disease: a study of 13 cases with alpha heavy-chain disease. Histopathology 17:7–17
Selik RM, Rabkin CS (1998) Cancer death rates associated with human immunodeficiency virus infection in the United States. J Natl Cancer Inst 90(17): 1300–1302
Serraino D, Carrieri P, Pradier,C, Bidoli E, Dorrucci M, Ghetti E, Shiesari A, Zucconi R, Pezzotti P, Dellamonica P, Franceschi S, Rezza G (1999) Risk of invasive cervical cancer among women with, or at risk for, HIV infection. Int J Cancer 82:334–337
Silvestri F, Pipan C, Barillari G, Zaja F, Fanin R, Infanti L, Russo D, Falasca E, Botta GA, Baccarani M (1996) Prevalence of Hepatitis C virus infection in patients with lymphoproliferative disorders. Blood 87:4296–4301
Sitas H, Bezwoda WR, Levin V, Ruff P, Kew MC, Hale MJ, Carrara H, Beral G, Fleming G, Odes R, Weaving A (2000) Association between human immunodeficiency virus type 1 infection and cancer in the black population of Johannesburg and Soweto, South Africa. Br J Cancer 75(11): 1704–1707
Swinnen LJ (2000) Posttransplant Lymphoproliferative Disorder. In: Goedert JJ ed. (2000) Infectious Causes of Cancer. Targets for Intervention. Humana Press, New Jersey pp. 63–76
Tabor E (1999) The epidemiology of virus transmission by plasma derivatives: clinical studies verifying the lack of transmission of hepatitis B and C viruses and HIV type 1. Transfussion 39:1160–1168
Thomas KK, Hughes JP, Kuypers JM, Kiviat NB, Lee SK, Adam DE, Koutsky LA (2000) Concurrent and sequential acquisition of different genital Human Papillomavirus types. J Infect Dis 182:1097–1102
Tokunaga M, Land CE, Uemura Y, Tokumode T, Tanaka S, Sato E (1993a) Epstein-Barr virus in gastric carcinoma. Am J Pathol 143(5): 1250–1254

Tokunaga M, Uemura Y, Tokudome T, Ishidate T, Masuda H, Ohazaka E, Kaneko K, Naoe S, Ito M, Okamura A et al. (1993b) Epstein-Barr virus related gastric cancer in Japan: a molecular patho-epidemiological study. Acta Pathol Lpn 43(10): 574–581

Vall Mayans M, de Sanjosé S (2000) El cáncer de cuello uterino y la influencia del VIH en su desarrollo en mujeres jovénes desfavorecidas socialmente. Med Clin 114: 656–657

van Damme P, Kne MA, Meheus A on behalf of the Viral Hepatitis Prevention Board (1997) Integration of hepatitis B vaccination into national immunisation programmes. BMJ 314:1033–1037

Uemura N, Okamoto S, Yamamoto S, Matsumura N, Yamaguchi S, Yamakido M, Taniyama K, Sasaki N, Schlemper RJ (2001) *Helicobacter Pylori* infection and the development of gastric cancer. N Engl J Med 345(11): 784–789

Walboomers JM, Jacobs MV, Manos MM, Bosch FX, Kummer JA, Shah KV, Snijders PJ, Peto J, Meijer CJ, Munoz N (1999) Human papillomavirus is a necessary cause of invasive cervical cancer worldwide. J Pathol 189(1): 12–19

Whitby D, Lluppi M, Barozzi P, Boshoff C, Weiss RA, Torelli G (1998) Human Herpesvirus 8 Seroprevalence in Blood Donors and Lymphoma Patients From Different Regions of Italy. J Natl Cancer Inst 90:395–397

Zucca E, Roggero E (1996) Biology and treatment of MALT lymphoma: the state-of-the-art in 1996. A workshop at the 6th International Conference on Malignant Lymphoma. Mucosa-Associated Lymphoid Tissue. Ann Oncol 7(8):787–792

CHAPTER 14

Xenobiotic Metabolism and Cancer Susceptibility

O. Pelkonen, K. Vähäkangas, and H. Raunio

A. Significance of Xenobiotic Metabolism in Carcinogenesis

Cancer formation is a very complex process involving changes in numerous genes (Akhurst and Balmain 1999; Sekido et al. 1999; Vähäkangas 2001). Any biological or mechanistic role of xenobiotic metabolizing genes (or rather, their products) in human cancer development must be considered against this basic principle. Consequently, research performed to date most probably gives only a very limited explanation of the associations between polymorphisms in xenobiotic metabolizing genes and individual susceptibility to cancer.

Most chemical carcinogens require metabolic activation for their carcinogenic effect. Customarily, metabolic activation has been linked with initiation, i.e., early phases, of the carcinogenic process. However, metabolic activation could play a role also in later phases of carcinogenesis and events following initiation give further chances for variation (Fig. 1).

Several lines of evidence indicate that metabolic activation and subsequent DNA binding of reactive metabolites is a necessary condition for chemical carcinogenesis. It is less clear, however, whether activation is a sufficient condition. Such steps as escape from repair (Friedberg et al 1995) and angiogenesis (deFlora et al. 2001; Dempke et al. 2001; Kuroi and Toi 2001) are required for the carcinogenic process to be completed. The most recent evidence for the importance of the activation comes from knockout mouse models. Mouse lines having disrupted genes encoding CYP1A2, CYP2E1, CYP1B1, microsomal epoxide hydrolase (mEH) and NADPH-quinone oxidoreductase have been established. None of these mice exhibit gross abnormal phenotypes, suggesting that the xenobiotic-metabolizing enzymes have no critical roles in mammalian development and physiological homeostasis. This explains why some of these genes are highly polymorphic in humans. In sharp contrast, these null mice do show marked difference in sensitivities to toxic outcomes including cancer formation, establishing the critical role of xenobiotic metabolism in chemical toxicities (Gonzalez and Kimura 2001).

There have been difficulties in extrapolating the results from the gene level to clinical significance. For enzyme activity, all levels, including the existence of the protein and the activity in enzyme assays, need to be studied before final conclusions can be made, because there may be no correlation

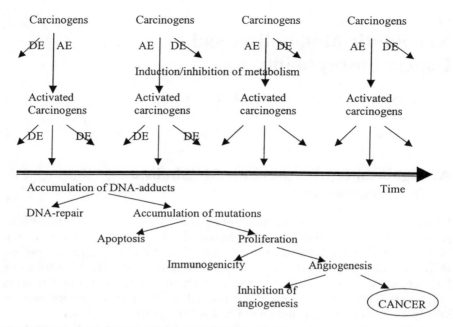

Fig. 1. Dynamic "rainfall" model of chemical carcinogenesis and the role of metabolism within. *AE*, activating enzyme; *DE*, deactivating enzyme

between mRNA and protein levels or protein levels with the enzyme activity (Williams 2001 and references within). In many cases, animal data precedes the human data. However, interspecies differences in metabolism cause difficulties in extrapolation from one species to another. A good example is tamoxifen which is a liver carcinogen in rat, but not in mouse regardless of similar metabolism and DNA binding, because the adducts accumulate only in rat which is also susceptible to the induction of cell proliferation by tamoxifen (Williams 2001).

The purpose of this chapter is to summarize the current knowledge about carcinogen metabolizing enzymes, metabolic activation, and DNA binding and to give examples of some of the more thoroughly characterized at-risk xenobiotic metabolizing genes. Emphasis is placed on the real or suspected biological links between the function of these genes and the outcomes studied. It should also be kept in mind that the activities of many xenobiotic-metabolizing enzymes depend not only on genotypes, but also vary due to externally caused enzyme induction or inhibition (Pelkonen et al. 1998).

B. Carcinogen Metabolism

Many carcinogens, including polycyclic aromatic hydrocarbons (PAHs), nitrosamines, aflatoxins and other mycotoxins, some alkylating agents and estrogens, are metabolized enzymatically to various metabolites, both reactive and detoxified. Both functionalization and conjugation reactions play a part in such an activation (GUENGERICH 2000; LANDI 2000). A variety of enzymes are involved (WILLIAMS and PHILLIPS 2000) of which cytochrome P450 (CYP) enzyme groups 1–3 are most important as xenobiotic metabolizing CYP forms (PELKONEN and RAUNIO 2000). Typically, oxidizing enzymes activate and conjugating enzymes detoxicate carcinogens and their metabolites. However, both oxidizing and conjugating enzymes can activate carcinogens to DNA binding metabolites (GUENGERICH 2000). For instance, in tamoxifen metabolism sulfotransferase-catalyzed formation of sulfate esters from α-hydroxytamoxifen is the activation step leading to DNA adducts (PHILLIPS 2001).

In addition to the well-known enzymes, like CYPs, GSTs and NATs, there are other enzymes that take part in carcinogen metabolism. WILLIAMS and PHILLIPS (2000) in their review on mammary expression of xenobiotic metabolizing enzymes pay attention to such enzymes as COMT inactivating catechol estrogens and lipoxygenase capable of aflatoxin B1 epoxidation in vitro. Myeloperoxidase, which can catalyze the activation of tobacco mutagens and environmental compounds to DNA-damaging metabolites, may be important in lung cancer etiology and is also polymorphic (WILLIAMS 2001). COX2, through the formation of endoperoxides, also catalyzes the activation of carcinogens (DEMPKE et al. 2001). Even minor, tissue-specific metabolic pathways may be very significant considering the toxicity of a compound. In the metabolism of benzo(a)pyrene, the best characterized PAH, the pathway leading to 7,8-diol-9,10-oxide (bay-region diolepoxide) represents only about 1% of the total metabolism and yet is the major activating pathway for the carcinogenic effect (PELKONEN and NEBERT 1982).

C. Significance of DNA Binding

According to the current understanding, DNA binding of activated carcinogens is essential for the carcinogenic effect (GELBOIN 1980; PELKONEN and NEBERT 1982; VÄHÄKANGAS and PELKONEN 1989; GUENGERICH 2000). It has been shown already in the seventies that the extent of DNA binding in rat liver correlates well with the potency of the carcinogenic effect in mouse skin (LUTZ 1979, in HEMMINKI et al. 2000). DNA adducts can be found in human tissues, also in the target tissue of the carcinogenic effect, and correlation between the number of adducts with the level of exposure can be found in molecular epidemiology studies (POIRIER et al. 2000; HEMMINKI et al. 2000). Although the relationship of DNA adducts and cancer is by no means simple, it is recognized that DNA adducts relate to genetic changes, which are the common denominator of malignant processes. However, the relationship between DNA adduct formation and human cancer risk awaits further studies for final conclusions (POIRIER et al. 2000).

It is notable that DNA adducts may be generated from internal processes in addition to the external carcinogens (GUENGERICH 2000). For instance, etheno-adducts can be from both internal (lipid peroxidation) and external (vinyl chloride, ethyl carbamate) sources (BARBIN 2000). Another example is the activation of estrogens to DNA-binding species (LIEHR 2000; WILLIAMS and PHILLIPS 2000). Furthermore, oxidation of arachidonic acid leads to highly reactive by-products capable of forming DNA adducts (DEMPKE et al. 2001).

Unrepaired DNA binding may lead to mutations and in a few cases muta-tions found in human cancer tissue within the TP53 gene, which is the most mutated in human cancers (HOLLSTEIN et al. 1991; GREENBLATT et al 1994; HERNANDEZ-BOUSSARD and HAINAUT 1998; HAINAUT and HOLLSTEIN 2000) clearly associate with exposure to an external carcinogen (HAINAUT and VÄHÄKANGAS 1997; HAINAUT and PFEIFER 2000; VÄHÄKANGAS 2001). A typical mutation in the TP53 gene can be found in the liver cancers from areas where aflatoxin contamination is common in food, while the same mutation is extremely rare in liver cancers from other geographical areas (OZTURK et al 1991). Another example is smoking-associated lung cancer where a typical mutation spectrum in TP53 gene can be identified (BENNETT et al. 1999; HAINAUT and PFEIFER 2001). DENNISSENKO and coworkers have shown that benzo(a)pyrene and other PAHs found in cigarette smoke bind preferentially to these hotspot codons of p53 where most smoking-associated mutations occur (DENNISSENKO et al. 1996; SMITH et al. 2000).

Level of DNA binding is determined by carcinogen activation, DNA repair, and the status of the gene (MILLER et al. 2001; INGELMAN-SUNDBERG 2001; BALAJEE and BOHR 2000). Actively transcribed genes are more prone to binding, but also to DNA repair. The importance of DNA repair in cancer is demonstrated by the higher cancer susceptibility in repair-deficient syndromes like Xeroderma pigmentosus and Cockayne syndrome (BALAJEE and BOHR 2000). Variation among healthy people has also been demonstrated e.g., in the activity of O6-methyltransferase (VÄHÄKANGAS et al. 1991). At the gene level, multiple SNPs have been described with potential effect on the function, although the number of studies is not sufficient for conclusions of their impor-tance in human disease (MILLER et al. 2001). DNA adducts may thus have sig-nificance as markers of exposure, unrepaired genotoxic dose and DNA repair capacity. It is also conceivable that adducts may serve as a marker of efficiency of chemoprevention.

Before DNA adducts can be used as markers, detection methods have to be validated for the specific purposes. Many methods sensitive enough for the detection of carcinogen adducts in human tissues exist, but all of the currently existing methods lack in some aspect when considering large scale molecular epidemiology studies (POIRIER et al. 2000; HEMMINKI et al. 2000).

D. Genetic Polymorphisms in Carcinogen Metabolism

Many important enzymes including CYPs (PELKONEN and RAUNIO 2000) as well as GSTs (LANDI 2000), sulfotransferases, and N-acetyl-transferases are polymorphic, potentially leading to individual variation in susceptibility (AUTRUP 2000, BOUCHARDY et al. 2001, PAVANELLO and CLONFERO 2000). Metabolic polymorphisms have an impact on the biologic indicators of genotoxic risk, although the findings are not consistent in case of some markers (PAVANELLO and CLONFERO 2000). The greatest impact from such low penetrance, polymorphic genes obviously comes from the combination of high activation and low deactivation capacities, maybe also combined with low DNA repair capacity (BALAJEE and BOHR 2000). This has been clearly shown, e.g., in studies pursuing lung cancer susceptibility (BENNETT et al. 1999; VÄHÄKANGAS 2001), where the most consistent results have been gained using combinations of polymorphisms, such as CYP1A1 and GSTM1 (BARTSCH et al. 2000; BOUCHARDY et al. 2001). High carcinogen activation by CYP1A1 combined with low detoxication by GSTM1 is one of the best known examples of combined polymorphisms probably affecting cancer susceptibility of smokers.

Many studies have shown that individuals with at risk alleles, e.g., CYP1A1*2 and/or GSTM1 null, have higher levels of carcinogen-DNA adducts and chromosomal aberrations in some tissues. The genotype influences also the type of mutations in critical genes (e.g., tumor suppressor genes; AUTRUP 2000, MILLER et al. 2001).

In addition to polymorphisms, more subtle SNPs may effect enzyme activity (WILLIAMS 2001). Induction and inhibition of carcinogen metabolism by exogenous compounds adds a further dimension to the variability in enzyme activity. There are several recent reviews addressing the role of genetic polymorphisms in the risk of developing different types of chemical caused cancers. Most of the human studies relate to cigarette smoke exposure, such as PAHs, nitrosamines, and aromatic amines (VINEIS et al. 1999; ANTTILA 1999; HIRVONEN 1999; AUTRUP 2000; BARTSCH et al. 2000; BOUCHARDY et al. 2001). The interaction between environment and xenobiotic-metabolizing genes in specific organ site cancers, such as those in the intestine (KIYOHARA 2000; MUCCI et al. 2001), head and neck (SCULLY et al. 2000), and breast (WEBER and NATHANSON 2000; THOMPSON and AMBROSONE 2000) have also been reviewed recently. This chapter describes some xenobiotic metabolizing genes in which polymorphic forms (at-risk alleles) have been associated with cancer risk. Selected genes are summarized in Table 1.

I. CYP1A1 and AHR

The role of CYP1A1 in cancer susceptibility has been studied for about 30 years. Theoretically, there are some very plausible biological reasons for a role of CYP1A1 in the genesis of tobacco smoke-elicited lung cancer: (a) the CYP1A1 enzyme catalyses the activation and inactivation of a large number of procarcinogens present in tobacco smoke, (b) CYP1A1 is found in catalytically active form in the human lung, (c) CYP1A1 is clearly inducible by cigarette smoking, (d) CYP1A1 appears to be hyperinducible in about 10% of Caucasian individuals. High inducibility of CYP1A1 has long

Table 1. A summary of selected xenobiotic-metabolizing genes, the main carcinogens metabolized, and possible association with cancer

Gene	Main carcinogens/ endogenous compounds metabolized	Association of polymorphisms with cancer	
		Yes	No
CYP, CYP1A1	PAHs	Lung, head and neck, esophagus[a], especially in Asians	Urinary tract, breast?
CYP1A2[b]	Aromatic and heterocyclic amines	Colon and rectum	Lung
CYP1B1	Estrogens, PAH dihydridiols, aromatic amines		Breast
CYP2A6	Nicotine, tobacco-specific nitrosamines	Lung	
CYP2D6	Tobacco-specific nitrosamines?	Lung[c], breast?	Head and neck, urinary tract
CYP2E1	Benzene, nitrosamines	Breast?	Lung, head and neck, urinary tract
CYP17	Conversion of cholesterol precursors to androgens, estrogens/ progestins		Breast?
CYP19		Breast?	
NAT	Aromatic and heterocyclic amines	Bladder, colon, breast?	Lung
GST[d]	Aflatoxin B1, nitro and nitroso hydrocarbons, PAHs, halogenated alkanes and alkenes	Lung, colon and rectum, bladder, head and neck?, breast?	
COMT	Catechol estrogens	Breast?	

Categorization into "Yes" or "No" groups is tentative pending further studies.
[a] Augmented by GST null genotype.
[b] No genetic polymorphism established.
[c] Phenotype-based studies show an association while genotype-based do not.
[d] At least five gene families.

been suspected to be a risk factor for lung cancer. Despite intense research, the causes of high inducibility phenotype in humans have not been fully characterized.

Several variant alleles of the CYP1A1 gene have been detected in various populations. Several nomenclature systems for these alleles have been introduced, but a consensus is forming that the designations assigned by the HUMAN

CYP ALLELE NOMENCLATURE COMMITTEE (www.imm.ki.se/cypalleles) should be used.

A meta-analysis was recently carried out by HOUSTON (2000) on the risk of lung cancer associated with the CYP1A1*2A (MspI) and CYP1A1*2B/C (exon 7-Val) alleles. In this analysis, the principal outcome measure was the odds ratio for the risk of lung cancer, using homozygosity of the wild-type allele (CYP1A1*1A) as the reference group. The odds ratio of lung cancer associated with the CYP1A1*2A combined and variant and homozygous genotypes were 1.09 (0.94–1.25) and 1.27 (0.91–1.77), respectively. The odds ratio of lung cancer associated with the CYP1A1*2B/C combined variant and homozygous genotypes were 1.16 (0.92–1.48) and 1.62 (0.93–2.82), respectively. The results do not support the role of variation in the CYP1A1 gene as a significant risk factor of lung cancer.

Also some recent studies in China (YIN et al. 2001), Taiwan (LIN et al. 2000), and Austria (GSUR et al. 2001) support the notion that CYP1A1 at-risk alleles alone are not sufficient to contribute to lung cancer incidence. There are several reports, however, that these two CYP1A1 alleles in combination with the GSTM1 0/0 genotype are associated with a significantly increased risk for lung cancer, especially squamous cell carcinoma in the Japanese population (BARTSCH et al. 2000; BOUCHARDY et al. 2001).

The aryl hydrocarbon receptor (AHR) is a ligand-activated nuclear transcription factor that regulates expression of CYP1A1, CYP1A2 and CYP1B1 as well as several genes encoding conjugating enzymes. The AHR mediates responses to toxic polynuclear aromatic hydrocarbons and numerous phytochemicals such as flavonoids and indole-3-carbinol. TCDD is a multisite carcinogen in several species and possibly in humans, whereas natural AHR ligands including carotenoids, indole-3-carbinol and flavonoids tend to protect against cancer. Consequently, selective modulators of the AHR are being actively investigated for their inhibitory actions on mammary and endometrial cancer development (SAFE 2001).

In mice, several polymorphic forms of the AHR are known, some of which have altered affinity for toxic and carcinogenic ligands. In contrast, remarkably little genetic variation has been detected in the human AHR gene (WONG et al. 2001). Despite some early reports to the contrary, hyperinducibility of CYP1A1 is not linked with the common AHR*2 (Arg554Lys) allele either in vitro (WONG et al. 2001) or in vivo (ANTTILA et al. 2001; SMITH et al. 2001). There is, however, a curious association between elevated CYP1A1 inducibility and the GSTM1 null allele (STUCKER et al. 2000), a finding that needs to be studied further.

II. CYP2A6

The interest in CYP2A6 has risen considerably after nicotine and some tobacco-specific nitrosamines were established as high-affinity substrates for this enzyme. Recently, the organization and structures of the CYP2A gene cluster and several polymorphic alleles of the CYP2A6 gene have been characterized. Two alleles with a point mutation and at least three different types of gene deletion, all leading to deficient gene function, have been found. The frequencies of these alleles vary considerably among different ethnic populations, the deletion alleles being most common in Asians (up to 20%) (PELKONEN et al. 2000; OSCARSON 2001; RAUNIO et al. 2001).

There is a biologically plausible link between CYP2A6 polymorphism and lung cancer predisposition. On one hand, CYP2A6 poor metabolizer phenotype could influence cigarette smoking habits, and on the other, an increased rate of procarcinogen activation could occur in CYP2A6 extensive metabolizers. Consistent with this hypothesis, a pilot case-control study (MIYAMOTO et al. 1999) in a Japanese population showed that the frequency of subjects homozygous for the CYP2A6 gene deletion was lower in lung cancer patients ($n = 492$) than in healthy control subjects ($n = 402$), with an odds ratio of 0.25 (95% CI 0.08–0.83). In an allele-based analysis, there was also a significant decrease in the odds ratio for the deletion allele (MIYAMOTO et al. 1999).

Several on-going studies in various ethnic groups address the putative link between CYP2A6 polymorphism and lung cancer. A case-control study in a French population (LORIOT et al. 2000) revealed no association between lung cancer incidence and CYP2A6 poor metabolizer genotypes.

A recent study (TAN et al. 2001) examined the relationship between the CYP2A6 gene deletion and susceptibility to lung and esophageal cancer in a Chinese population. The allele frequency of the CYP2A6*4 deletion was 8.6% among controls compared with 8.4% among cases with esophageal squamous cell carcinoma ($p = 0.29$) or 13.2% among cases with lung cancer ($p < 0.01$). Individuals who harbored at least one CYP2A6*4 deletion allele were at a twofold increased risk of developing lung cancer (95% CI 1.2–3.2) compared with those without a defective CYP2A6 allele. The overall risk of esophageal cancer did not appear to be associated with this CYP2A6 genetic polymorphism The distribution of CYP2A6 genotype frequency was not significantly different ($p = 0.40$) between smokers and nonsmokers in this study population (TAN et al. 2001).

Findings of novel mutations of the CYP2A6 gene impairing its promoter activity (PITARQUE et al. 2001) and altering stability and activity of the CYP2A6 protein (ARIYOSHI et al. 2001) add a new level of complexity to the studies on the association of CYP2A6 genotype and cancer susceptibility.

III. CYP2D6

The CYP2D6 enzyme catalyses the oxidative metabolism of numerous clinically used drugs. However, virtually no mutagenic and procarcinogenic compound is a high-affinity substrate to CYP2D6, and its expression in the human lung tissue is ambiguous (HUKKANEN et al. 2001).

Several independent studies indicate that the CYP2D6 metabolic status is a secondary factor in the risk of developing lung cancer. Phenotyping-based studies of lung cancer have consistently shown an increased risk associated with the extensive metabolizer phenotype, with an OR of 1.3 (95% CI 1.0–1.6) in a meta-analysis (VINEIS et al. 1999). The majority of genotyping studies, however, do not reveal such an association. This is probably due to the fact that only a few inactivating mutations are analyzed simultaneously in these studies (LAFOREST et al. 2000).

An interesting line of research studies the influence of CYP2D6 status on smoking behavior. A strong interaction between the level of CYP2D6 activity and smoking consumption has been reported (BOUCHARDY et al. 1996), with lung cancer risk being associated with high CYP2D6 enzyme activity only among the heaviest smokers. Rapid CYP2D6 phenotype may increase the probability of being addicted to smoking (SAARIKOSKI et al. 2000). A significantly increased frequency of carriers of the CYP2D6 gene duplication was recently found among lung and larynx cancer patients (13%), as compared with healthy controls (6.9%) (AGUNDEZ et al. 2001).

IV. GST

GST genes are expressed in virtually all tissues and organs. Polymorphisms have been identified in GSTM1, GSTM3, GSTP1, and GSTT1 genes (HAYES and STRANGE 2000). The protein products of these genes catalyze the detoxification of a large number of reactive, mutagenic, and procarcinogenic compounds (Table 1). This is achieved by neutralization of their electrophilic center by the SH group of the conjugated glutathione. Many GST genes are inducible by cell-specific environmental and endogenous agents.

Numerous studies have addressed several alleles of the polymorphic GST genes as risk factors in many types of cancer. A meta-analysis (VINEIS et al. 1999) showed that carriers of the GSTM1 null genotype had 1.2-fold and 1.5-fold increased risk of lung cancer in Caucasians and Asians, respectively. The effect of this polymorphism is greatest among heavy smokers. Data is insufficient for GSTM3 and GSTT1 to draw definitive conclusions (RESZKA and WASOWICZ 2001).

Very recent findings support the view that certain combinations of GST genotypes contribute to individual breast cancer risk (MITRUNEN et al. 2001) and that interindividual differences in activity of GSTs that prevent therapy-generated reactive oxidant damage may have an important impact on breast cancer recurrence and overall survival (AMBROSONE et al. 2001). The overall conclusion is that as single factors, some GST polymorphisms are moderate risk factors and that they are often synergistic factors together with other at-risk genes or other risk factors, such as heavy smoking.

V. N-Acetyltransferases

Two N-Acetyltransferases (NAT) enzymes, NAT1 and NAT2, are polymorphic and catalyze both N-acetylation (usually deactivation) and O-acetylation (usually activation) of aromatic and heterocyclic amine carcinogens. NAT1, but not NAT2 is found in lungs. There are several studies suggesting a role for NAT1 and NAT2 in various cancers. Associations between slow NAT2 acetylator genotypes and urinary bladder cancer and between rapid NAT2 acetylator genotypes and colorectal cancer are the most consistently reported (VINEIS et al. 1999). The individual risks associated with NAT1 and/or NAT2 acetylator genotypes are small, but they increase when considered in conjunction with other susceptibility genes (HEIN et al. 2000; MILLER et al. 2001). Because of the relatively high frequency of some NAT1 and NAT2 genotypes in the population, the attributable cancer risk may be high.

NAT2 has been a target of a number of studies examining its role in bladder cancer risk caused by cigarette smoking and occupational exposure to arylamine carcinogens. Two recent surveys (GREEN et al. 2000; MARCUS et al. 2000) examined several case-control studies on the association between NAT2 polymorphism and bladder cancer risk. The published evidence suggests that NAT2 slow acetylator phenotype or genotype may be associated with a small increase in bladder cancer risk. Due to the possibility of selective publication of results from studies that found an excessive risk, the current evidence is not sufficient to conclude that there is a real increase in risk. When NAT2 and CYP1A2 rapid metabolizer phenotypes were combined, a significant increased risk (OR 2.8) has been detected among consumers of well-done meat (KIYOHARA 2000).

VI. Other Genes

CYP1B1 and mEH knock-out mouse models convincingly link these enzymes with chemical carcinogenesis (GONZALEZ and KIMURA 2001). The respective genes are well conserved in human population, and no clear-cut associations between several variant alleles of these genes and cancer formation have been established.

CYP2E1 enzyme metabolizes mostly low-molecular weight compounds such as N-nitrosamines, ethanol, benzene, and styrene. Of the several polymorphic forms found in the CYP2E1 gene, none of the respective enzymes differ significantly from the wild-type one (INGELMAN-SUNDBERG 2001). Consequently, no convincing links between CYP2E1 genotypes and any type of cancer have emerged to date.

CYP17, CYP19 and catechol-O-methyl transferase (COMT) are all enzymes involved in estradiol biosynthesis and catabolism. In addition to metabolizing numerous suspected mammary carcinogens, CYP1A1 and CYP1B1 possess estradiol hydroxylating activity. All of these enzymes are expressed in human breast tissue. There are reports linking specific alleles of these genes with breast cancer development, but so far, with the possible exception of CYP1B1, the evidence is inconclusive for single gene loci (THOMPSON and AMBROSONE 2000; WEBER and NATHANSON 2000; WILLIAMS and PHILLIPS 2000; KRISTENSEN et al. 2001). Using a multifactor-dimensionality reduction method, RITCHIE et al. (2001) were able to reveal that a combination of four loci (at risk-alleles of CYP1A1, CYP1B1 and COMT) was significantly associated with risk for sporadic breast cancer.

WILLIAMS (2001) points to the fact that carcinogen activating sulfotransferases and peroxidases have wider substrate specificities than NAT, activating N-hydroxylated heterocyclic amines, aromatic amines and polycyclic aromatic hydrocarbons, of which the first two groups are also activated by NAT. In humans, ten SULT genes coding for sulphotransferases are known and genetic polymorphisms have been described in three of these genes with two having functional consequences (GLATT 2000; GLATT et al. 2000, 2001). The His-Arg213 polymorphism of SULT1A1 seems especially important because it decreases the activation considerably in bacterial expression system (GLATT et al. 2000). On basis of this and the fact that SULT isoforms are expressed in mammalian tissue, WILLIAMS (2001) suggests that SULT may be important in breast cancer etiology.

E. Xenobiotic-Metabolizing Enzymes and Chemoprevention

Due to their role in the chemical carcinogenesis process, xenobiotic-metabolizing enzymes are intriguing targets to be modulated. Cancer chemoprevention, i.e., the administration of nontoxic chemicals or dietary components to prevent cancer or slow down its progression, is an attractive concept, which is currently very actively researched. PUBMED gave 753 entries during the last 2 years with search words "chemoprevention AND cancer".

Before any chemoprevention protocols can be realized, the patterns of changes on the expression of CYP and conjugating enzymes caused by putative chemopreventive agents need to be elucidated. Recently, transgenic mice have been created in which agents affecting CYP1A1 and GSTA1 gene expression in different tissues can be studied in vivo (HENDERSON et al. 2000). Such models will greatly aid in the study of modulation patterns of CYP and conjugating enzyme expression.

I. Anticarcinogenic Chemicals Affecting Metabolism-Related Phenomena

Because xenobiotic metabolism play such an important role in carcinogen activation and detoxication, a considerable number of investigations has been published on chemicals that increase detoxication, decrease activation, or otherwise change balance of various enzymes favoring detoxication (WOLF et al. 1996). Animal experiments demonstrate clearly that chemical-induced carcinogenesis is clearly attenuated by the treatment of animals before, during, or following the exposure to a carcinogenic chemical (GREENWALD 2001). The puzzle of tamoxifen being as carcinogenic in male rat liver as in female rat liver although the sulfotransferase activating alpha-hydroxytamoxifen the basal activity is much higher in female rat can be explained by a higher inducibility in males (Phillips 2001). Flavonoids present a good example of inhibition of carcinogen activating enzymes, like CYP1A1, CYP1A2, and COX2, with putative chemoprevention potential (Heo et al. 2001).

Recently, considerable progress has been achieved in unraveling the mechanisms of regulation of cytoprotective genes, including xenobiotic-metabolizing genes (Wolf 2001). It seems that a number of transcription factors convey signals of environmental insults and oxidative stress to increased expression of appropriate genes, with the result of enhanced protection of cells against chemicals and oxidants. The elucidation of exact mechanisms will probably lead to a more efficient development of cancer chemopreventive agents. However, usefulness of cancer chemopreventive agents will be largely determined by safety considerations, similarly to any chemical substances used for preventive purposes.

II. Prevention of Binding of Reactive Intermediates

Inhibition of DNA binding also inhibits cancer formation (Wattenberg 1985). A large number of substances which prevent the binding of reactive intermediates to DNA have been described during the last 30 years (Greenwald 2001). For instance, El-Bayoumy (2001) presents evidence that one of the mechanisms of the chemoprotective effect of selenium against cancer is inhibition of the formation of covalent carcinogen-DNA adducts, although also suppression of consequences of covalent binding may be another mechanism of action.

III. Scavenging of Radical By-Products of Metabolism

CYP enzymes produce oxygen radicals as by-products of oxidation and these radicals have been implicated to contribute to genotoxicity and carcinogenicity. In experimental animals, harmful consequences of oxygen radicals can be prevented by scavenging agents, for example glutathione and thiols, but the role of oxidative stress in human cancer is currently still undefined, although strongly implicated (Wolf 2001).

IV. Inhibition/Downregulation of Carcinogen-Induced Expression of Cancer Markers

It is demonstrated in a number of experimental cancer as well as in certain human tumors that CYP and other xenobiotic metabolizing enzymes are upregulated. The pathophysiological functions, if any, of these upregulated enzymes are currently unknown. However, it is very interesting that COX-2, although not exactly a xenobiotic metabolizing enzyme, is upregulated in intestinal and other tumors, and its inhibition by nonsteroidal anti-inflammatory drugs prevents or attenuates the development of cancer in genetically susceptible individuals.

F. Identification of Individuals at Increased Risk Because of Genotype

In clinical settings it has been widely accepted that identification of variant geno/phenotypes, for example poor and ultrarapid metabolizers due to CYP2D6 gene polymorphisms would lead to more efficient and targeted therapy, although the actual widespread application of pharmacogenetic principles has been waiting for quick and cheap techniques to study genetic variants of actual patients. With respect to chemical carcinogenesis, the situation is less clear as discussed above. However, at least theoretically, it should be of importance to identify at risk genotypes, because many interventions would be possible and beneficial. For example, at risk individuals could be persuaded to avoid hazardous exposure, possibly through intensive smoking cessation programs. Another potentially beneficial approach might be to recruit at risk people to chemoprevention trials by appropriate drugs or to screening programs. These approaches would become more efficient by using intermediary risk markers, rather than cancer as an endpoint, for the assessment of proof of concept, long before the actual emergence of manifest cancer.

G. Conclusions

Despite all the hopes (and hype) regarding anticarcinogenic chemical and nutrients, it has to be kept in mind that the most important preventive measure is the prevention of exposure to carcinogens and modifying chemicals. However, although cancer is theoretically largely a preventable disease, in practice the prevention by excluding carcinogenic chemicals cannot be completely achieved and we would need approaches to prevent the effects of carcinogenic exposures and protect genetically susceptible individuals. At this point both of these approaches are largely at the experimental stage. Although cancer chemoprevention has experienced considerable advances, it is not yet an established option. With respect to protecting individuals, at this point we cannot identify with certainty any specific relationship between a CYP risk allele and cancer development. A lot more research is needed to establish the functional consequences of polymorphisms of CYP and other xenobiotic-metabolizing enzymes (INGELMAN-SUNDBERG 2001).

References

Agundez JA, Gallardo L, Ledesma MC, Lozano L, Rodriguez-Lescure A, Pontes JC, Iglesias-Moreno MC, Poch J, Ladero JM, Benitez J (2001) Functionally active duplications of the CYP2D6 gene are more prevalent among larynx and lung cancer patients. Oncology 61:59–63

Akhurst RJ, Balmain A (1999) Genetic events and the role of TGFbeta in epithelial tumour progression. J Pathol 187:82–90

Anttila S (1999) Modification of lung cancer risk by host factors involved in the activation and detoxification of tobacco-derived carcinogens. Recent Res Devel Cancer 1:321–339

Ambrosone CB, Sweeney C, Coles BF, Thompson PA, McClure GY, Korourian S, Fares MY, Stone A, Kadlubar FF, Hutchins LF (2001) Polymorphisms in glutathione S-transferases (GSTM1 and GSTT1) and survival after treatment for breast cancer. Cancer Res 61:7130–7135

Anttila S, Tuominen P, Hirvonen A, Nurminen M, Karjalainen A, Hankinson O, Elovaara E (2001) CYP1A1 levels in lung tissue of tobacco smokers and polymorphisms of CYP1A1 and aromatic hydrocarbon receptor. Pharmacogenetics 11:501–509

Ariyoshi N, Sawamura Y, Kamataki T (2001) A novel single nucleotide polymorphism altering stability and activity of CYP2A6. Biochem Biophys Res Commun 281:810–814

Autrup H (2000) Genetic polymorphisms in human xenobiotica metabolizing enzymes as susceptibility factors in toxic response. Mutation Res 464:65–76

Balajee AS, Bohr VA (2000) Genomic heterogeneity of nucleotide excision repair. Gene 250:15–30

Barbin A (2000) Etheno-adduct-forming chemicals: from mutagenicity testing to tumor mutation spectra. Mutat Res 462:55–69

Bartsch H, Nair U, Risch A, Rojas M, Wikman H, Alexandrov K (2000) Genetic polymorphisms of CYP genes, alone or in combination, as a risk modifier of tobacco-related cancers. Cancer Epidem Biomark Prev 9:3–28

Bennett WP, Hussain SP, Vähäkangas KH, Khan MA, Shields PG, Harris CC (1999) Molecular epidemiology of human cancer risk: Gene-environment interactions and p53 mutation spectrum in human lung cancer. J Pathol 187:8–18.

Bouchardy C, Benhamou S, Dayer P (1996) The effect of tobacco on lung cancer risk depends on CYP2D6 activity. Cancer Res 56:251–253

Bouchardy C, Benhamou S, Jourenkova N, Dayer, Hirvonen A (2001) Metabolic genetic polymorphisms and susceptibility to lung cancer. Lung Cancer 32:109–112

DeFlora S, Izzotti A, D'Agostini F, Balansky RM, Noona D, Albini A (2001) Multiple points of intervention of cancer and other mutation-related diseases. Mutat Res 480–481:9–22

DempkeW, Rie C, Grothey A, Schmoll H-J (2001) Cyclooxygenase-2:a novel target for cancer chemotherapy. J Cancer Res Clin Oncol 127:411–417

Denissenko MF, Pao A, Tang M, Pfeifer GP (1996) Preferential formation of benzo[a]pyrene adducts at lung cancer mutational hotspots in P53. Science 274:430–432

El-Bayoumy K (2001) The protective role of selenium on genetic damage and on cancer. Mutat Res 475:123–139

Gelboin HV (1980) Benzo[alpha]pyrene metabolism, activation and carcinogenesis: role and regulation of mixed-function oxidases and related enzymes. Physiol Rev 60:1107–1166

Glatt H (2000) Sulfotransferases in the bioactivation of xenobiotics. Chem Biol Interact 129:141–170

Glatt H, Boeing H, Engelke CE, Ma L, Kuhlow A, Pabel U, Pomlun D, Teubner W, Meinl W (2001) Human cytosolic sulphotransferases: genetics, characteristics, toxicological aspects. Mutat Res 482:27–40

Glatt H, Engelke CE, Pabel U, Teubner W, Jones AL, Coughtrie MW, Andrae U, Falany CN, Meinl W (2000) Sufotransferases: genetics and role in toxicology. Toxicol Lett 112–113:341–348

Gonzalez FJ, Kimura S (2001) Understanding the role of xenobiotic-metabolism in chemical carcinogenesis using gene knockout mice. Mutat Res 477:79–87

Green J, Banks E, Berrington A, Darby S, Deo H, Newton R (2000) N-acetyltransferase 2 and bladder cancer: an overview and consideration of the evidence for gene-environment interaction. Br J Cancer 83:412–417

Greenblatt MS, Bennett WP, Hollstein M, Harris CC (1994) Mutations in the p53 tumor suppressor gene: clues to cancer etiology and molecular pathogenesis. Cancer Res 54:4855–4878

Greenwald P (2001) From carcinogenesis to clinical interventions for cancer prevention. Toxicology 166:37–45.

Gsur A, Haidinger G, Hollaus P, Herbacek I, Madersbacher S, Trieb K, Pridun N, Mohn-Staudner A, Vetter N, Vutuc C, Micksche M (2001) Genetic polymorphisms of CYP1A1 and GSTM1 and lung cancer risk. Anticancer Res 21:2237–2242

Guengerich FP (2000) Metabolism of chemical carcinogens. Carcinogenesis 21:345–351

Hainaut P, Hollstein M (2000) p53 and human cancer: the first ten thousand mutations. Adv Cancer Res 77:81–137

Hainaut P, Pfeifer GP (2001) Patterns of p53 G→T transversions in lung cancers reflect the primary mutagenic signature of DNA-damage by tobacco smoke. Carcinogenesis 22:367–374

Hainaut P, Vahakangas K (1997) p53 as a sensor of carcinogenic exposures: mechanisms of p53 protein induction and lessons from p53 gene mutations. Pathol Biol (Paris) 45:833–844

Hayes JD, Strange RC (2000) Glutathione S-transferase polymorphisms and their biological consequences. Pharmacology 61:154–166

Hein DW, Doll MA, Fretland AJ, Leff MA, Webb SJ, Xiao GH, Devanaboyina US, Nangju NA, Feng Y (2000) Molecular genetics and epidemiology of the NAT1 and NAT2 acetylation polymorphisms. Cancer Epidemiol Biomarkers Prev 9:29–42

Hemminki K, Koskinen M, Rajaniemi H, Zhao C (2000) DNA adducts, mutations and cancer 2000. Regul Toxicol Pharmacol 32:264–275

Henderson CJ, Sahraouei A, Wolf CR (2000) Cytochrome P450s and chemoprevention. Biochem Soc Trans 28:42–46

Heo MY, Sohn SJ, Au WW (2001) Anti-genotoxicity of galancin as a cancer chemopreventive agent candidate. Mutat Res 488:135–150

Hernandez-Boussard TM, Hainaut P (1998) A specific spectrum of p53 mutations in lung cancer from smokers: review of mutations compiled in the IARC p53 database. Environ Health Perspect 106:385–91

Hirvonen A (1999) Polymorphisms of xenobiotic-metabolizing enzymes and susceptibility to cancer. Environ Health Perspect 107 [Suppl 1]: 37–47

Hollstein M, Sidransky D, Vogelstein B, Harris CC (1991) p53 mutations in human cancers. Science 253:49–53

Houlston RS (2000) CYP1A1 polymorphisms and lung cancer risk: a meta-analysis. Pharmacogenetics 10:105–114

Hukkanen J, Pelkonen O, Raunio H (2001) Expression of xenobiotic-metabolizing enzymes in human pulmonary tissue: possible role susceptibility for ILD. Eur Resp J 18 [Suppl 32]: 122S–126S

Ingelman-Sundberg M (2001) Genetic susceptibility to adverse effects of drugs and environmental toxicants. The role of the CYP family of enzymes. Mutat Res 482: 11–19

Ingelman-Sundberg M (2001) Genetic variability in susceptibility and response to toxicants. Toxicol Lett 120:259–268

Kiyohara C (2000) Genetic polymorphism of enzymes involved in xenobiotic metabolism and the risk of colorectal cancer. J Epidemiol 10:349–360

Kuroi K, Toi M (2001) Circulating angiogenesis regulators in cancer patients. Int J Biol Markers 16:5–26

Laforest L, Wikman H, Benhamou S, Saarikoski ST, Bouchardy C, Hirvonen A, Dayer P, Husgafvel-Pursiainen K (2000) CYP2D6 gene polymorphism in Caucasian smokers: lung cancer susceptibility and phenotype-genotype relationships. Eur J Cancer 36:1825–1832

268   O. PELKONEN et al.

Landi S (2000) Mammalian class theta GST and differential susceptibility to carcinogens: a review. Mutat Res 463:247–283

Lazarus P, Park JY. Metabolizing enzyme genotype and risk for upper aerodigestive tract cancer. Oral Oncol 2000, 36:421–31

Liehr JG (2000) Role of DNA adducts in hormonal carcinogenesis. Regul Toxicol Pharmacol 32:276–282

Lin P, Wang SL, Wang HJ, Chen KW, Lee HS, Tsai KJ, Chen CY, Lee H (2000) Association of CYP1A1 and microsomal epoxide hydrolase polymorphisms with lung squamous cell carcinoma. Br J Cancer 82:852–857

Loriot MA, Rebuissou S, Oscarson M, Cenee S, Miyamoto M, Ariyoshi N, Kamataki T, Hemon D, Beaune P, Stucker I (2000) Genetic polymorphisms of cytochrome P450 2A6 in a case-control study on lung cancer in a French population. Pharmacogenetics 11:39–44

Marcus PM, Vineis P, Rothman N (2000) NAT2 slow acetylation and bladder cancer risk: a meta-analysis of 22 case-control studies conducted in the general population. Pharmacogenetics 10:115–122

Miller MC, Mohrenweiser HW, Bell DA (2001) Genetic variability in susceptibility and response to toxicants. Toxicol Lett 120:269–280

Mitrunen K, Jourenkova N, Kataja V, Eskelinen M, Kosma VM, Benhamou S, Vainio H, Uusitupa M, Hirvonen A (2001) Glutathione S-transferase M1, M3, P1, and T1 genetic polymorphisms and susceptibility to breast cancer. Cancer Epidemiol Biomarkers Prev 10:229–236

Miyamoto M, Umetsu Y, Dosaka-Akita H, Sawamura Y, Yokota J, Kunitoh H, Nemeto N, Sato K, Ariyoshi N, Kamataki T (1999) CYP2A6 gene deletion reduces susceptibility to lung cancer. Biochem Biophys Res Commun 261:658–60

Mucci LA, Wedren S, Tamimi RM, Trichopoulos D, Adami HO (2001) The role of gene-environment interaction in the aetiology of human cancer: examples from cancers of the large bowel, lung and breast. J Intern Med 249:477–493

Nebert DW, Roe AL (2001) Ethnic and genetic differences in metabolism genes and risk of toxicity and cancer. Sci Total Environ 274:93–102

Ozturk M (1991) p53 mutation in hepatocellular carcinoma after aflatoxin exposure. Lancet 338:1356–1359

Pavanello S, Clonfero E (2000) Biological indicators of genotoxic risk and metabolic polymorphisms. Mutat Res 463:285–308

Pelkonen O, Nebert DW (1982) Metabolism of polycyclic aromatic hydrocarbons: Etiologic Role in carcinogenesis. Pharmacol Rev 34:189–222

Pelkonen O, Rautio A, Raunio H, Pasanen M (2000) CYP2A6:a human coumarin 7-hydroxylase. Toxicology 144:139–147

Pelkonen O, Taavitsainen P, Rautio A, Raunio H, Mäenpää J (1998) Inhibition and induction of human cytochrome P450 (CYP) enzymes. Xenobiotica 28:1203–1253

Phillips DH (2001) Understanding the genotoxicity of tamoxifen. Carcinogenesis 22: 839–849

Pitarque M, von Richter O, Oke B, Berkkan H, Oscarson M, Ingelman-Sunberg M (2001) Identification of a single nucleotide polymorphism in the TATA box of the CYP2A6 gene: impairment of its promoter activity. Biochem Biophys Res Commun 284:455–460

Poirier MC, Santella R, Weston A (2000) Carcinogen macromolecular adducts and their measurement. Carcinogenesis 21:353–359

Raunio H, Gullsten H, Rautio A, Pelkonen O (2001) Polymorphisms of CYP2A6 and its practical consequences. Br J Clin Pharmacol 52:357–363

Reszka E, Wasowicz W (2001) Significance of genetic polymorphisms in glutathione S-transferase multigene family and lung cancer risk. Int J Occup Med Environ Health 14:99–113

Ritchie MD, Hahn LW, Roodi N, Bailey LR, Dupont WD, Parl FF, Moore JH (2001) Multifactor-dimensionality reduction reveals high-order interactions among estrogen-metabolism genes in sporadic breast cancer. Am J Hum Genet 69:138–147

Saarikoski ST, Sata F, Husgafvel-Pursiainen K, Rautalahti M, Haukka J, Impivaara O, Jarvisalo J, Vainio H, Hirvonen A (2000) CYP2D6 ultrarapid metabolizer genotype as a potential modifier of smoking behaviour. Pharmacogenetics 10:5–10

Safe S (2001) Molecular biology of the Ah receptor and its role in carcinogenesis. Toxicol Lett 120:1–7

Scully C, Field JK, Tanzawa H (2000) Genetic aberrations in oral or head and neck squamous cell carcinoma (SCCHN): 1. Carcinogen metabolism, DNA repair and cell cycle control. Oral Oncol 36:256–263.

Sekido Y, Fong KM, Minna JD (1998) Progress in understanding the molecular pathogenesis of human lung cancer. Biochim Biophys Acta 1378:F21–F59

Smith GB, Harper PA, Wong JM, Lam MS, Reid KR, Petsikas D, Massey TE (2001) Human lung microsomal cytochrome P450 (CYP1A1) activities: impact of smoking status and CYP1A1, aryl hydrocarbon receptor, and glutathione S-transferase M1 genetic polymorphisms. Cancer Epidemiol Biomarkers Prev 10:839–853

Smith LE, Denissenko MF, Bennett WP, Li H, Amin S, Tang M, Pfeifer GP (2000) Targeting of lung cancer mutational hotspots by polycyclic aromatic hydrocarbons. J Natl Cancer Inst 92:803–811

Stucker I, Jacquet M, de Waziers I, Cenee S, Beaune P, Kremers P, Hemon D (2000) Relation between inducibility of CYP1A1, GSTM1 and lung cancer in a French population. Pharmacogenetics 10:617–627

Tan W, Chen GF, Xing DY, Song CY, Kadlubar FF, Lin DX (2001) Frequency of CYP2A6 gene deletion and its relation to risk of lung and esophageal cancer in the Chinese population. Int J Cancer 95:96–101

Vähäkangas K (2002) Molecular epidemiology of human cancer risk: gene-environment interactions and p53 mutation spectrum in human lung cancer. In Lung Cancer vol. 1: Molecular Pathology Methods and Reviews, Methods in Molecular Medicine vol 74 (ed. B. Driscoll), Humana Press, Totowa, New Jersey, pp. 43–59

Vähäkangas K, Pelkonen O (1989) Host variations in carcinogen metabolism and DNA repair. In Lynch, H. T. and Hirayama, T., editors. Genetic Epidemiology of Cancer, CRC Press, Boca Raton

Vähäkangas K, Trivers GE, Plummer S, Hayes RB, Krokan H, Rowe M, Swartz RP, Yeager H Jr, Harris CC (1991) O(6)-methylguanine-DNA methyltransferase and uracil DNA glycosylase in human broncho-alveolar lavage cells and peripheral blood mononuclear cells from tobacco smokers and non-smokers. Carcinogenesis 12:1389–1394

Vineis P, Malats N, Lang M, d'Errico N, Caporaso N, Cuzick J, Boffetta P (Editors) (1999) Metabolic Polymorphisms and Susceptibility to Cancer. IARC Scientific Publications No. 148

Wattenberg LW (1985) Chemoprevention of cancer. Cancer Res 45:1–8

Weber BL, Nathason KL (2000) Low penetrance genes associated with increased risk for breast cancer. Eur J Cancer 36:1193–1199

Williams JA (2001) Single nucleotide polymorphisms, metabolic activation and environmental carcinogenesis: why molecular epidemiologists should think about enzyme expression. Carcinogenesis 22:209–214

Williams JA, Phillips DH (2000) Mammary expression of xenobiotic metabolising enzymes and their potential role in breast cancer. Cancer Res 60:4667–4677

Wolf CR (2001) Chemoprevention: Increased potential to bear fruit. Proc natl Acad Sci USA 98:2941–2943

Wong JM, Harper PA, Meyer UA, Bock KW, Morike K, Lagueux J, Ayotte P, Tyndale RF, Sellers EM, Manchester DK, Okey AB (2001) Ethnic variability in the allelic distribution of human aryl hydrocarbon receptor codon 554 and assessment of variant receptor function in vitro. Pharmacogenetics 11:85–94

Yin L, Pu Y, Liu T, Tung Y, Chen K, Lin P (2001) Genetic polymorphisms of NAD(P)H quinone oxidoreductase, CYP1A1 and microsomal epoxide hydrolase and lung cancer risk in Nanjing, China. Lung Cancer 33:133–41

CHAPTER 15

Animal Models for Mechanistic Cancer Research

ZHAO-QI WANG

A. Introduction

Cancers are due to the actions of combined genetic mutations and environmental factors that induce inappropriate activation or inactivation of specific genes leading to neoplastic transformation. Epidemiological cancer studies in humans as well as basic research using cultured cells and experimental animals strongly suggest that the transition of a normal cell into a tumor cell with metastatic potential is a multistep process. This process is manifested by distinguishable histological changes, ranging from normal tissue to hyperplasia with highly proliferating cells, to dysplasia and finally, to solid tumors. Molecular and genetic studies have demonstrated that each step of this process is based on sequential genetic changes that can cause chromosomal aberrations, telomere dysfunction and alterations in individual genes, such as tumor suppressor genes, cell cycle regulators and oncogenes, as well as genes in cell death pathways and cell adhesion (Fig. 1). It is now generally accepted that cancer is a disease of our genes and that the activation of oncogenes, the loss of function of tumor suppressor genes and the altered expression of genes controlling cell proliferation and death, as well as cell adhesion and migration are all implicated in the development of tumors (VOGELSTEIN and KINZLER 1998). Oncogene products regulate normal cell proliferation and differentiation and include transcription factors, growth factors and their receptors, as well as those mediating growth signals. Tumor suppressor genes encode proteins that function in DNA damage repair and response, and in cell cycle control, and loss of their function leads to uncontrolled cell proliferation. While tumor suppressor genes are likely to be directly involved in growth inhibition, many "tumor susceptibility genes" are likely to have a more passive role in tumor growth. Their inactivation in a cell leads to an increased rate of mutation in other genes (e.g., oncogenes, tumor suppressor genes) and genomic stability, which only indirectly promotes cell proliferation. Apoptosis, or programmed cell death, is a physiological event by which multicellular eukaryotic organisms eliminate unwanted cells and can be induced by cell cycle checkpoints usually controlled by tumor suppressor gene products that detect cells containing "unacceptable damage" in physiological and pathological circumstances. Therefore, the inhibition of apoptosis or promoting cell proliferation is frequently an essential step in the process of tumor development.

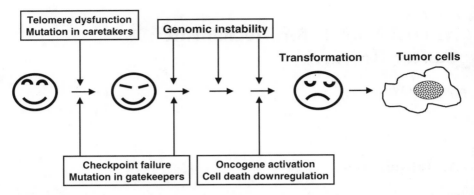

Fig. 1. Multistep process of tumor development. The transformation of a normal cell into a tumor cell involves genetic changes in genes operative in telomere function, DNA repair, and genomic stabilization ("caretakers"), cell cycle checkpoints ("gate-keepers") as well as oncogenes.

The continuing uncertainty about the molecular basis of the genetic and epigenetic changes involved in human cancer is a challenge for scientists and clinicians in cancer research. This uncertainty is due, at least partly, to the limited availability of human material for genetic studies and the lack of tools for dissecting the individual steps of carcinogenesis. These questions can only be addressed by using an animal model system, in which the various steps of tumor initiation and progression can be genetically analyzed. The possibility of investigating the function of potential cancer predisposing genes by mouse models has a great advantage over any in vitro system, such as cell culture. This is because tumor development in vivo is very complex and involves features not easily reproduced in a Petri dish, such as the host immune response, cell–cell and cell–matrix interactions, as well as the influence of the environment. Use of experimental animals has been a powerful tool for exploring the environmental factors associated with a high risk of carcino-genesis in humans. The assessment of the carcinogenicity of chemical com-pounds has been largely based on long-term rodent bioassays (IARC MONOGRAPHS 1999). Rodent models are also very useful in studying the action mechanism of carcinogens. Specific biomarkers of exposure to genotoxic car-cinogens (DNA adducts) or of biological effects (mutation spectra), can be identified in rodents and subsequently used for risk assessment in humans. Extensive research has shown clearly that these chemicals specifically induce alterations in specific genes, including oncogenes, tumor suppressor genes, and genes involved in regulation of cell death pathways. Therefore, studies using animal models are an essential and necessary step to translate basic mecha-nistic understanding into tools for human cancer prevention and treatment. This information has been invaluable for research scientists, clinicians, and pharmaceutical companies in the development of strategies and tools to fight cancer. This chapter attempts to present examples of studies using genetically modified mice as models for human cancer as well as for the mechanistic understanding of human cancers.

B. Genetically Modified Mice to Study Tumor Development

The two major genetic approaches, namely gain-of-function and loss-of-function studies, are commonly used to generate animal models for the molecular analysis of tumor development (ADAMS and CORY 1991; FOWLIS and BALMAIN 1993; JACKS 1996; WAGNER and WANG 2000).

1. Genes of interest can be overexpressed or inappropriately expressed in mice following DNA-microinjection into mouse zygotes. Lines of mice generated by this technique which express foreign genes are termed "transgenic" and the transgenes can either be expressed in specific tissues at specific developmental stages using tissue- and developmentally-specific promoters, or expressed in a wide range of tissues if an ubiquitous promoter is used. This gain-of-function approach has been used extensively to over-express oncogenes, growth factors/receptors and dominant negative mutant genes, and thereby a large number of lines of transgenic mice with a heritable predisposition to develop specific cancers have been produced (MERLINO 1994).

2. The second approach is to inactivate a specific gene using gene targeting technology in embryonic stem (ES) cells which are then used to generate mice with loss of function mutations, the so-called "knock-out" mice. This strategy is used for studying the normal biological function of individual genes and often to test the function of the cancer-associated genes in tumor development. However, many gene knock-out studies did not give a definitive answer regarding their tumor-relevant functions, as the absence of these molecules caused embryonic lethality due to their essential function in fundamental cellular processes, such as DNA replication, cell cycle progression and cell death. To overcome this problem, "conditional" knock-out strategies have been developed to specifically delete the gene in a time- and tissue-specific manner (RAJEWSKY et al. 1996; SIBILIA and WAGNER 1996).

A refinement of the standard transgenic or knock-out approach is to generate mice that develop tissue- or stage-specific tumors. A broad range of tumor types can now be generated in mice by regulated expression of "relevant" genes and they often recapitulate the ontogeny of tumorigenesis through a series of reproducible temporal and histological stages that are accessible to molecular analysis and which are similar or identical to human cancers. However, despite these points of similarity, there are several significant differences between murine and human cancers – as there are between mice and man – which must be taken into consideration. For example, the life span of mice, the size differences as well as differences in body temperature, and also certain aspects of metabolism and the particular genetics of individual mouse strains, may all influence the quality of a specific mouse model for cancer. Nevertheless, mouse models have clearly been useful thus far and provide a powerful tool for understanding the molecular mechanisms of tumorigenesis. Since genetically modified mice are also instrumental for dissecting gene function in normal developmental processes, the comparative study of gene function in development and in disease provides valuable insights into the genetic networks operating in complex biological processes.

C. Mouse Models for Human Tumors

A large number of genetically modified mice has been generated for cancer research and better model systems using novel strategies to regulate the onset and the cell-type specific expression of oncogenes and to selectively inactivate a tumor suppressor gene, have offered the possibility to study their fundamental function in normal and tumor development. Ideally, one would want to have a mouse model for every major human cancer, such as lung, breast, colon-rectum, prostate, esophagus, stomach, liver, lymphoma, cervix, ovary, and brain. Numerous attempts are being made in this direction, although presently only a limited collection of mouse models is available, which has already been summarized elsewhere (FOWLIS and BALMAIN 1993; MERLINO 1994; WAGNER and WANG 2000). Due to limitation of space, we will briefly discuss mouse models with three organ sites which resemble those of human cancers and which provide some molecular insights into the mechanisms of cancer development. In addition, we will also present several models in which the function of tumor suppressor or tumor susceptibility genes has been well studied.

I. Skin Cancer

Mouse skin has been used as a model for human squamous cancer for decades and has provided the definition of tumor initiation, promotion and malignant conversion (BROWN and BALMAIN 1995). To generate a mouse model for understanding the mechanism underlying this malignancy, transgenic mice have been generated using keratin promoter driven H-*ras* because this oncogene is often activated in chemically-induced mouse skin tumors. Indeed, mice over-expressing this oncogene develop epidermal hyperplasia and papillomas (BAILLEUL et al. 1990). Mice carrying the v-H-*ras* oncogene fused to the δ-globin promoter develop papillomas at areas of epidermal abrasion (LEDER et al. 1990). They were tested for their ability to respond to carcinogen exposure, such as benzoyl peroxide (BPO), dimethylbenz[*a*]anthracene (DMBA) and 12-*O*-tetradecanoylphorbol-13-acetate (TPA), 2-butanol peroxide (2-BUP), phenol, acetic acid, and aceton. The results showed that BPO, 2-BUP, and TPA promote skin tumor formation, whereas the other chemicals tested are not carcinogenic (Spalding et al. 1993). Mice from another transgenic line expressing human c-Ha-*ras* were also found to be susceptible to treatment with various types of carcinogens, such as 4-nitroquinoline-1-oxide (4NQO), *N,N*-diethylnitrosamine (DEN), *N*-methyl-*N*-nitrosourea (MNU), *N*-methyl-*N'*nitro-*N*-nitrosoguruanidine (MNNG) and methylazoxymethanol (MAM) (Yamamoto et al. 1996). These studies confirm the in vivo carcinogenic effect of some carcinogens previously classified as potential risk factors for humans.

A well-studied model whereby different stages of squamous cell carcinoma (SCC) develop reproducibly is that which utilizes mice expressing viral oncogenes such as E6 and E7 of human papillomavirus type 16 under the control of the human keratin14 promoter (Arbeit et al. 1994). In these mice, skin keratinocytes faithfully recapitulate the stages of SCC development in humans, from hyperproliferation to the premalignant lesion (dependent on the genetic background) with upregulation of FGFs and VEGF as well as the angiogenic switch to highly vascularized malignant carcinomas, reminiscent of human cervical cancers (Coussens et al. 1996).

Sunlight (UVB) is a strong risk factor in human basal cell carcinoma (BCC), a common skin cancer. Patients of xeroderma pigmentosum (XP) are susceptible to UV-induced skin cancers because genes affected in this disease are involved in nucleotide excision repair. Inactivation of XPC and XPA genes in mice established a mouse model for this human disease as homozygous mice are highly susceptible to UV- and chemical carcinogen-induced skin carcinogenesis (Sands et al. 1995; de Vries et al. 1995). In addition, the Cockayne syndrome B molecule is associated with transcription-coupled repair in human cells and mice lacking the gene are predisposed to skin cancer upon UV exposure (van der Host et al. 1997). These models mimic human skin cancer development and provide insights into the molecular mechanism of this disease.

The "patched" (*Ptc*) gene, which plays a central role in vertebrate development, seems to be responsible for basal cell nevus syndrome (BCNS), since mice carrying a mutation in this gene are highly susceptible to various cancers, predominantly BCCs of the skin (Gailani and Bale 1997). Transgenic mice overexpressing the ligand for PTC, Sonic hedgehog (Shh), which inactivates PTC, develop BCCs which mimic many features of BCNS (Oro et al. 1997), suggesting that PTC is a tumor suppressor molecule which plays a specific role in skin carcinogenesis. However, disruption of the *Ptc* gene in exon 1 and 2, or in exon 6 and 7, results in lethality in homozygous embryos. Heterozygous mutant mice survived and did not reproduce the skin pathology, but developed some defects reminiscent of BCNS patients, such as cerebellar medulloblastomas and rhabdomyosarcomas (Goodrich et al. 1997; Hahn et al. 1998). In addition, defects in mammary gland development have been observed in *Ptc* heterozygous mice (Lewis et al. 1999). Nevertheless, these

studies revealed that mutations in *Ptc* predispose animals to tumor development, an experimental evidence for human cancer.

II. Breast Cancer

Cancer of the breast is one of the most frequent causes of death in women
and there has been a great deal of effort to generate mouse models to
study the mechanism of this disease. This includes attempts in early days to
overexpress oncogenes and, recently, work on the inactivation of breast-
cancer-susceptible genes.

1. Overexpressing Oncogenes in Mice

Regulatory elements of the mouse mammary tumor virus (MMTV-LTR)
directs expression of genes to the mammary gland throughout the life span,
whereas the whey acidic protein (WAP) promoter is only activated during the
lactation period. Transgenic mice expressing either the *myc* or *ras* oncoprotein
from the MMTV-LTR or WAP promoter develop well-differentiated carcinomas of the mammary gland, usually several months after pregnancy and lactation (MERLINO 1994). MMTV-*myc*- and MMTV-*ras*-induced tumors appear
rapidly and at a high frequency (STEWART et al. 1984; SINN et al. 1987) and are
accelerated in MMTV-*myc*/MMTV-*ras* double transgenics, indicating that a
common pathway is affected. Besides these oncogenes, growth factors and
their receptors are often involved in epithelial cell transformation in human
carcinomas. The ectopic expression of TGFα and its receptors, EGF receptor
(EGFR) and HER2 in mice, also results in a high frequency of adenocarcinomas of the mammary gland (MULLER et al. 1988; BOUCHARD et al. 1989;
MATSUI et al 1990; SANDGREN et al. 1990; JHAPPAN et al. 1990). Moreover,
although activation of *Wnt*-1 and *Fgf* 3 alone under the MMTV promoter did
not render mice susceptible to significant mammary carcinomas, transgenic
mice expressing these two molecules exhibited accelerated tumor formation
(KWAN et al. 1992), and p53 deficiency accelerated mammary tumorigenesis in
Wnt-1 transgenic mice (DONEHOWER et al. 1995). Finally, mice overexpressing
cyclin D1, a cell-cycle-related gene which is amplified or overexpressed in
many human breast cancers (SHERR and ROBERTS 1995), develop mammary
gland hyperplasia and carcinoma (WANG et al. 1994). Interestingly, mice
lacking cyclin D1 are protected from *neu* and *ras* activation-induced breast
cancer (YU et al. 2001). These studies have provided many important new
insights for this tumor type by overexpressing oncogenes, growth factors, and
growth factor receptors or altering cell cycle related genes.

2. Mice Carrying Disrupted Breast Cancer Susceptibility Genes *BRCA*1 and *BRCA*2

Identification of breast cancer susceptibility genes such as *BRCA*1 and
*BRCA*2 have greatly advanced our understanding of this tumor type (MIKI et
al. 1994; WOOSTER et al. 1995). Mutation in *BRCA*1 and *BRCA*2 predisposes

individuals to breast and ovarian cancers and biochemical studies have demonstrated that these genes are involved in DNA damage response (ZHANG et al. 1998). Functional studies using animal models aiming to elucidate the function of these molecules were not satisfactory since null mutations of *BRCA1* and *BRCA2* in mice result in embryonic lethality (HAKEM et al. 1996; SHARAN et al. 1997; LUDWIG et al. 1997). Therefore, the involvement of these molecules in particular tumor types is unclear. In order to study their role in cancer development, efforts were made to produce viable mice by introducing a truncation mutation into the genes. Mice truncated with the BRCA2 protein exhibit numerous spontaneous chromosomal abnormalities and are prone to lymphoma development (CONNOR et al. 1997; FRIEDMAN 1998). The lack of breast tumors in these mice could be due to a short life span and the disease symptoms associated with lethal thymic lymphoma. To overcome such a problem and to generate models for breast cancer, a conditional knock-out strategy has been applied to inactivate *BRCA2*, and mice with conditional deletion of *BRCA2* and *p53* presented a high frequency of breast cancer development (JONKER 2001). Similarly, mice with specific mammary gland disruption in exon 11 of *BRCA1* showed that mammary tumors (XU et al. 1999) can be enhanced by the mutation of *p53*, causing a decrease in apoptosis and cell cycle checkpoint control (XU et al. 2001). All these studies confirmed that genetic factors *BRCA1* and *BRCA2* are indeed involved in human breast cancer, most likely in a p53 dependent manner.

III. Liver Cancer

Liver cancer, such as hepatocellular carcinoma (HCC), is a major tumor burden in developing countries and the major risk factor, besides alcohol and diet, is attributable to infection with hepatitis B and C viruses and liver injury (BUENDIA 2000). During the infection and development period of HCC, multiple genetic events occur. Several promoters were used to overexpress oncogenes in the liver such as the albumin gene enhancer and promoter, as well as the inducible metallothionein (MT) promoter. Directed expression of SV40 T antigen, *myc* and *ras* by the albumin promoter in transgenic mice causes liver tumors within a few months of age (SANDGREN et al. 1989). Although TGFα expression by the MT promoter induces hepatocarcinomas with a longer latency in transgenic mice (1 year, JHAPPAN et al. 1990), it dramatically enhances *myc* and SV40 T antigen-induced tumorigenesis (SANDGREN et al. 1993). A similar finding was obtained when albumin-TGFα transgenic mice were crossed with albumin-*myc* transgenic mice (MURAKAMI et al. 1993). These data once more indicate that activation of several oncogenes is required for neoplastic transformation in hepatocytes. Since liver cancer in humans has a high incidence in association with human hepatitis B virus (HBV) infection, it was important to demonstrate that overexpression of HBV in mice also induced various steps of liver cancer (CHISARI et al. 1989). In addition, double transgenic mice showed that TGFα cooperates with HBV in liver tumorigenesis (JAKUBCZAK et al. 1997), indicating a synergistic effect of growth factor signalling and viral infection. Some liver carcinogens, such as aflatoxin and diethylnitrosamine (DEN) are thought to mutate some genes which, together with viral infection-induced mutations, may be important in the etiology of liver cancer. Mice overexpressing HBV were used to test this hypothesis by exposing them to aflatoxins and DEN. These transgenic mice develop an increased frequency of liver cancer (SELL et al. 1991; SLAGLE et al. 1996). Therefore, these studies provide experimental evidence for the synergistic effect between environmental carcinogens and HBV infection.

Targeted disruption of specific genes in mice has not been successful in generating models for liver cancer and only a few examples of these mice develop liver tumors. Inactivation of gap junction molecule connexin 32 in mice causes these mice to develop a high frequency of liver cancer (TEMME et al. 1997). These mice are also susceptible to DEN-induced liver tumor development (TEMME et al. 1997). These data suggest that the presence of functional gap junction can inhibit the development of spontaneous and chemically induced liver tumors. p53 is a tumor suppressor which is often mutated in humans. Mice homozygous and heterozygous for *p53* develop mainly lymphomas and sarcomas (see below) and these mice showed a high susceptibility to DEN-induced liver cancer (KEMP et al. 1995). Finally, the point mutation in the p53 gene (codon 246) increased the carcinogenic action of aflatoxin B and hepatitis B infection in these mice (GHERBRANIOUS and SELL 1998a,b).

IV. Disruption of the Genes That Are Responsible for DNA Repair and Genomic Stability

Loss of genomic integrity resulting from defects in molecules that are involved in DNA damage response, repair, and recombination after exposure to endogenous and environmental insults, plays an important role in human tumor development (LENGAUER et al. 1998). The relation of these genes to tumor and disease susceptibility is an important area of cancer research. For the majority of tumor suppressor or DNA repair genes, mainly mouse knockout models have been produced (JACKS 1996). These contribute to a better understanding of the mechanisms underlying tumor formation and also to the pathways that regulate DNA repair and genomic stability. The outcome of these mouse studies vary: some mimic the relevant human disease fairly closely, while others display increased tumor susceptibilities to a different range of tumors. Many of these studies provide no clear answer to the tumor suppressors' role in tumor development because deletion of the gene induced early embryonic lethality. The different physiology, genetic predisposition, life span, and "lifestyle" between mouse and man may account for the unexpected results. A few outstanding examples from the analysis of mice with disrupted genes responsible for DNA repair, genomic stability, or tumor suppressors are briefly discussed below.

1. Mice Deficient in p53

The most thoroughly characterized knock-out mouse in cancer research is the mouse that contains the disrupted *p53* gene (DONEHOWER 1996). In addition to its biochemical role as a putative transcription factor, the physiological function of p53 has been elucidated using mice lacking p53. The mice are viable but develop a variety of tumor types, including a high frequency of lymphomas, soft tissue sarcoma and rare osteosarcomas, brain tumors, and carcinomas within 3–6 months of age. Interestingly, and in parallel with observations of humans with a germline *p53* mutation, mice with one wild-type allele also develop tumors, albeit at a relatively long latency (18 months). The results from the analysis of these mutant mice have confirmed the tumor suppressing function of p53 (DONEHOWER 1996).

The *p53* knock-out mouse model has been extensively used to study the potential of various carcinogens for causing tumors. For example, dimethylnitrosamine (DMN), a liver carcinogen, induces susceptibility in *p53* heterozygous mice for liver hemangiosarcoma formation (HARVEY et al. 1993). Radiation treatment of *p53*-deficient mice enhances lymphoma development in both heterozygous and homozygous mutant mice (KEMP et al. 1994). In addition, when a *p53* null mutation was introduced into mice overexpressing the K10-*ras* transgene, a *p53* mutation was identified as a critical genetic factor in tumor progression, but not in tumor initiation, in the classic skin carcinogenesis model using DMBA/TPA (KEMP et al. 1993).

Interestingly, recent studies have demonstrated that loss of p53 is a major limiting step in carcinogenesis induced by mutations in other genes that are involved in DNA repair and genomic stability. For example, mice without telomerase or with short telomeres are prone to carcinogenesis (RUDOLPH et al. 1999) and this can be enhanced by the deficient checkpoints mediated by p53 (CHIN et al. 1999; ARTANDI et al. 2000). Moreover, although mice with disrupted Ku80, a DNA binding subunit of DNA dependent protein kinase (DNA-PK), rarely develop tumors, mutation of p53 rendered these mice susceptible to a high frequency of pro-B-cell lymphoma, involving specific chromosomal translocations between amplified c-*myc* and the IgH locus (DIFILIPPANTONIO et al. 2000; LIM et al. 2000). These data suggest that genes responsible for DNA repair or genomic stability cooperate with p53 mutation in suppressing tumor development. Finally, studies on cooperation of p53 with breast cancer susceptible genes *BRCA1* and *BRCA2* (see Sect. C.II.) have demonstrated that disruption of the p53 pathway is pivotal in *BRCA*-associated breast cancer development (XU et al. 2001; JONKER et al. 2001).

2. Mice with Inactivated DNA Repair Genes

Mutations of DNA repair genes are shown to be important contributors to tumor development. Some of these genes were originally isolated from inherited human diseases which are prone to tumor development and are perturbed in human cancers. Knock-out studies have strengthened the notion that these genes display biochemical characteristics similar to tumor suppressor genes and are involved in tumorigenesis. Several studies showing the involvement of these genes in cancer development have been discussed in previous sections (see Sects. C.I., C.II.) and additional examples are discussed below.

a) Mismatch Repair Genes

Inactivation of the mismatch repair gene *Msh2* in mice predisposes them to lymphoma formation due to an aberrant recombination (DE WIND et al. 1995). Further characterization of *Msh2* mutant mice in an immune deficient background revealed that this gene also plays a role in colon cancer development (DE WIND et al. 1998). In addition, if the *Msh2* null mutation is introduced into *Min*/+ mice heterozygous for a germ line mutation of the *Apc* gene, these double-mutant mice develop many colonic aberrant crypt foci and, rapidly, a greater number of adenomas (REITMAIR et al. 1996). Mutation of another mismatch repair gene, *MLH1*, is often observed in human nonpolyposis colon cancer (HNPCC) (BRONNER et al. 1994). Mice deficient for *MLH1* are susceptible to intestinal cancer (PROLLA et al. 1998). Although mice with disrupted *PMS2*, another mismatch repair gene, only develop sarcoma and lymphoma (BAKER et al. 1995; PROLLA et al. 1998), when this null mutation was introduced into *Min* mice, accelerated intestinal tumors developed in these double-mutant mice (BAKER et al. 1998), mimicking human hereditary nonpolyposis colorectal cancer. These studies demonstrate a general involvement of these mismatch repair genes in colon cancer and an additional role in lymphoid tumor development.

b) Disruption of PARP-1

Poly(ADP-ribose) polymerase (PARP-1) binds to DNA strand breaks after exposure to DNA damaging agents, and is proposed to play a multifunctional role in a range of cellular processes including DNA repair and recombination, proliferation and cell death, stress response, as well as the maintenance of chromosomal stability (LINDAHL et al. 1995; HERCEG and WANG 2001). While PARP-1$^{-/-}$ mice develop normally, they are hypersensitive to high doses (8 Gy) of whole-body radiation (WANG et al. 1995; MENISSIER-DE MURCIA et al. 1997; WANG et al. 1997; TONG et al. 2000). PARP-1$^{-/-}$ cells exhibit telomere dysfunction and high levels of chromosomal instability, including elevated sister chromatid exchange (SCE) and more micronuclei, as well as loss or gain of chromosomes (MENISSIER-DE MURCIA et al. 1997; WANG et al. 1997; D'ADDA DI FAGAGNA et al. 1999; SIMBULAN-ROSENTHAL et al. 1999; TONG et al. 2001), indicating the importance of PARP-1 in the maintenance of telomere function and genomic integrity. Despite a late onset of tumor development, the absence of PARP-1 in an 129/Sv genetic background renders these mice susceptible to a high incidence of tumors, mainly adenomas and carcinomas (Tong and Wang, unpublished data), consistent with involvement of PARP-1 in genomic stability and DNA damage response. More importantly, together with other mutations, PARP-1 deficiency promotes tumor formation in various tumorigenesis models (see below). When PARP-1 deficiency was introduced into a p53 null background, the tumor spectrum of PARP-1$^{-/-}$p53$^{-/-}$ mice was wider than in p53$^{-/-}$ controls and included brain tumors, carcinomas of the colon, pancreas, skin, and liver. p53$^{+/-}$ mice with a PARP-1-deficient background also developed a high frequency of mammary gland carcinomas and brain tumors, reminiscent of the Li-Fraumeni syndrome in humans (TONG et al. 2001).

c) Genes Responsible for DNA Double-Strand Break Repair

The ataxia telangiectasia mutated gene (*ATM*) has been shown to be involved in cell cycle regulation, meiotic recombination, DNA damage checkpoints, and telomere length monitoring. Mice with a null mutation in the *ATM* gene develop thymic lymphoblastic tumors at 2–4 months of age and exhibit an acute hypersensitivity to γ-radiation (BARLOW et al. 1996). DNA-PK is a molecule responsible for DNA double-strand break repair and specific V(D)J recombination (SMITH and JACKSON 1999). The inactivation of the catalytic subunit of this gene (DNA-PKcs) in mice results in a high susceptibility to tumor development (JHAPPAN et al. 1997). Disruption of Ku70, a DNA-binding subunit of DNA-PK, results in development of the T-cell lymphoma at a mean age of 6 months (LI et al. 1998). Moreover, in server-combined immune deficient (SCID) mice, in which DNA-PKcs is mutated, PARP-1 deficiency partially rescues T-cell development and these mice succumb to thymic lymphoma, most likely due to increased uncontrolled anomalous V(D)J recombination (MORRISON et al. 1997), suggesting a cooperative function of these two molecules in tumor development. XRCC4 is another nonhomologous endjoining protein employed in DNA double-strand break repair and in V(D)J recombination. Although *XRCC4* null mutant mice die at the embryonic stage, *p53* null mutation rescues the lethality, but the doubly mutant mice succumb to B-cell lymphoma due to specific chromosomal translocation involving the c-*myc* oncogene and IgH locus (GAO et al. 2000).

D. Genetic Tools for Molecular Epidemiological and Environmental Carcinogenesis Studies

Cancers are the consequence of activation or inactivation of specific genes leading to neoplastic transformation. Genetic mutations can occur spontaneously or as a result of exposure to environmental factors. Apart from the powerful application of transgenic and knockout mice in dissecting the molecular mechanism of multistage carcinogenesis, one of the most important principles underlying the use of these genetically susceptible animals is as targets for environment-genome interactions.

The p53 protein is dysfunctional or absent in the majority of human tumors, primarily due to single point mutations in the gene (VOGELSTEIN and KINZLER 1992). Up to the present, standard laboratory mouse strains used in animal cancer tests have been employed to induce *p53* mutations for com-

parison with published human tumor *p53* spectra (HOLLSTEIN et al. 1999), or
to test the efficacy of new p53-targeting drugs, but human/mouse species differences call into question the predictive value of such experiments. Thus,
genetically engineered mice in which a "humanized" *p53* gene, expressed at
physiological levels, would complement existing in vivo test systems and would
be of potential interest in preclinical testing of the p53-modulating drugs under
development.

A human p53 knock-in (*Hupki*) mouse in which exons 4–9 of the endogenous mouse *p53* alleles were replaced with the homologous, normal human
p53 sequences has been generated. These mice, harboring a p53 core domain
identical to that of humans, retain various p53 cellular functions (LUO et al.
2001a). This "humanized" mouse provides a unique tool for examining spontaneous and induced mutations in human *p53* gene sequences in vivo. One
such application is to test sunlight as an etiological agent contributing to
human nonmelanoma skin cancer. The *p53* gene is usually mutated in these
tumors, and the mutations have a "UV signature", single or tandem transitions
at dipyrimidine sequences in the DNA binding domain (DBD). When epidermal cells of *Hupki* mice are irradiated in vivo with a single acute dose of
UVB light, they accumulate UV photoproducts at the same locations of the
p53 gene as human cells. DNA preparations from sections of chronically irradiated *Hupki* epidermis harbor C to T and CC to TT mutations at two mutation hotspots identified in human skin cancer, one at codons 278–279, and one
at codons 247–248, which are the most frequent UVB-associated mutation
sites in humans. *Hupki* keratinocytes harboring these *p53* mutations thus syn-
thesize p53 protein with an aberrant DBD identical in amino acid sequence
to the mutant p53 molecules in human tumors (LUO et al. 2001b).

Further genetic refinement may be needed to optimize this approach, as
the *Hupki* strain can be combined with other genetically modified mouse
strains which would be able to test specific genetic pathways in response to
various carcinogens. The *Hupki* mouse or its derivatives will pave the way for
preclinical in vivo testing of new pharmaceuticals designed to restore/enhance
(human) p53 tumor suppressor DNA binding/transcription activation functions, or drugs designed to temporarily hamper these functions in order to
ameliorate the side effects of chemotherapy (FOSTER et al. 1999; KOMAROV et
al. 1999). In addition, it would be of interest to validate this model as a potential target for therapeutic molecules that modulate p53 activity (SELIVANOVA
et al. 1998; RODRIGUEZ et al. 1999).

E. Perspectives

These mouse models have taught us about how, and by which molecular mechanisms cancer-related genes affect human cancer initiation, promote tumor
progression and facilitate metastasis. Moreover, studies on these animal
models have identified important molecular bases and key events in the devel-

opment of human cancer, such as oncogene activation, the maintenance of genomic stability, cell cycle control, and the balance between proliferation and apoptosis in cells. We have also gained enormous knowledge of how cancer suppressor or susceptibility genes function in normal development and in differentiation of the organism. However, the current mouse model systems have their limitations and cannot address every type of problem. This is because cancer starts as a single cell phenomenon and the development of a tumor from this single transformed cell will depend to a large extent on its interactions with its environment. Some of these limitations may be partially overcome by the use of improved, more selective gene modification techniques, or by the development of different mouse models specifically designed to answer different questions. Further development is the great demand among the scientific community to generate animal models that parallel the ways that human cancers develop, progress and respond to therapy or preventive agents. For the future, our goals must be to turn the cancer knowledge gained from mouse studies into clinical applications. Ultimately, these animal models will be used to test new approaches for diagnosis and to explore the cancer-gene derived molecular targets necessary to foster new developments for the prevention and possible cure of cancer.

Acknowledgments. I apologize to those whose work I could not cite due to space restrictions. I am very grateful to Dr. Wei-Min Tong for his critical comments and Mrs. E. El-Akroud for editing the manuscript. Research in Dr. Zhao-Qi Wang's laboratory is supported by the Association for International Cancer Research, UK and by the Association pour la Recherche contre le Cancer, France.

References

Adams JM, Cory S (1991) Transgenic models of tumor development. Science 254: 1161–1167

Arbeit JM, Munger K, Howley PM, Hanahan D (1994) Progressive squamous epithelial neoplasia in K14-human papillomavirus type 16 transgenic mice. J Virol 68: 4358–4368

Artandi SE, Chang S, Lee SL, Alson S, Gottlieb GJ, Chin L, DePinho RA (2000) Telomere dysfunction promotes nonreciprocal translocations and epithelial cancers in mice. Nature 406:641–645

Bailleul B, Surani MA, White S, Barton SC, Brown K, Blessing M, Jorcano J, Balmain A (1990) Skin hyperkeratosis and papilloma formation in transgenic mice expressing a ras oncogene from a suprabasal keratin promoter. Cell 62:697–708

Baker SM, Bronner CE, Zhang L, Plug AW, Robatzek M, Warren G, Elliott EA, Yu J, Ashley T, Arnheim N, et al. (1995) Male mice defective in the DNA mismatch repair gene PMS2 exhibit abnormal chromosome synapsis in meiosis. Cell 82: 309–319

Baker SM, Harris AC, Tsao JL, Flath TJ, Bronner CE, Gordon M, Shibata D, Liskay RM (1998) Enhanced intestinal adenomatous polyp formation in Pms2-/-;Min mice. Cancer Res 58:1087–1089

Barlow C, Hirotsune S, Paylor R, Liyanage M, Eckhaus M, Collins F, Shiloh Y, Crawley JN, Ried T, Tagle D, Wynshaw-Boris A (1996) Atm-deficient mice: a paradigm of ataxia telangiectasia. Cell 86:159–171

284 Z.-Q. WANG

Bouchard L, Lamarre L, Tremblay PJ, Jolicoeur P (1989) Stochastic appearance of mammary tumors in transgenic mice carrying the MMTV/c-neu oncogene. Cell 57: 931–936

Bronner CE, Baker SM, Morrison PT, Warren G, Smith LG, Lescoe MK, Kane M, Earabino C, Lipford J, Lindblom A, et al. (1994) Mutation in the DNA mismatch repair gene homologue hMLH1 is associated with hereditary nonpolyposis colon cancer. Nature 368:258–261

Brown K, Balmain A (1995) Transgenic mice and squamous multistage skin carcinogenesis. Cancer Metastasis Rev 14:113–124

Buendia MA (2000) Genetics of hepatocellular carcinoma. Semin Cancer Biol 10: 185–200

Chin L, Artandi SE, Shen Q, Tam A, Lee SL, Gottlieb GJ, Greider CW, DePinho RA (1999) p53 deficiency rescues the adverse effects of telomere loss and cooperates with telomere dysfunction to accelerate carcinogenesis. Cell 97:527–538

Chisari FV, Klopchin K, Moriyama T, Pasquinelli C, Dunsford HA, Sell S, Pinkert CA, Brinster RL, Palmiter RD (1989) Molecular pathogenesis of hepatocellular carcinoma in hepatitis B virus transgenic mice. Cell 59:1145–1156

Connor F, Bertwistle D, Mee PJ, Ross GM, Swift S, Grigorieva E, Tybulewicz VL, Ashworth A (1997) Tumorigenesis and a DNA repair defect in mice with a truncating Brca2 mutation. Nat Genet 17:423–430

Coussens LM, Hanahan D, Arbeit JM (1996) Genetic predisposition and parameters of malignant progression in K14-HPV16 transgenic mice. Am J Pathol 149: 1899–1917

d'Adda di Fagagna F, Hande MP, Tong WM, Lansdorp PM, Wang Z-Q, Jackson SP (1999) Functions of poly(ADP-ribose) polymerase in controlling telomere length and chromosomal stability. Nat Genet 23:76–80

de Vries A, van Oostrom CT, Hofhuis FM, Dortant PM, Berg RJ, de Gruijl FR, Wester PW, van Kreijl CF, Capel PJ, van Steeg H, Verbeek SJ (1995) Increased susceptibility to ultraviolet-B and carcinogens of mice lacking the DNA excision repair gene XPA. Nature 377:169–173

de Wind N, Dekker M, Berns A, Radman M, te Riele H (1995) Inactivation of the mouse Msh2 gene results in mismatch repair deficiency, methylation tolerance, hyperrecombination, and predisposition to cancer. Cell 82:321–330

de Wind N, Dekker M, van Rossum A, van der Valk M, te Riele H (1998) Mouse models for hereditary nonpolyposis colorectal cancer. Cancer Res 58:248–255

Difilippantonio MJ, Zhu J, Chen HT, Meffre E, Nussenzweig MC, Max EE, Ried T, Nussenzweig A (2000) DNA repair protein Ku80 suppresses chromosomal aberrations and malignant transformation. Nature 404:510–514

Donehower LA (1996) The p53-deficient mouse: a model for basic and applied cancer studies. Semin Cancer Biol 7:269–278

Donehower LA, Godley LA, Aldaz CM, Pyle R, Shi YP, Pinkel D, Gray J, Bradley A, Medina D, Varmus HE (1995) Deficiency of p53 accelerates mammary tumorigenesis in Wnt-1 transgenic mice and promotes chromosomal instability. Genes Dev 9:882–895

Foster BA, Coffey A, Morin MJ, Rastinejad F (1999) Pharmacological rescue of mutant p53 conformation and function. Science 286:2507–2510

Fowlis DJ, Balmain A (1993) Oncogenes and tumour suppressor genes in transgenic mouse models of neoplasia. Eur J Cancer 29A: 638–645

Friedman LS, Thistlethwaite FC, Patel KJ, Yu VP, Lee H, Venkitaraman AR, Abel KJ, Carlton MB, Hunter SM, Colledge WH, Evans MJ, Ponder BA (1998) Thymic lymphomas in mice with a truncating mutation in Brca2. Cancer Res 58:1338–1343

Gailani MR, Bale AE (1997) Developmental genes and cancer: role of patched in basal cell carcinoma of the skin. J Natl Cancer Inst 89:1103–1109

Gao Y, Ferguson DO, Xie W, Manis JP, Sekiguchi J, Frank KM, Chaudhuri J, Horner J, DePinho RA, Alt FW (2000) Interplay of p53 and DNA-repair protein XRCC4 in tumorigenesis, genomic stability and development. Nature 404:897–900

Ghebranious N, Sell S (1998a) Hepatitis B injury, male gender, aflatoxin, and p53 expression each contribute to hepatocarcinogenesis in transgenic mice. Hepatology 27:383–391

Ghebranious N, Sell S (1998b) The mouse equivalent of the human p53ser249 mutation p53ser246 enhances aflatoxin hepatocarcinogenesis in hepatitis B surface antigen transgenic and p53 heterozygous null mice. Hepatology 27:967–973

Goodrich LV, Milenkovic L, Higgins KM, Scott MP (1997) Altered neural cell fates and medulloblastoma in mouse patched mutants. Science 277:1109–1113

Hahn H, Wojnowski L, Zimmer AM, Hall J, Miller G, Zimmer A (1998) Rhabdomyosarcomas and radiation hypersensitivity in a mouse model of Gorlin syndrome. Nat Med 4:619–622

Hakem R, de la Pompa JL, Sirard C, Mo R, Woo M, Hakem A, Wakeham A, Potter J, Reitmair A, Billia F, Firpo E, Hui CC, Roberts J, Rossant J, Mak TW (1996) The tumor suppressor gene Brca1 is required for embryonic cellular proliferation in the mouse. Cell 85:1009–1023

Harvey M, McArthur MJ, Montgomery CA Jr, Butel JS, Bradley A, Donehower LA (1993) Spontaneous and carcinogen-induced tumorigenesis in p53-deficient mice. Nat Genet 5:225–229

Herceg Z, Wang Z-Q (2001) Functions of poly(ADP-ribose) polymerase (PARP-1) in DNA repair, genomic integrity and cell death. Mut Res 477:97–110

Hollstein M, Hergenhahn M, Yang Q, Bartsch H, Wang Z-Q, Hainaut P (1999) New approaches to understanding p53 gene tumor mutation spectra. Mut Res 431:199–209

IARC Monographs on No.71. (1999) "The Evaluation of Carcinogenic Risks to Humans", IARC, Lyon

Jacks T (1996) Tumor suppressor gene mutations in mice. Annu Rev Genet 30:603–636

Jakubczak JL, Chisari FV, Merlino G (1997) Synergy between transforming growth factor alpha and hepatitis B virus surface antigen in hepatocellular proliferation and carcinogenesis. Cancer Res 57:3606–3611

Jhappan C, Morse HC 3rd, Fleischmann RD, Gottesman MM, Merlino G (1997) DNA-PKcs: a T-cell tumour suppressor encoded at the mouse scid locus. Nat Genet 17:483–486

Jhappan C, Stahle C, Harkins RN, Fausto N, Smith GH, Merlino GT (1990) TGF alpha overexpression in transgenic mice induces liver neoplasia and abnormal development of the mammary gland and pancreas. Cell 61:1137–1146

Jonkers J, Meuwissen R, van Der Gulden H, Peterse H, van Der Valk M, Berns A (2001) Synergistic tumor suppressor activity of BRCA2 and p53 in a conditional mouse model for breast cancer. Nat Genet 29:418–425

Kemp CJ (1995) Hepatocarcinogenesis in p53-deficient mice. Mol Carcinog 12:132–136

Kemp CJ, Donehower LA, Bradley A, Balmain A (1993) Reduction of p53 gene dosage does not increase initiation or promotion but enhances malignant progression of chemically induced skin tumors. Cell 74:813–822

Kemp CJ, Wheldon T, Balmain A (1994) p53-deficient mice are extremely susceptible to radiation-induced tumorigenesis. Nat Genet 8:66–69

Komarov PG, Komarova EA, Kondratov RV, Christov-Tselkov K, Coon JS, Chernov MV, Gudkov AV (1999) A chemical inhibitor of p53 that protects mice from the side effects of cancer therapy. Science 285:1733–1737

Kwan H, Pecenka V, Tsukamoto A, Parslow TG, Guzman R, Lin TP, Muller WJ, Lee FS, Leder P, Varmus HE (1992) Transgenes expressing the Wnt-1 and int-2 proto-oncogenes cooperate during mammary carcinogenesis in doubly transgenic mice. Mol Cell Biol 12:147–154

Leder A, Kuo A, Cardiff RD, Sinn E, Leder P (1990) v-Ha-ras transgene abrogates the initiation step in mouse skin tumorigenesis: effects of phorbol esters and retinoic acid. Proc Natl Acad Sci USA 87:9178–9182

Lengauer C, Kinzler KW, Vogelstein B (1998) Genetic instabilities in human cancers. Nature 396:643–649

Lewis MT, Ross S, Strickland PA, Sugnet CW, Jimenez E, Scott MP, Daniel CW (1999) Defects in mouse mammary gland development caused by conditional haploin-sufficiency of Patched-1. Development 126:5181–5193

Li GC, Ouyang H, Li X, Nagasawa H, Little JB, Chen DJ, Ling CC, Fuks Z, Cordon-Cardo C (1998) Ku70:a candidate tumor suppressor gene for murine T cell lym-phoma. Mol Cell 2:1–8

Lim DS, Vogel H, Willerford DM, Sands AT, Platt KA, Hasty P (2000) Analysis of Ku80-mutant mice and cells with deficient levels of p53. Mol Cell Biol 20:3772–3780

Lindahl T, Satoh MS, Poirier GG, Klungland A (1995) Post-translational modification of poly(ADP-ribose) polymerase induced by DNA strand breaks. Trends Biochem Sci 20:405–411

Ludwig T, Chapman DL, Papaioannou VE, Efstratiadis A (1997) Targeted mutations of breast cancer susceptibility gene homologs in mice: lethal phenotypes of Brca1, Brca2, Brca1/Brca2, Brca1/p53, and Brca2/p53 nullizygous embryos. Genes Dev 11:1226–1241

Luo JL, Tong W-M, Yoon J-H, Hergenhahn M, Koomagi R, Yang Q, Galendo D, Pfeifer GP, Wang Z-Q, Hollstein M (2001b) UV-induced DNA damage and mutations in Hupki (human p53 knock-in) mice recapitulate p53 patterns in sun-exposed human skin. Cancer Res 61:8158–8163

Luo JL, Yang Q, Tong W-M, Hergenhahn M, Wang Z-Q, Hollstein M (2001a) Knock-in mice with a chimeric human/murine p53 gene develop normally and show wild-type p53 responses to DNA damaging agents: a new biomedical research tool. Oncogene 20:320–328

Matsui Y, Halter SA, Holt JT, Hogan BL, Coffey RJ (1990) Development of mammary hyperplasia and neoplasia in MMTV-TGF alpha transgenic mice. Cell 61:1147–1155

Menessier-de Murcia J, Niedergang C, Trucco C, Ricoul M, Dutrillaux B, Mark M, Oliver FJ, Masson M, Dierich A, LeMeur M, Walztinger C, Chambon P, de Murcia G (1997) Requirement of poly (ADP-ribose) in recovery from DNA damage in mice and in cells. Proc Natl Acad Sci USA 94:7303–7307

Merlino G (1994) Transgenic mice as models for tumorigenesis. Cancer Invest 12:203–213

Miki Y, Swensen J, Shattuck-Eidens D, Futreal PA, Harshman K, Tavtigian S, Liu Q, Cochran C, Bennett LM, Ding W, et al. (1994) A strong candidate for the breast and ovarian cancer susceptibility gene BRCA1. Science 266:66–71

Morrison C, Smith GC, Stingl L, Jackson SP, Wagner EF, Wang Z-Q (1997) Genetic interaction between PARP and DNA-PK in V(D)J recombination and tumorige-nesis. Nat Genet 17:479–482

Muller WJ, Sinn E, Pattengale PK, Wallace R, Leder P (1988) Single-step induction of mammary adenocarcinoma in transgenic mice bearing the activated c-neu onco-gene. Cell 54:105–115

Murakami H, Sanderson ND, Nagy P, Marino PA, Merlino G, Thorgeirsson SS (1993) Transgenic mouse model for synergistic effects of nuclear oncogenes and growth factors in tumorigenesis: interaction of c-myc and transforming growth factor alpha in hepatic oncogenesis. Cancer Res 53:1719–1723

Oro AE, Higgins KM, Hu Z, Bonifas JM, Epstein EH Jr, Scott MP (1997) Basal cell carcinomas in mice overexpressing sonic hedgehog. Science 276:817–821

Prolla TA, Baker SM, Harris AC, Tsao JL, Yao X, Bronner CE, Zheng B, Gordon M, Reneker J, Arnheim N, Shibata D, Bradley A, Liskay RM (1998) Tumour suscep-tibility and spontaneous mutation in mice deficient in Mlh1, Pms1 and Pms2 DNA mismatch repair. Nat Genet 18:276–279

Rajewsky K, Gu H, Kuhn R, Betz UA, Muller W, Roes J, and Schwenk F (1996) Con-ditional gene targeting. J Clin Invest 98:600–603

Reitmair AH, Cai JC, Bjerknes M, Redston M, Cheng H, Pind MT, Hay K, Mitri A, Bapat BV, Mak TW, Gallinger S (1996) MSH2 deficiency contributes to acceler-ated APC-mediated intestinal tumorigenesis. Cancer Res 56:2922–2926

Rodriguez MS, Desterro JM, Lain S, Midgley CA, Lane DP, Hay RT (1999) SUMO-1 modification activates the transcriptional response of p53. EMBO J 18:6455–6461

Rudolph K, Chang S, Lee HW, Blasco M, Gottlieb GJ, Greider CW, DePinho RA (1999) Longevity, stress response, and cancer in aging telomerase-deficient mice. Cell 96:701–712

Sandgren EP, Luetteke NC, Palmiter RD, Brinster RL, Lee DC (1990) Overexpression of TGF alpha in transgenic mice: induction of epithelial hyperplasia, pancreatic metaplasia, and carcinoma of the breast. Cell 61:1121–1135

Sandgren EP, Luetteke NC, Qiu TH, Palmiter RD, Brinster RL, Lee DC (1993) Transforming growth factor alpha dramatically enhances oncogene-induced carcinogenesis in transgenic mouse pancreas and liver. Mol Cell Biol 13:320–330

Sandgren EP, Quaife CJ, Pinkert CA, Palmiter RD, Brinster RL (1989) Oncogene-induced liver neoplasia in transgenic mice. Oncogene 4:715–724

Sands AT, Abuin A, Sanchez A, Conti CJ, Bradley A (1995) High susceptibility to ultraviolet-induced carcinogenesis in mice lacking XPC. Nature 377:162–165

Selivanova G, Kawasaki T, Ryabchenko L, Wiman KG (1998) Reactivation of mutant p53:a new strategy for cancer therapy. Semin Cancer Biol 8:369–378

Sell S, Hunt JM, Dunsford HA, Chisari FV (1991) Synergy between hepatitis B virus expression and chemical hepatocarcinogens in transgenic mice. Cancer Res 51: 1278–1285

Sharan SK, Morimatsu M, Albrecht U, Lim DS, Regel E, Dinh C, Sands A, Eichele G, Hasty P, Bradley A (1997) Embryonic lethality and radiation hypersensitivity mediated by Rad51 in mice lacking Brca2. Nature 386:804–810

Sherr CJ, Roberts JM (1995) Inhibitors of mammalian G1 cyclin-dependent kinases. Genes Dev 9:1149–1163

Sibilia M, Wagner EF (1996) Transgenic animals. European Review 4:371–391

Simbulan-Rosenthal CM, Haddad BR, Rosenthal DS, Weaver Z, Coleman A, Luo R, Young HM, Wang Z-Q, Ried T, Smulson ME (1999) Chromosomal aberrations in PARP$^{-/-}$ mice: Genome stabilization in immortalized cells by reintroduction of PARP cDNA. Proc Natl Acad Sci USA 96:13191–13196

Sinn E, Muller W, Pattengale P, Tepler I, Wallace R, Leder P (1987) Coexpression of MMTV/v-Ha-ras and MMTV/c-myc genes in transgenic mice: synergistic action of oncogenes in vivo. Cell 49:465–475

Slagle BL, Lee TH, Medina D, Finegold MJ, Butel JS (1996) Increased sensitivity to the hepatocarcinogen diethylnitrosamine in transgenic mice carrying the hepatitis B virus X gene. Mol Carcinog 15:261–269

Smith GCM, Jackson SP (1999) The DNA-dependent protein kinase. Genes Dev 13: 916–934

Spalding JW, Momma J, Elwell MR, Tennant RW (1993) Chemically induced skin carcinogenesis in a transgenic mouse line (TG.AC) carrying a v-Ha-ras gene. Carcinogenesis 14:1335–1341

Stewart TA, Pattengale PK, Leder P (1984) Spontaneous mammary adenocarcinomas in transgenic mice that carry and express MTV/myc fusion genes. Cell 38:627–637

Temme A, Buchmann A, Gabriel HD, Nelles E, Schwarz M, Willecke K (1997) High incidence of spontaneous and chemically induced liver tumors in mice deficient for connexin32. Curr Biol 7:713–716

Tong W-M, Galendo D, Wang Z-Q (2000) Role of DNA break-sensing molecule poly(ADP-ribose) polymerase (PARP) in cellular function and radiation toxicity. Cold Spring Harb Symp Quant Biol 65:583–591

Tong W-M, Hande MP, Lansdorp PM, Wang Z-Q (2001) DNA strand break-sensing molecule poly(ADP-ribose) polymerase cooperates with p53 in telomere function, chromosome stability, and tumor suppression. Mol Cell Biol 21:4046–4054

van der Horst GT, van Steeg H, Berg RJ, van Gool AJ, de Wit J, Weeda G, Morreau H, Beems RB, van Kreijl CF, de Gruijl FR, Bootsma D, Hoeijmakers JH (1997) Defective transcription-coupled repair in Cockayne syndrome B mice is associated with skin cancer predisposition. Cell 89:425–435

Vogelstein B, Kinzler KW (1992) p53 function and dysfunction. Cell 70:523–526
Vogelstein B, Kinzler KW (ed) (1998) The genetic basis of human cancer. McGraw-Hill, New York St. Louis San Francisco Auckland Bogota Caracas Lisbon London Madrid Mexico City Milan Montreal New Delhi San Juna Singapore Sydney Tokyo Toronto
Wagner EF, Wang Z-Q (1999) Genetically modified mice as tools for cancer research. In: "Development-Genetics, Epigenetics and Environmental Regulation", Russo E, Cove D, Edgar L, Jaenisch R, Salamini F (eds), Chapter 30, Springer-Verlag Berlin Heidelberg New York, pp 471–485
Wang TC, Cardiff RD, Zukerberg L, Lees E, Arnold A, Schmidt EV (1994) Mammary hyperplasia and carcinoma in MMTV-cyclin D1 transgenic mice. Nature 369: 669–671
Wang Z-Q, Auer B, Stingl L, Berghammer H, Haidacher D, Schweiger M, Wagner EF (1995) Mice lacking ADPRT and poly(ADP-ribosyl)ation develop normally but are susceptible to skin disease. Genes Dev 9:509–520
Wang Z-Q, Stingl L, Morrison C, Jantsch M, Los M, Schulze-Osthoff K, Wagner EF (1997) PARP is important for genomic stability but dispensable in apoptosis. Genes Dev 11:2347–2358
Wooster R, Bignell G, Lancaster J, Swift S, Seal S, Mangion J, Collins N, Gregory S, Gumbs C, Micklem G (1995) Identification of the breast cancer susceptibility gene BRCA2. Nature 378:789–792
Xu X, Qiao W, Linke SP, Cao L, Li WM, Furth PA, Harris CC, Deng CX (2001) Genetic interactions between tumor suppressors Brca1 and p53 in apoptosis, cell cycle and tumorigenesis. Nat Genet 28:266–271
Xu X, Wagner KU, Larson D, Weaver Z, Li C, Ried T, Hennighausen L, Wynshaw-Boris A, Deng CX (1999) Conditional mutation of Brca1 in mammary epithelial cells results in blunted ductal morphogenesis and tumour formation. Nat Genet 22: 37–43
Yamamoto S, Mitsumori K, Kodama Y, Matsunuma N, Manabe S, Okamiya H, Suzuki H, Fukuda T, Sakamaki Y, Sunaga M, Nomura G, Hioki K, Wakana S, Nomura T, Hayashi Y (1996) Rapid induction of more malignant tumors by various genotoxic carcinogens in transgenic mice harboring a human prototype c-Ha-ras gene than in control nontransgenic mice. Carcinogenesis 17:2455–2461
Yu Q, Geng Y, Sicinski P (2001) Specific protection against breast cancers by cyclin D1 ablation. Nature 411:1017–1021
Zhang H, Tombline G, Weber BL (1998) BRCA1, BRCA2, and DNA damage response: collision or collusion? Cell 92:433–436

New Promising Chemopreventive Agents and Mechanisms

C. Gerhäuser and N. Frank

A. Introduction

The development of cancer is a multistage process which is generally divided into initiation, promotion and progression phases. In the initiation phase, a carcinogen, either directly or after metabolic activation to a reactive molecule, interacts with intracellular macromolecules (DNA, proteins). This may cause DNA damage, which, if not repaired, can result in mutations and genetic damage. These mutations eventually lead to an altered expression of oncogenes and tumor suppressor genes or, e.g., continuous activation of protein kinases during the promotion phase, and finally result in modified cell structure, uncontrolled cell proliferation, tumor growth, and metastases in the progression phase. This cascade of events offers a variety of targets for chemopreventive intervention to prevent or inhibit the slow process of cellular changes from early genetic lesions to tumor development.

As indicated in Fig. 1, well-established molecular mechanisms of chemoprevention include modulation of drug metabolism, antioxidant, radical-scavenging, anti-inflammatory, antitumor promoting and antiproliferative activities, as well as induction of terminal cell differentiation and apoptosis of cancer-prone cells.

B. Chemopreventive Agent Development

Isolation of active chemopreventive agents from plants based on activity-guided fractionation using in vivo animal models is not feasible due to time and cost factors. Moreover, the complexity of reactions in a whole organism complicates the interpretation and elucidation of biological mechanisms. Therefore, a complementary series of defined cell- and enzyme-based in vitro marker systems relevant for inhibition of carcinogenesis in vivo at the initiation, promotion and progression stage has been set up (Table 1).

Taken together, these test systems allow fast (within days), sensitive, and cost effective identification of promising lead compounds and plant extracts and have been utilized for activity-guided isolation of active principles (Gerhauser et al., in press). To date, a total of more than 2,200 samples (plant constituents and synthetic analogs, extracts from various biological sources including medicinal plants, dietary components, mosses, marine bacteria and

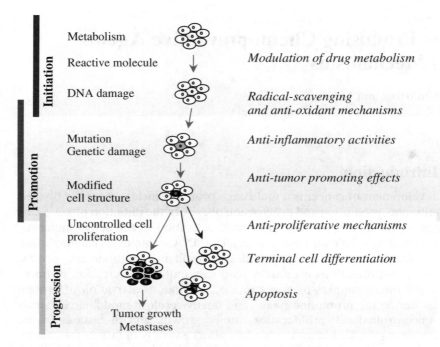

Fig. 1. Cellular carcinogenesis (*left*) and mechanisms relevant for cancer prevention (*right*)

fungi, and subfractions thereof) have been tested for biological activities in subsets of the bioassay systems described in Table 1.

A drawback of in vitro investigations is the identification of false positive leads, i.e., compounds which show activity in vitro, but fail to inhibit carcinogenesis in vivo. Therefore, we have established an organ culture model using mouse mammary glands (MMOC) as a link between short-term in vitro and long-term in vivo carcinogenesis models. This system combines the advantages of an in vitro system (feasibility and handling, compound requirements, duration of the experimental procedure) with the complex cellular, metabolic, and developmental conditions present in an entire organ (Mehta 2000). Results in the MMOC model have been shown previously to demonstrate good correlation with the outcome of long-term carcinogenesis models (Steele et al. 1996).

Based on in vitro bioassay data, promising compounds and a series of optimized structures were selected for further detailed analyses (Fig. 2).

I. Xanthohumol

Hop resin, derived from the cones of *Humulus lupulus* L., is rich in prenylated flavonoids (Stevens et al. 1997) and represents a good source of phenolic com-

Table 1. Bioassay systems for the identification of potential chemopreventive agents

Anti-initiation mechanisms: modulation of carcinogen metabolizing systems
  Inhibition of Cyp 1A activity in homogenates of β-naphthoflavone-induced H4IIE
  rat hepatoma cells (CRESPI et al. 1997)
  Induction of Cyp 1A activity in intact Hepa 1c1c7 murine hepatoma cells
  (according to CRESPI et al. 1997)
  Induction of NAD(P)H:quinone oxidoreductase (QR) activity in cultured Hepa
  1c1c7 cells (PROCHASKA and SANTAMARIA 1988; GERHAUSER et al. 1997)

Anti-initiating mechanisms: radical scavenging and antioxidant capacity
  Determination of free radical scavenging activity by reaction with 1,1-diphenyl-2-
  picrylhydrazyl (DPPH) free radicals (VAN AMSTERDAM et al. 1992)
  Analysis of hydroxyl (OH*)- and peroxyl (ROO*)-radical scavenging capacity in
  the oxygen radical absorbance capacity (ORAC) assay (PRIOR and CAO 1999)
  Scavenging of superoxide anion radicals, generated in xanthine oxidase system
  (X/XO) (UKEDA et al. 1997)
  Scavenging of superoxide anion radicals after stimulation of differentiated HL-60
  cells with 12-O-tetradecanoyl phorbol-13-acetate (TPA) (PICK and MIZEL 1981)
  Induction of glutathione levels in cellular systems (GERHAUSER et al. 1997;
  RIDNOUR et al. 1999)

Antitumor promoting mechanisms
  Inhibition of cyclooxygenase (Cox) 1 activity using sheep seminal vesicle
  microsomes (JANG et al. 1997)
  Inhibition of human recombinant Cox-2 activity (KUHL et al. 1984)
  Inhibition of soybean lipoxygenase 1 activity (BEN-AZIZ et al. 1970)
  Inhibition of lipopolysaccharide (LPS)-mediated inducible nitric oxide synthase
  (iNOS) induction in Raw 264.7 murine macrophage cell culture (HEISS et al.
  2001)
  Inhibition of TPA-mediated induction of ornithine decarboxylase in cultured 308
  murine keratinocytes (GERHAUSER et al. 1995)
  Assessment of estrogenic and antiestrogenic properties in Ishikawa human
  endometrium cancer cell culture via the estrogen-dependent induction of
  alkaline phosphatase (ALP) activity (LITTLEFIELD et al. 1990; MARKIEWICZ et al.
  1992)
  Inhibition of human recombinant aromatase (Cyp19) activity (STRESSER et al.
  2000)

Antiproliferative mechanisms relevant for the inhibition of tumor progression
  Inhibition of DNA polymerase α (PENGSUPARP et al. 1996)
  Induction of terminal cell differentiation in human (HL-60) or murine (MELC)
  leukemia cell lines (SUH et al. 1995; RICHON et al. 1996)

pounds in beer. Recently, prenylflavonoids from hop were shown to modulate drug metabolism in vitro by inhibition of various cytochrome P450 enzymes and by induction of NAD(P)H:quinone oxidoreductase (QR) activity; further, antioxidant and cytotoxic activities were described (HENDERSON et al. 2000; MIRANDA et al. 1999, 2000a,b). Therefore, a hop extract was subjected to activity-guided fractionation and yielded a major component, the prenylated chalcone xanthohumol (2′,4,4′-trihydroxy-3′-prenyl-6′-methoxychalcone, Fig. 2), its cyclization product, the isoflavanone isoxanthohumol and a series of related compounds (GERHAUSER et al. 2002). In subsequent bioassay tests

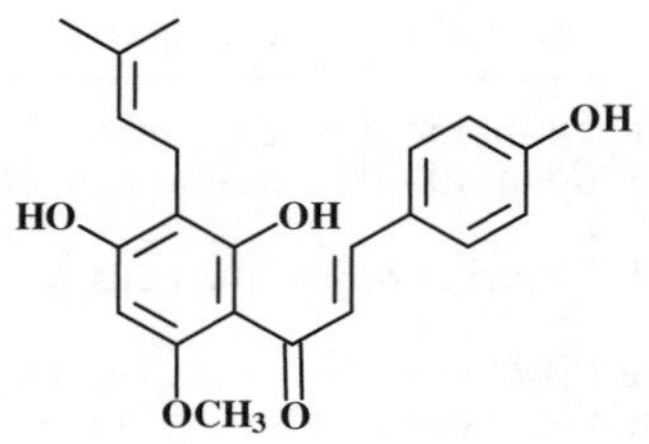

Xanthohumol 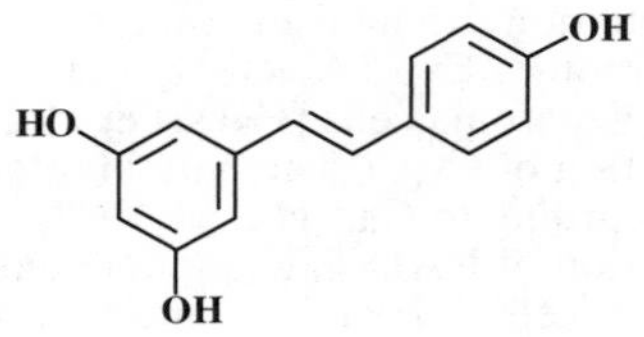   Resveratrol

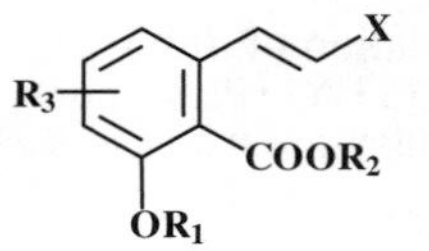

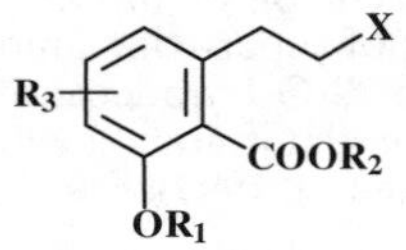

Lunularic acid-derived bibenzyls

X=Aryl, Heteroaryl, R_1, R_2 = H, CH_3, C_2H_5,

R_3 = OH, Br, AcO

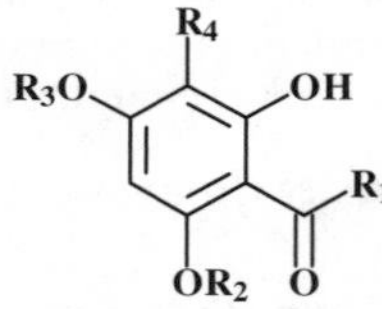

Acylphloroglucinol   Acylphloroglucinol

Monomer, R_1 = Acyl   Dimer, R_1 = Acyl

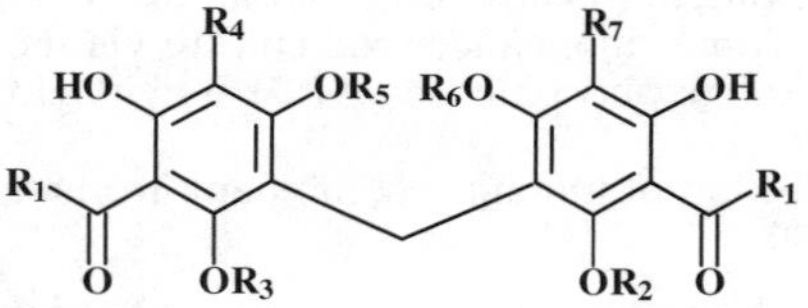

R_2, R_3, R_4 = H, CH_3 R_2, R_3, R_4, R_5, R_6, R_7 = H, CH_3

Fig. 2. Chemical structures of xanthohumol, resveratrol, lunularic acid-derived biben-zyls, and mono- and dimeric acylphloroglucinols

(described in Table 1), chemopreventive activities of xanthohumol were compared with those of the well known chemopreventive agent resveratrol, a tri-hydroxy stilbene found in grapes and red wine (Fig. 2). The results are summarized in Table 2.

Indicative of chemopreventive potential in the initiation phase, xantho-humol was found to potently inhibit phase 1 Cyp1A activity in a competitive

Table 2. Comparison of bioassay results of xanthohumol and resveratrol

	Xanthohumol	Resveratrol
Anti-initiation mechanisms		
Inhibition of Cyp1A activity (IC_{50})	$0.02\,\mu M$	$0.23\,\mu M$
Induction of QR activity in Hepa1c1c7 (CD)	$1.7\,\mu M$	$23.8\,\mu M$
Inhibition of Hepa1c1c7 cell proliferation (IC_{50})	$7.4\,\mu M$	$29.4\,\mu M$
$ORAC_{OH}$ (units)	8.9	3.2
$ORAC_{ROO}$ (units)	2.9	2.1
Superoxide anion radical scavenging (HL-60)	$2.6\,\mu M$	$>100\ (29)$[a]
Superoxide anion radical scavenging (X/XO)	$27.7\,\mu M$	$>100\ (50)$[a]
Antitumor promoting mechanisms		
Inhibition of Cox-1 activity (IC_{50})	$16.6\,\mu M$	$1.6\,\mu M$
Inhibition of Cox-2 activity (IC_{50})	$41.5\,\mu M$	$32.2\,\mu M$[b]
Inhibition of iNOS induction (IC_{50})	$12.9\,\mu M$	$31.7\,\mu M$
Inhibition of E2-induced ALP activity in the Ishikawa cell line (antiestrogenic potential) (IC_{50})	$6.6\,\mu M$	$18.5\,\mu M$[c]
Inhibition of TPA-mediated ODC induction (IC_{50})	$>10\,\mu M\ (31)$[a]	$>10\,\mu M\ (0)$[a]
Antiproliferative mechanisms		
Inhibition of DNA polymerase α activity	$23.0\,\mu M$	$>500\,\mu M\ (37)$[a]
Cell cycle arrest (MDA-MB 435 cell line)	S phase	S phase[d]
Differentiation of cultured HL-60 cells		
NBT reduction (granulocytic lineage)	$6.25\,\mu M$: 37.2%[e]	ED_{50}: $11\,\mu M$[f]
NSE staining (monocytic/macrophagic lineage)	$6.25\,\mu M$: 44.8%[e]	ED_{50}: $19\,\mu M$[f]
Inhibition of cell proliferation (IC_{50})	$3.7\,\mu M$	$18\,\mu M$[f]
MMOC (IC_{50})	$0.02\,\mu M$	$4.2\,\mu M$

[a] Values in parenthesis indicate the percentage of inhibition at the indicated concentration.
[b] From WAFFO-TEGUO et al. 2001.
[c] Concomitant induction of ALP activity in the absence of 17β-estradiol is indicative of estrogenic activity.
[d] From HSIEH et al. 1999.
[e] Percentage of positive cells at the indicated concentration.
[f] ED_{50}: Halfmaximal effective dose, according to JANG et al. 1997.

manner, with a halfmaximal inhibitory concentration (IC_{50}) of $0.02\,\mu M$. This is of relevance for chemoprevention as Cyp1A activity contributes to the metabolic activation of certain carcinogens. Resveratrol was about tenfold less active. Xanthohumol was also identified as a monofunctional inducer of QR activity, with a CD value (concentration required to double the specific activity of QR) of $1.7\,\mu M$. QR activity is often induced coordinately with phase 2 enzymes like glutathione S-transferases (GSTs), which generally conjugate activated xenobiotics to endogenous ligands and thus facilitate their detoxification. These activities were consistent with earlier reports. As an additional indication of anti-initiating potential, the antioxidant capacity of xanthohumol was investigated. Xanthohumol at a concentration of $1\,\mu M$ was 8.9-fold and

2.9-fold more potent than the reference compound Trolox, a water-soluble vitamin E analog, in scavenging OH*- and ROO* radicals, respectively. Also, it dose-dependently inhibited superoxide anion radical production in the xanthine/xanthine oxidase (X/XO) system, and by TPA-stimulated HL-60 leukemia cells differentiated to granulocytes. Resveratrol was inactive in both systems up to a concentration of $100\,\mu$M.

With respect to mechanisms involved in the prevention of tumor promotion, xanthohumol demonstrated anti-inflammatory potential by inhibition of Cox-1 and -2 activity, but resveratrol was significantly more potent in inhibiting Cox-1 activity. Both compounds weakly prevented NO release by LPS-stimulated Raw 264.7 murine macrophages. Further, xanthohumol efficiently inhibited estrogen-mediated induction of alkaline phosphatase (ALP) activity in the Ishikawa cell line, indicative of antiestrogenic mechanisms, without possessing intrinsic estrogenic potential. In this system, resveratrol demonstrated activities consistent with mixed estrogen/antiestrogen properties. Both compounds were inactive in inhibiting phorbol ester-induced ODC activity in 308 murine keratinocytes up to $10\,\mu$M.

Antiproliferative mechanisms of xanthohumol to prevent carcinogenesis in the progression phase included inhibition of human recombinant DNA polymerase α, cell cycle arrest of cultured MDA-MB-435 breast cancer cells in the S phase at 10 and $20\,\mu$M, and induction of apoptosis in 14.9% of attached cells after an incubation of 48 h at $25\,\mu$M. Although resveratrol was inactive in the DNA polymerase α system, it has been reported to arrest various cancer cell lines in S phase, including the estrogen receptor negative MDA-MB-435 cell line (HSIEH et al. 1999; JOE et al. 2002). As an additional mechanisms to control hyperproliferation of cancer cells, both xanthohumol and resveratrol induced terminal cell differentiation in HL-60 cell culture.

Importantly, in the MMOC model, xanthohumol prevented preneoplastic mammary lesion formation 200-fold more efficiently than resveratrol, with an IC$_{50}$ value of $0.02\,\mu$M, presumably due to a combination of the preventive mechanisms described in this section (GERHAUSER et al. 2001). Currently, further studies on metabolism, bioavailability, safety, and efficacy in a rat mammary tumor model are ongoing. Our present data provide promising evidence for novel possible applications of xanthohumol and hop products with respect to cancer prevention, and further investigations are warranted.

II. Lunularic Acid-Derived Bibenzyls

Bibenzyles are found in nature in mosses, like *Polytrichum pallidisetum* (*Polytrichaceae*) (ZHENG et al. 1994), or in the South African tree *Combretum caffrum* (*Combretaceae*) (PETTIT et al. 1988). Combretastatins have been described as inhibitors of tumor vasculature and as antimitotic compounds through a tubulin-binding mechanism and were shown to inhibit tumor cell growth in vitro (PETTIT et al. 1995). Moscatilin, a natural bibenzyl compound isolated from an orchid from China, *Dendrobium nobile* (*Orchidaceae*), exerted antimutagenic activity (MIYAZAWA et al. 1999), whereas bifluranol, a synthetic fluorinated bibenzyl, was found to be antiprostatic (DEKANSKI 1980). Liverworts (*Hepaticae*) are a unique source of bibenzyl derivatives of the lunularic acid type (Fig. 2). These compounds display structural similarities with resveratrol, and analogs can be synthesized easily in large quantities (ZINSMEISTER et al. 1991).

Screening of a series of more than 100 natural and synthetic bibenzyls for potential chemopreventive activity led to their identification as potent *modulators of phase 1 and phase 2 metabolizing enzymes* (Gerhauser et al., in preparation). CD values for the induction of QR activity in Hepa 1c1c7 cell culture were in the range of 0.03–51 μM, depending on the substitution of the ring systems. As an example, EC-252, a synthetic derivative with a bromo-substituted thiophene ring system, with a CD value of 0.06 μM induced QR activity 1.4- to 6.6-fold in a concentration range of 0.016–1.0 μM. Active compounds were additionally tested in cultured BP^{r}c1 cells, a mutant cell line derived from Hepa 1c1c7 with defective Ah (aryl-hydrocarbon)-receptor/ ARNT (Ah-receptor nuclear translocator protein)-mediated transcriptional activation of Ah-receptor-dependent enzymes. Lack of QR-inducing potential in the BP^{r}c1 cell line indicated that the mechanism of induction of these compounds might involve interaction with the Ah-receptor, activation of the xenobiotic responsive element (XRE) and potential to additionally induce Ah-receptor dependent phase 1 enzymes. In transient transfection experiments with QR-chloramphenicol acetyltransferase plasmid constructs, QR induction was confirmed to involve activation of the XRE. Subsequently, dose-dependent *induction of Cyp1A activity* in cultured Hepa 1c1c7 cells could be demonstrated, although the compounds have no structural similarity to known ligands of the Ah-receptor (e.g., polychlorinated biphenyls, polyaromatic aryl-hydrocarbons). Since induction of Cyp1A might result in the activation of pro-carcinogens, potential *to inhibit Cyp1A activity* was investigated. Interestingly, selected compounds were identified as potent inhibitors of Cyp1A enzyme activity using lysates of β-naphthoflavone-induced H4IIE rat hepatoma cells and 3-cyano-7-ethoxy-coumarin (CEC) as a substrate. Most potent compounds resulted in IC$_{50}$ values of about 0.1 μM. EC-252 as a model compound demonstrated competitive inhibition of Cyp1A activity with respect to the substrate CEC, which was determined by Lineweaver-Burk-, Dixon- and Cornish-Bowden plots of the results of kinetic experiments.

The bibenzyl core motive is commonly found in many ligands of the estrogen receptor (ER). Consistently, resveratrol was identified as an ER receptor super-agonist and demonstrated estrogenic and antiestrogenic properties in Ishikawa cell culture (see Sect. B.I.) and mammary cancer models (BHAT et al. 2001). When selected lunularic acid derivatives were analyzed in the Ishikawa cell line, hydrogen-substitution at R$_1$ in combination with a (hydroxyl-substituted) phenyl ring in position X resulted in mixed estrogenic and antiestrogenic activities, whereas heteroaryl substitution in X (e.g., in EC-252) led to pure antiestrogenic potential. These effects might be due to direct (ant)agonistic interaction with the ER. Also, Ah-receptor ligand-mediated inhibition of estrogen-induced gene expression has been described (Wormke et al. 2000) and might contribute to the observed antiestrogenic response. Further activities of bibenzyl derivatives included scavenging of DPPH free radicals and anti-inflammatory mechanisms (inhibition of Cox-1 activity and LPS-induced NO production). The activity profile strongly depended on type and pattern of substitution of the bibenzyl structure.

In recent investigations, EC-252 was found to inhibit DMBA-induced preneoplastic lesions in the MMOC model with an IC_{50} value of 0.19μM (Gerhauser et al. 2000). EC-252 was further identified as an extremely potent inhibitor of benzo(a)pyrene-mediated transformation of primary rat tracheal epithelial (RTE) cells (based on Steele et al. 1990), with an IC_{50} value less than 0.01μM. Similar to the results obtained in the MMOC model, positive results in the RTE assay have a >70% correlation with the results obtained in long-term in vivo chemoprevention models (Steele et al. 1996). These results will be of importance for further investigation of in vivo efficacy.

III. Acylphloroglucinol Derivatives

Ferns of the genus *Dryopteris* are a rich source of acylphloroglucinols (Widen et al. 2001). The chemical structure of acylphloroglucinol mono- and dimeres is shown in Fig. 2. Acylphloroglucinols are also common constituents of *Eucalyptus* species and exhibit a wide range of biological activities (Ghisalberti 1996). In the area of carcinogenesis, inhibition of TPA-induced activation of Epstein-Barr virus (Takasaki et al. 1990) as well as antiviral activity against the vesicular stomatitis virus (Chiba et al. 1992) has been reported. The authors could demonstrate that the acyl chain length played an essential role for the biological activity. Also, a strong inhibitory effect on mouse skin (Takasaki et al. 1995) and mouse pulmonary (Takasaki et al. 2000) tumor promotion was detected, and the dimeric compounds aspidin and desaspidin were found to inhibit papilloma formation in the two stage mouse skin model (Kapadia et al. 1996).

We tested about 50 mono-, di-, tri- and tetrameric acylphloroglucinol derivatives in our bioassay systems. Several compounds were identified as potent inhibitors of Cox-1 activity (Gerhauser et al., in preparation). The monomeric synthetic derivative isoaspidinol (R_1 = propyl, R_2, R_4 = methyl, R_3 = H, Haapalainen and Widen 1970) was identified as the most potent inhibitor of Cox-1 activity of this series, with an IC_{50} value of 2.3μM. For comparison, the unsubstituted phloroglucinol (1,3,5-trihydroxybenzene) inhibited Cox-1 activity with an IC_{50} value of 3.8μM. Interestingly, replacement of the 4-hydroxyl-group of isoaspidinol (R_3 = H) by a 4-methoxy-group in methyl-butyryl-phloroglucinol-4,6-dimethylether (R_3 = CH_3) significantly reduced the inhibitory potential (12% *versus* 99% inhibition at a test concentration of 100μM, respectively). The isomeric compounds o-desaspidinol B and desaspidinol B (R_1 = propyl, R_2 = methyl, R_3, R_4 = H), which lack the methyl-group at position 3, were slightly less active than isoaspidinol, with IC_{50} values of about $10\,\mu M$. Substitution of the butyryl- by a propionyl- (desaspidinol P) or an acetyl-side chain (desaspidinol A) further reduced the inhibitory activity (IC_{50} values: $17.3\,\mu M$ and $28.6\,\mu M$, respectively). Selected dimeric compounds tested were moderately active, with IC_{50} values in the range of $15-37\,\mu M$, whereas tri- and tetrameric aclyphloroglucinols were generally not active (IC_{50} values $>50\,\mu M$).

In addition to assessing Cox-1 inhibitory potential, isoaspidinol and phlorogucinol were tested using human recombinant Cox-2 as an enzyme source. Whereas isoaspidinol was inactive in inhibiting Cox-2 activity at concentrations up to $100\,\mu M$, phloroglucinol was identified as a dual Cox-1 and -2 inhibitor with an IC_{50} value for Cox-2 of $7.2\,\mu M$. Both compounds were further tested in the MMOC model. At a test concentration of $10\,\mu M$, phloroglucinol inhibited preneoplastic lesion formation by 47% in comparison with the solvent control. Isoaspidinol was more active, and we could demonstrate dose-dependent inhibition in a concentration range of $0.01-50\,\mu M$, with an IC_{50} value of $3.4\,\mu M$.

Further activities mainly observed with dimeric acylphloroglucionols included scavenging of DPPH stable radicals and inhibitory effects on TPA-induced ODC activity and LPS-mediated iNOS induction. Overall, dimerization also increased cytotoxicity. Therefore, we will focus our further investigations on the most interesting monomers.

C. Novel Mechanisms of Chemopreventive Agents

In addition to identification of candidate chemopreventive agents, in vitro test systems are important for the elucidation of their mechanism of action. This will allow the efficient development of most promising compounds for in vivo application. Based on their profile of biological activities in the in vitro test panel, sulforaphane and ellagic acid (Fig. 3) were selected for comprehensive mechanistic investigations.

I. NF-κB as a Molecular Target of Sulforaphane

Sulforaphane (1-isothiocyanato-(4R)methylsulfinyl)butane) is a naturally occurring isothiocyanate found as a precursor glucosinolate in cruciferous vegetables like broccoli (ZHANG et al. 1992). Interestingly, bioavailability in humans after ingestion of fresh broccoli was about three times higher than from cooked broccoli (CONAWAY et al. 2000). Sulforaphane inhibits chemically induced mammary tumors in rats (ZHANG et al. 1994), preneoplastic lesions in MMOC (GERHAUSER et al. 1997), and was found to prevent azoxymethane-induced colonic aberrant crypt foci in rats (CHUNG et al. 2000). This anticarcinogenic activity has been mainly attributed to inhibitory effects on various cytochrome P450 isoenzymes (BARCELO et al. 1996; MAHEO et al. 1997; BARCELO

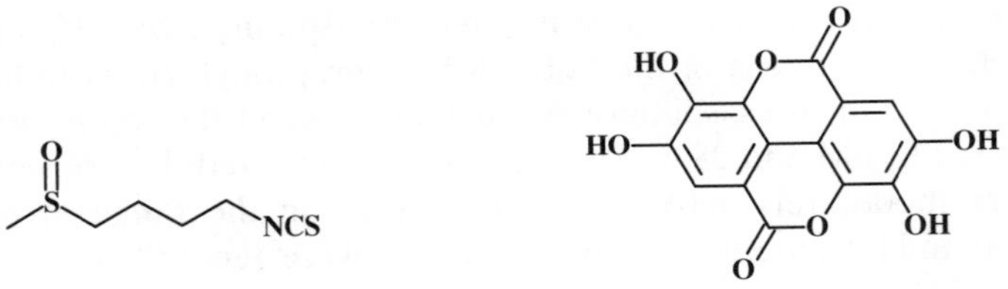

Sulforaphane　　　　　　　　　　Ellagic acid

Fig. 3. Chemical structures of sulforaphane and ellagic acid

et al. 1998) concomitantly with potent induction of phase 2 drug-metabolizing enzymes (Zhang et al. 1992; Gerhauser et al. 1997) and of the multidrug resistance-associated protein 2 (MRP2) transporter pump (Payen et al. 2001). Recently, sulforaphane was also shown to inhibit TPA-induced ODC activity, to induce cell differentiation in the HL-60 human leukemia cell line (Lee et al. 1999), and to initiate cell cycle arrest and apoptosis in human colon cancer cell lines and in T-cell leukemia (Gamet-Payrastre et al. 2000; Bonnesen et al. 2001; Fimognari et al. 2002).

Aiming to investigate so far unknown anti-inflammatory mechanisms of sulforaphane, we have demonstrated a potent decrease in LPS-induced secretion of proinflammatory and procarcinogenic signaling factors in cultured Raw 264.7 macrophages after sulforaphane-treatment, i.e., nitric oxide (NO), prostaglandin E_2 and tumor necrosis factor α, with IC_{50} values of 0.7 μM, 1.4 μM, and 7.8 μM, respectively. Inhibition of increased NO levels was measurable when sulforaphane was added either simultaneously with or up to 4 h post LPS treatment. Direct interaction of sulforaphane with NO could be excluded. When the NO-donor SIN-1 was used as an exogenous source of NO, sulforaphane did not lower nitrite levels determined by the Griess reaction. In addition, sulforaphane was unable to directly inhibit iNOS or Cox-1 enzymatic activity. Rather, western blot and RT-PCR analyses revealed a sulforaphane-mediated dose- and time-dependent decrease of LPS-stimulated iNOS and Cox-2 protein expression and iNOS mRNA induction. Electrophoretic mobility shift assay (EMSA) analyses pointed to a reversible and thiol-dependent inhibition of DNA binding of transcription factor NF-κB upon sulforaphane treatment, whereas DNA binding of AP-1 and NF-IL6 (C/EBPβ) was not impaired. Other than resveratrol (Holmes-McNary and Baldwin 2000), sulforaphane did not inhibit the IκB kinase-mediated phosphorylation and subsequent degradation of IκB (inhibitor of NF-κB), which is a prerequisite for NF-κB activation. Also, nuclear translocation of NF-κB was not impaired. Since isothiocyanates easily react with sulfhydryl groups by dithiocarbamate formation, we rather speculate that modulation of essential thiol groups of NF-κB subunits or of factors involved in the redox regulation of NF-κB DNA binding, including glutathione (GSH) and the redox modulators thioredoxin and Ref-1, contributes to the inhibitory mechanism of sulforaphane (HEISS et al. 2001).

We have identified NF-κB as an important target for anti-inflammatory activities of sulforaphane, and further studies are warranted to elucidate the relevance of these properties for sulforaphane-mediated cancer chemopreventive efficacy.

II. Novel Antioxidant Mechanisms of Ellagic Acid

Ellagic acid (4,4',5,5',6,6'-hexahydrodiphenic acid 2,6,2',6'-dilactone) is a widely distributed phenolic compound found in berries, nuts, tea, red wine, and various medicinal plants. The average intake of ellagic acid in men is up to 5.2 mg/day (RADTKE et al. 1998). Ellagic acid has been demonstrated to inhibit tumor growth in animal models, induced by various chemical carcinogens, including polycyclic aromatic hydrocarbons, N-nitrosamines, aflatoxins and aromatic amines (SAN and CHAN 1987; PERCHELLET et al. 1992; TANAKA et al. 1993; DOW et al. 1994; BARCH et al. 1996; STONER and MORSE 1997). In these studies, ellagic acid was identified as an effective chemopreventive agent against rodent colon, skin, tongue, lung, liver, and esophageal carcinogenesis. Several mechanisms have been proposed to explain the broad antimutagenic and anticarcinogenic effects of ellagic acid, including the inhibition of cytochrome P450 isoenzymes, and the induction of the phase 2 detoxification enzymes including GSTs, QR, and UDP glucuronosyltransferase (AHN et al. 1996). Ellagic acid applied topically to mouse skin effectively inhibited TPA-induced ODC activity, H_2O_2 production, and DNA synthesis (CASTONGUAY et al. 1997). It also induced cell cycle G_1 arrest and apoptosis by increasing p21 levels via a p53-independent mechanism in cervical carcinoma cells (NARAYANAN et al. 1999). Further, ellagic acid was identified as a potent inhibitor of the catalytic activities of both DNA topoisomerases I and II, although it did not trap the enzyme-DNA reaction intermediate and was therefore not regarded as a topoisomerase poison (CONSTANTINOU et al. 1995).

With respect to antioxidant activity, ellagic acid potently scavenged H_2O_2-derived reactive oxygen species, prevented H_2O_2- or bleomycin-induced DNA damage in CHO cells and potently inhibited the formation of 8-oxo-2'-deoxyguanosine (8-oxodG) in a Cu^{2+}-mediated Fenton-type reaction (COZZI et al. 1995; FESTA et al. 2001; SRINIVASAN et al. 2002). Based on these reports, we aimed to investigate whether ellagic acid acted mainly as a direct antioxidant, based on its polyphenol structure, or might activate additional intracellular antioxidant mechanisms. In the ORAC assay, ellagic acid exhibited a high scavenging capacity against different physiologically relevant reactive species, including ROO*, OH*, and Cu^{2+}, and enhanced significantly the antioxidant activities of both the protein and nonprotein fractions of human hepatocellular carcinoma cells HUH-7 cells against ROO* and OH* radicals. It significantly increased total intracellular thiol levels and moderately elevated the GSH/GSSG ratio. The increase in total thiols was not only due to elevated

GSH levels, but mainly due to thiol-containing proteins, which might include enzymes like catalase, glutathione peroxidase and thioredoxin reductase, or cysteine-rich proteins like metallothioneins (MT).

Human metallothioneins (hMTs) are a conserved family of heavy metal-binding proteins that participate in detoxification of transition metals such as Cd and Zn and protect against oxidative stress. Since MT isoforms have been reported to belong to the antioxidant responsive element (ARE)-regulated family of genes (CAMPAGNE et al. 2000) and MT was inducible by genistein-treatment of cultured Caco-2 human colon carcinoma cells (KUO and LEAVITT 1999), the influence of ellagic acid on MT expression was further investigated. Using ELISA and RT-PCR techniques, EA was shown to moderately induce MT protein levels and to fivefold upregulate MT-1a mRNA expression in HUH-7 cells, whereas MT-2a mRNA levels were about 50% reduced. Transcriptional regulation of MT expression involves the activation of metal response elements (MRE), which are present in multiple copies in the proximal promoters of MT genes, by the MRE-binding transcription factor-1 (MTF-1). In EMSA analyses we could demonstrate that ellagic acid differentially up-and downregulated DNA binding of MTF-1 and of transcription factor Sp1 to MREs (a–d), whereas AP-1 DNA binding was not influenced. In addition, ellagic acid treatment time- and dose-dependently enhanced the activities of essential cellular antioxidant enzymes including catalase, glutathione peroxidase and thioredoxin reductase. As a consequence, chemically induced lipid peroxidation in HUH-7 cells, determined as malondialdehyde levels, was effectively prevented by ellagic acid treatment. Taken together, our studies support the role of ellagic acid as a cancer chemopreventive agent acting by multiple antioxidant mechanisms (GAMAL-ELDEEN et al. 2001).

D. Conclusion

In the present report we could demonstrate that identification and evaluation of novel potential chemopreventive agents through a bioassay test panel is feasible. Activity-guided fractionation allowed the determination of active principles and lead compounds from plant extracts. Verification of in vitro results by an ex vivo model (MMOC) further improves the predictive value for animal experiments and for human use. The elucidation of chemopreventive mechanisms of novel, but also of known chemopreventive agents should allow a more target-oriented and therefore more effective use, and optimization by structural modifications. Overall, chemopreventive mechanisms and their relevance for preventive efficacy should be demonstrated from simple in vitro systems to complex animal models and studies in humans.

References

Ahn D, Putt D, Kresty L, Stoner GD, Fromm D, Hollenberg PF (1996) The effects of dietary ellagic acid on rat hepatic and esophageal mucosal cytochromes P450 and phase II enzymes. Carcinogenesis 17:821–828

Barcelo S, Gardiner JM, Gescher A, Chipman JK (1996) CYP2E1-mediated mechanism of antigenotoxicity of the broccoli constituent sulforaphane. Carcinogenesis 17:277–282

Barcelo S, Mace K, Pfeifer AM, Chipman JK (1998) Production of DNA strand breaks by N-nitrosodimethylamine and 2-amino-3-methylimidazo[4,5-f]quinoline in THLE cells expressing human CYP isoenzymes and inhibition by sulforaphane. Mutat Res 402:111–120

Barch DH, Rundhaugen LM, Stoner GD, Pillay NS, Rosche WA (1996) Structure-function relationships of the dietary anticarcinogen ellagic acid. Carcinogenesis 17:265–269

Ben Aziz A, Grossman S, Ascarelli I, Budowski P (1970) Linoleate oxidation induced by lipoxygenase and heme proteins: a direct spectrophotometric assay. Anal Biochem 34:88–100

Bhat KP, Lantvit D, Christov K, Mehta RG, Moon RC, Pezzuto JM (2001) Estrogenic and antiestrogenic properties of resveratrol in mammary tumor models. Cancer Res 61:7456–7463

Bonnesen C, Eggleston IM, Hayes JD (2001) Dietary indoles and isothiocyanates that are generated from cruciferous vegetables can both stimulate apoptosis and confer protection against DNA damage in human colon cell lines. Cancer Res 61: 6120–6130

Campagne MV, Thibodeaux H, van Bruggen N, Cairns B, Lowe DG (2000) Increased binding activity at an antioxidant-responsive element in the metallothionein-1 promoter and rapid induction of metallothionein-1 and -2 in response to cerebral ischemia and reperfusion. J Neurosci 20:5200–5207

Castonguay A, Gali H, Perchellet EM, Gao XM, Boukharta M, Jalbert G, Okuda T, Yoshida T, Hatano T, Perchellet J-P (1997) Antitumorigenic and antipromoting activities of ellagic acid, ellagitannins and oligomeric anthocyanin and procyanidin. Int J Oncol 10:367–373

Chiba K, Takakuwa T, Tada M, Yoshii T (1992) Inhibitory effect of acylphloroglucinol derivatives on the replication of vesicular stomatitis virus. Biosci Biotechnol Biochem 56:1769–1772

Chung FL, Conaway CC, Rao CV, Reddy BS (2000) Chemoprevention of colonic aberrant crypt foci in Fischer rats by sulforaphane and phenethyl isothiocyanate. Carcinogenesis 21:2287–2291

Conaway CC, Getahun SM, Liebes LL, Pusateri DJ, Topham DK, Botero-Omary M, Chung FL (2000) Disposition of glucosinolates and sulforaphane in humans after ingestion of steamed and fresh broccoli. Nutr Cancer 38:168–178

Constantinou A, Stoner GD, Mehta R, Rao K, Runyan C, Moon R (1995) The dietary anticancer agent ellagic acid is a potent inhibitor of DNA topoisomerases in vitro. Nutr Cancer 23:121–130

Cozzi R, Ricordy R, Bartolini F, Ramadori L, Perticone P, De Salvia R (1995) Taurine and ellagic acid: two differently-acting natural antioxidants. Environ Mol Mutagen 26:248–254

Crespi CL, Miller VP, Penman, BW (1997) Microtiter plate assays for inhibition of human, drug-metabolizing cytochromes P450. Anal Biochem 248:188–190

Dekanski JB (1980) Antiprostatic activity of bifluranol, a fluorinated bibenzyl. Br J Pharmacol 71:11–16

Dow LR, Chou TT, Bechle MB, Goddard C, Larson RE (1994) Identification of tricyclic analogs related to ellagic acid as potent/selective tyrosine protein kinase inhibitors. J Med Chem 37:224–231

Festa F, Aglitti T, Duranti G, Ricordy R, Perticone P, Cozzi R (2001) Strong antioxidant activity of ellagic acid in mammalian cells in vitro revealed by the comet assay. Anticancer Res 21(6A):3903–3908

Fimognari C, Nusse M, Cesari R, Iori R, Cantelli-Forti G, Hrelia P (2002) Growth inhibition, cell-cycle arrest and apoptosis in human T-cell leukemia by the isothiocyanate sulforaphane. Carcinogenesis 23:581–586

Gamet-Payrastre L, Li P, Lumeau S, Cassar G, Dupont MA, Chevolleau S, Gasc N, Tulliez J, Terce F (2000) Sulforaphane, a naturally occurring isothiocyanate, induces cell cycle arrest and apoptosis in HT29 human colon cancer cells. Cancer Res 60:1426–1433

Gamal-Eldeen A, Gerhäuser C, Frank N, Bartsch H (2001) Ellagic acid induces antioxidant mechanisms in cultured human hepatocellular carcinoma cells HUH-7. J Cancer Res Clin Oncol 127:S34

Gerhauser C, Alt A, Heiss E, Gamal-Eldeen A, Klimo K, Knauft J, Neumann I, Scherf H-R, Frank N, Bartsch H, Becker H (2001) Xanthohumol from hop (*Humulus lupulus*) as a novel potential cancer chemopreventive agent. Proc Am Assoc Cancer Res 42:18

Gerhauser C, Alt A, Heiss E, Gamal-Eldeen A, Klimo K, Knauft J, Neumann I, Scherf H-R, Frank N, Bartsch H, Becker H (2002) Cancer Chemopreventive Activity of Xanthohumol, a Natural Product derived from Hop. Molecular Cancer Therapeutics 1:959–969

Gerhäuser C, Heiss E, Klimo K, Neumann I, Becker H, Eicher Th, Bartsch H (2000) Bibenzyl derivatives as novel lead compounds in chemoprevention. Proc Am Assoc Cancer Res 41:412

Gerhäuser C, Klimo K, Heiss E, Neumann I, Gamal Eldeen A, Knauft J, Liu G, Sitthimonchai S, Frank N (2002) Mechanism-based in vitro Screening of Potential Cancer Chemopreventive Agents. Mutation Research (Fundamental and Molecular Mechanisms of Mutagenesis) (in press)

Gerhauser C, Mar W, Lee SK, Suh N, Luo Y, Kosmeder J, Luyengi L, Fong HH, Kinghorn AD, Moriarty RM, Mehta RG, Constantinou A, Moon RC, Pezzuto JM (1995) Rotenoids mediate potent cancer chemopreventive activity through transcriptional regulation of ornithine decarboxylase. Nat Med 1:260–266

Gerhauser C, You M, Liu J, Moriarty RM, Hawthorne M, Mehta RG, Moon RC, Pezzuto JM (1997) Cancer chemopreventive potential of sulforamate, a novel analogue of sulforaphane that induces phase 2 drug-metabolizing enzymes. Cancer Res 57:272–278

Ghisalberti EL (1996) Bioactive acylphloroglucinol derivatives from *Eucalyptus* species. Phytochem 41:7–22

Haapalainen L, Widen CJ (1970) Thin-layer chromatographic separation of phloroglucinol derivatives from *Dryopteris* ferns at different pH values. Farm Aikak 79: 161–173

Heiss E, Herhaus C, Klimo K, Bartsch H, Gerhauser C (2001) Nuclear factor-κB is a molecular target for sulforaphane-mediated antiinflammatory mechanisms. J Biol Chem 276:32008–32015

Henderson MC, Miranda CL, Stevens JF, Deinzer ML, Buhler DR (2000) In vitro inhibition of human P450 enzymes by prenylated flavonoids from hop *Humulus lupulus*. Xenobiotica 30:235–251

Holmes-McNary M, Baldwin AS Jr (2000) Chemopreventive properties of transresveratrol are associated with inhibition of activation of the IkappaB kinase. Cancer Res 60:3477–3483

Hsieh TC, Burfeind P, Laud K, Backer JM, Traganos F, Darzynkiewicz Z, Wu JM (1999) Cell cycle effects and control of gene expression by resveratrol in human breast carcinoma cell lines with different metastatic potentials. Int J Oncol 15:245–252

Jang M, Cai L, Udeani GO, Slowing KV, Thomas CF, Beecher CW, Fong HH, Farnsworth NR, Kinghorn AD, Mehta RG, Moon RC, Pezzuto JM (1997) Cancer chemopreventive activity of resveratrol, a natural product derived from grapes. Science 275:218–220

Joe AK, Liu H, Suzui M, Vural ME, Xiao D, Weinstein IB (2002) Resveratrol induces growth inhibition, S-phase arrest, apoptosis, and changes in biomarker expression in several human cancer cell lines. Clin Cancer Res 8:893–903

Kapadia GJ, Tokuda H, Konoshima T, Takasaki M, Takayasu J, Nishino H (1996) Anti-tumor promoting activity of *Dryopteris* phlorophenone derivatives. Cancer Lett 105:161–165

Kuhl P, Shiloh R, Jha H, Murawski U, Zilliken F (1984) 6,7,4'-Trihydroxyisoflavan: a potent and selective inhibitor of 5-lipoxygenase in human and porcine peripheral blood leukocytes. Prostaglandins 28:783–804

Kuo SM, Leavitt PS (1999) Genistein increases metallothionein expression in human intestinal cells, Caco-2. Biochem Cell Biol 77:79–88

Lee SK, Song L, Mata-Greenwood E, Kelloff GJ, Steele VE, Pezzuto JM (1999) Modulation of in vitro biomarkers of the carcinogenic process by chemopreventive agents. Anticancer Res 19:35–44

Littlefield BA, Gurpide E, Markiewicz L, McKinley B, Hochberg, RB (1990) A simple and sensitive microtiter plate estrogen bioassay based on stimulation of alkaline phosphatase in Ishikawa cells: estrogenic action of delta 5 adrenal steroids. Endocrinology 127:2757–2762

Maheo K, Morel F, Langouet S, Kramer H, Le Ferrec E, Ketterer B, Guillouzo A (1997) Inhibition of cytochromes P-450 and induction of glutathione S-transferases by sulforaphane in primary human and rat hepatocytes. Cancer Res 57:3649–3652

Markiewicz L, Hochberg RB, Gurpide E (1992) Intrinsic estrogenicity of some progestagenic drugs. J Steroid Biochem Mol Biol 41:53–58

Mehta RG (2000) Experimental basis for the prevention of breast cancer. Eur J Cancer 36:1275–1282

Miranda CL, Stevens JF, Helmrich A, Henderson MC, Rodriguez RJ, Yang YH, Deinzer ML, Barnes DW, Buhler DR (1999) Antiproliferative and cytotoxic effects of prenylated flavonoids from hop (*Humulus lupulus*) in human cancer cell lines. Food Chem Toxicol 37:271–285

Miranda CL, Aponso GL, Stevens JF, Deinzer ML, Buhler DR (2000a) Prenylated chalcones and flavanones as inducers of quinone reductase in mouse Hepa 1c1c7 cells. Cancer Lett 149:21–29

Miranda CL, Stevens JF, Ivanov V, McCall M, Frei B, Deinzer ML, Buhler DR (2000b) Antioxidant and prooxidant actions of prenylated and nonprenylated chalcones and flavanones in vitro. J Agric Food Chem 48:3876–3884

Miyazawa M, Shimamura H, Nakamura S, Sugiura W, Kosaka H, Kameoka H (1999) Moscatilin from Dendrobium nobile, a naturally occurring bibenzyl compound with potential antimutagenic activity. J Agric Food Chem 47:2163–2167

Narayanan BA, Geoffroy O, Willingham MC, Re GG, Nixon DW (1999) p53/p21 (WAF1/CIP1) Expression and its possible role in G1 arrest and apoptosis in ellagic acid treated cancer cells. Cancer Lett 136:215–221

Payen L, Courtois A, Loewert M, Guillouzo A, Fardel O (2001) Reactive oxygen species-related induction of multidrug resistance-associated protein 2 expression in primary hepatocytes exposed to sulforaphane. Biochem Biophys Res Commun 282:257–263

Pengsuparp T, Serit M, Hughes SH, Soejarto DD, Pezzuto JM (1996) Specific inhibition of human immunodeficiency virus type 1 reverse transcriptase mediated by soulattrolide, a coumarin isolated from the latex of *Calophyllum teysmannii*. J Nat Prod 59:839–842

Perchellet JP, Gali HU, Perchellet EM, Klish DS, Armbrust AD (1992) Antitumor promoting activities of tannin acid, ellagic acid, and several gallic acid derivatives in mouse skin. Basic Life Sci 59:783–801

Pettit GR, Singh SB, Boyd MR, Hamel E, Pettit RK, Schmidt JM, Hogan F (1995) Antineoplastic agents. 291. Isolation and synthesis of combretastatins A-4, A-5, and A-6(1a). J Med Chem 38:1666–1672

Pettit GR, Singh SB, Schmidt JM, Niven ML, Hamel E, Lin CM (1988) Isolation, structure, synthesis, and antimitotic properties of combretastatins B-3 and B-4 from Combretum caffrum. J Nat Prod 51:517–527

Pick E, Mizel D (1981) Rapid microassays for the measurement of superoxide and hydrogen peroxide production by macrophages in culture using an automatic enzyme immunoassay reader. J Immunol Methods 46:211–226

Prior RL, Cao G (1999) In vivo total antioxidant capacity: comparison of different analytical methods. Free Radic Biol Med 27:1173–1181

Prochaska HJ, Santamaria AB (1988) Direct measurement of NAD(P)H:quinone reductase from cells cultured in microtiter wells: a screening assay for anticarcinogenic enzyme inducers. Anal Biochem 169:328–336

Radtke J, Linseisen J, Wolfram G (1998) Phenolic acid intake of adults in a Bavarian subgroup of the national food consumption survey. Zeitschrift für Ernährungswissenschaft 37:190–197

Richon VM, Webb Y, Merger R, Sheppard T, Jursic B, Ngo L, Civoli F, Breslow R, Rifkind RA, Marks PA (1996) Second generation hybrid polar compounds are potent inducers of transformed cell differentiation. Proc Natl Acad Sci USA 93:5705–5708

Ridnour LA, Winters RA, Ercal N, Spitz DR (1999) Measurement of glutathione, glutathione disulfide, and other thiols in mammalian cell and tissue homogenates using high-performance liquid chromatography separation of N-(1-pyrenyl) maleimide derivatives. Methods Enzymol 299:258–267

San RHC, Chan RIM (1987) Inhibitory effect of phenolic compounds on aflatoxin B1 metabolism and induced mutagenesis. Mutat Res 177:229–239

Srinivasan P, Vadhanam MV, Arif JM, Gupta RC (2002) A rapid screening assay for antioxidant potential of natural and synthetic agents in vitro. Int J Oncol 20: 983–986

Steele VE, Kelloff GJ, Wilkinson BP, Arnold JT (1990) Inhibition of transformation in cultured rat tracheal epithelial cells by potential chemopreventive agents. Cancer Res 50:2068–2074

Steele VE, Sharma S, Mehta R, Elmore E, Redpath L, Rudd C, Bagheri D, Sigman CC, Kelloff GJ (1996) Use of in vitro assays to predict the efficacy of chemopreventive agents in whole animals. J Cell Biochem Suppl 26:29–53

Stevens JF, Ivancic M, Hsu VL, Deinzer ML (1997) Prenylflavonoids from Humulus lupulus, Phytochemistry 44:1575–1585

Stoner GD, Morse AM (1997) Isothiocyanates and plant polyphenols as inhibitors of lung and esophageal cancer. Cancer Lett 114:113–119

Stresser DM, Turner SD, McNamara J, Stocker P, Miller VP, Crespi CL, Patten CJ (2000) A high-throughput screen to identify inhibitors of aromatase (CYP19). Anal Biochem 284:427–430

Suh N, Luyengi L, Fong HH, Kinghorn AD, Pezzuto JM (1995) Discovery of natural product chemopreventive agents utilizing HL-60 cell differentiation as a model. Anticancer Res 15:233–239

Takasaki M, Konoshima T, Etoh H, Pal-Singh I, Tokuda H, Nishino H (2000) Cancer chemopreventive activity of euglobal-G1 from leaves of Eucalyptus grandis. Cancer Lett 155:61–65

Takasaki M, Konoshima T, Kozuka M, Tokuda H (1995) Antitumor-promoting activities of euglobals from Eucalyptus plants. Biol Pharm Bull 18:435–438

Takasaki M, Konoshima T, Shingu T, Tokuda H, Nishino H, Iwashima A, Kozuka M (1990) Structures of euglobal-G1, -G2, and -G3 from Eucalyptus grandis, three new inhibitors of Epstein-Barr virus activation. Chem Pharm Bull (Tokyo) 38: 1444–1446

Tanaka T, Kojima T, Kawamori T, Wang A, Suzui M, Okamoto K, Mori H (1993) Inhibition of 4-nitroquinoline-1-oxide-induced rat tongue carcinogenesis by the naturally occurring plant phenolics caffeic, ellagic, chlorogenic and ferulic acids. Carcinogenesis 14:1321–1325

Ukeda H, Maeda S, Ishii T, Sawamura M (1997) Spectrophotometric assay for superoxide dismutase based on tetrazolium salt 3',1-(phenylamino)-carbonyl-3,4-tetrazolium]-bis(4-methoxy-6-nitro)benzenesulfonic acid hydrate reduction by xanthine-xanthine oxidase. Anal Biochem 251:206–209

van Amsterdam FT, Roveri A, Maiorino M, Ratti E, Ursini F (1992) Lacidipine: a dihydropyridine calcium antagonist with antioxidant activity. Free Radic Biol Med 12:183–187

Waffo-Teguo P, Hawthorne ME, Cuendet M, Merillon JM, Kinghorn AD, Pezzuto JM, Mehta RG (2001) Potential cancer-chemopreventive activities of wine stilbenoids and flavans extracted from grape (Vitis vinifera) cell cultures. Nutr Cancer 40: 173–179

Widen CJ, Fraser-Jenkins CR, Reichstein T, Sarvela J (2001) A survey of phenolic compounds in Dryopteris and related fern genera. Part III. Ann Bot Fennici 38:99–138

Wormke M, Castro-Rivera E, Chen I, Safe S (2000) Estrogen and aryl hydrocarbon receptor expression and crosstalk in human Ishikawa endometrial cancer cells. J Steroid Biochem Mol Biol 72:197–207

Zhang Y, Kensler TW, Cho CG, Posner GH, Talalay P (1994) Anticarcinogenic activities of sulforaphane and structurally related synthetic norbornyl isothiocyanates. Proc Natl Acad Sci U S A 91:3147–3150

Zhang Y, Talalay P, Cho CG, Posner GH (1992) A major inducer of anticarcinogenic protective enzymes from broccoli: isolation and elucidation of structure. Proc Natl Acad Sci U S A 89:2399–2403

Zheng GQ, Ho DK, Elder PJ, Stephens RE, Cottrell CE, Cassady JM (1994) Ohioensins and pallidisetins: novel cytotoxic agents from the moss Polytrichum pallidisetum. J Nat Prod 57:32–41

Zinsmeister HD, Becker H, Eicher Th (1991) Bryophytes, a source of biologically active naturally occurring material? Angew Chem Int Edn Engl 30:130–147

CHAPTER 17

Molecular Epidemiology in Cancer Prevention

C.P. WILD

A. Introduction

A major goal of cancer epidemiology is to provide evidence from population-based studies for the implementation of public health measures to reduce cancer morbidity and mortality. Molecular epidemiology provides laboratory-based tools with which to better achieve this goal. The types of laboratory measure incorporated into cancer epidemiology are varied and include measures of environmental or endogenous exposures, genetic or other host factors influencing susceptibility to disease and surrogate markers for the disease itself. The measurement of these biological events ("biomarkers"), which are on or related to the carcinogenic pathway, can contribute to primary, secondary, and tertiary cancer prevention strategies (Fig. 1).

In identifying environmental risk factors and the individuals sensitive to those factors molecular epidemiology contributes directly to cancer prevention. However, molecular epidemiology can make a further contribution by permitting a more informative examination of molecular mechanisms underlying disease. Rapid technological developments promise the power to examine all stages of the cancer process, including the role of genes and interactions with environmental factors. This contribution is valuable both in establishing a causal association between exposure and disease through the demonstration of biological plausibility, but also in providing the mechanistic understanding needed for specific prevention strategies. This is particularly relevant in the case of chemoprevention using dietary and pharmaceutical agents. Furthermore, biomarkers may be used in chemoprevention trials as surrogate endpoints for cancer. The understanding of molecular and cellular alterations during carcinogenesis also promises biomarkers that could be used in surveillance programs leading to earlier detection of malignancy with more effective treatment and disease management. Finally, such biomarkers occurring during the disease process may also be useful in monitoring response to therapy and eventual disease recurrence although these are not considered in detail here. The different possibilities, summarized in Fig. 1, are developed below with examples.

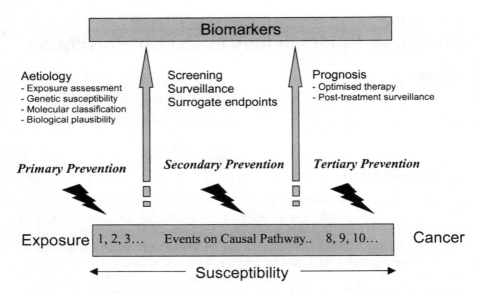

Fig. 1. The schema illustrates the different areas where molecular epidemiology through the application of biomarkers can contribute to cancer prevention

B. Etiology

I. Assessment of Environmental Exposures

Rapid changes in cancer incidence over time and studies of migrant populations imply that the large variations in cancer incidence seen worldwide are, for the most part, due to environmental rather than genetic factors (IARC 1990; PETO 2001). Carcinogenic substances in the environment have been recognized for at least 250 years, but it is over the last 70 years or so that epidemiology has identified major environmental risk factors. These include tobacco smoke, occupational hazards, high-levels of ionizing radiation, and a number of specific infections. Exposures associated with large increases in risk [e.g., hepatitis B virus (HBV) and hepatocellular carcinoma (HCC), tobacco smoking and lung cancer] have probably, for the most part, been identified. The focus is now on modest risks associated with more ubiquitous exposures such as low levels of ionizing radiation, nonionizing radiation, various aspects of dietary intake, endogenous and exogenous hormone exposures, and other lifestyle factors (PETO 2001).

In the past, because the identified causes of human cancer were often associated with the type of large increases in risk mentioned above, epidemiological studies did not need to rely on laboratory measures for exposure assessment. For example, in the 1930s and 1940s, epidemiological evidence associated tobacco smoke with increased lung cancer risk but pathology reports were the only laboratory contribution (MULLER 1939; SCHAIRER and

SCHONIGER 1943). However, environmental exposures conferring lower risks are difficult to identify without precise exposure measurement. For example, the role of environmental tobacco smoke (ETS) in human cancer is much more difficult to assess than the role of smoking per se. With biomarkers, however, TANG et al. (1999) showed an increase in 4-aminobiphenyl- and polycyclic aromatic hydrocarbon-DNA adducts in the peripheral blood cells of preschool children of mothers and other household members who smoked. This observation adds to the biological plausibility of ETS being associated with an increased risk of cancer, in addition to providing a method sensitive enough to quantify this exposure. Without appropriate biomarkers of this type the problem of misclassification of exposure will continue to hinder epidemiology.

Another example where exposure biomarkers have been valuable in studying an environmental chemical carcinogen is that of the aflatoxins (MONTESANO et al. 1997; WILD and HALL 2000). Aflatoxins contaminate foods as a result of fungal infestation in hot, humid conditions and their heterogeneity in any given commodity makes representative sampling of foods, and therefore exposure estimation, difficult. Similarly, because diets in many high exposure countries are relatively uniform, dietary questionnaires using foods frequently contaminated with toxin as a surrogate for aflatoxin exposure are largely uninformative. Urinary and blood-based biomarkers have yielded a number of significant advances, including a better understanding of geographical and temporal patterns of exposure (MONTESANO et al. 1997; WILD et al. 2000) and demonstration of associations between exposure and HCC risk (QIAN et al. 1994; WANG et al. 1996). In a nested case-control study in China (QIAN et al. 1994), a significant increase in relative risk of HCC was associated with a positive biomarker result (presence of urinary aflatoxins) but not with a dietary assessment of foods likely to be contaminated with aflatoxins. Equally, biomarkers have been a key to understanding the molecular mechanisms of aflatoxin carcinogenesis and their interaction with HBV (WILD and HALL 1999). The relevance of this to cancer prevention strategies is discussed below (see Sect. E).

There are other examples where elevations in biomarkers have been linked to increased cancer risk. BONASSI and colleagues (BONASSI et al. 2000) demonstrated that individuals with elevated chromosomal aberrations in peripheral blood cells at the time of recruitment were at higher risk of developing cancer at any site. In the examples of chromosomal aberrations and aflatoxin, the biomarkers were applied in nested case-control studies within the context of prospective cohort studies with biological samples banked prior to disease onset. One of the concerns in case-control studies conducted at the time of cancer diagnosis is that the biomarker level will be affected by the disease state in cases giving a biased picture of the difference between cases and controls. For example, in studies of HCC there is a possibility that HCC or associated cirrhosis and liver disease affects hepatic metabolism of aflatoxin and hence biomarker levels (HALL and WILD 1992). Despite these concerns there are instances where DNA adducts have differentiated exposure levels in case-control studies. The ^{32}P-post-labeling method has been used to measure "bulky" DNA adducts resulting from exposure to aromatic hydrocarbons with higher levels found in bladder cancer cases than controls (PELUSO et al. 2000). In this study peripheral blood cells were used as the source of DNA and it can be argued that these cells are relatively unaffected by cancer in the bladder. Each situation must therefore be considered carefully with regard to what is known about the absorption, distribution, and metabolism of the agent under study.

The above discussion implicitly draws attention to outstanding challenges to the development of exposure biomarkers, namely the need to account for the temporal variation in level of exposure and the varying impact of exposure at different periods in the natural history of the disease (Fig. 2). This situation differs, for example, from a genetic polymorphism, which remains constant over an individual's life span.

Exposure biomarkers therefore need to take account of the effect of the variable and cumulative lifetime exposures, e.g., to tobacco carcinogens in smokers, which undoubtedly play a part in the multiple genetic alterations observed in the development of a given malignancy. With infectious agents, e.g., HBV, evidence of prior exposure, in the form of serum antibodies to viral antigens, persists and is easily measured. For chemical exposures, the situation is more complex. In rare cases, such as pesticide residues in body fat and blood (STELLMAN et al. 1998) the markers persist over months or years. However, in the majority of instances the half-life of the biomarker will be relatively short and provide information on exposure only from a few days through to a few months, whereas the relevant period for disease etiology may be years or decades. Biomarkers of longer-term past exposure would therefore represent a major advance for epidemiology. One exciting development has been the obser-

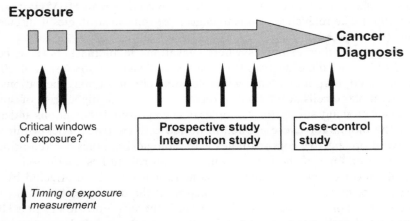

Fig. 2. The timing of biomarker measurements is presented in the context of the natural history of cancer development and the design of epidemiological studies

vation that a specific mutation in codon 249 of the p53 gene is associated with aflatoxin exposure and can be detected in plasma samples (KIRK et al. 2000; JACKSON et al. 2001). This biomarker was detected not only in HCC patients but also some with cirrhosis and some with no clinically diagnosed liver disease in The Gambia, an area of high aflatoxin exposure. This raises the possibility that, in addition to indicating the presence of HCC, the biomarker could reflect cumulative aflatoxin exposure at earlier stages in the disease process.

Whilst the limited life span of biomarkers restricts past exposure assessment, it should be noted that a biomarker responding rapidly to changing exposures can be an advantage when monitoring the impact of intervention strategies, e.g., antismoking programs (MACLURE et al. 1990) or for evaluating chemoprevention strategies (see Sect. E).

In addition to considering the ability of a biomarker to integrate dose over time, it is important to recognize that in some circumstances the exposure may be crucial only at a specific period of time; childhood infection with HBV, for example, is critical for development of chronic infection and HCC in adulthood (WILD and HALL 1999). In another example, YU et al. (1988) suggested that the risk of nasopharyngeal carcinoma was particularly linked to salted fish intake in the weaning period and early childhood compared to intakes in adult life. The important exposure may occur even earlier, namely in utero. The possible etiological roles of a variety of factors acting at this critical time in human development is receiving increasing attention (ANDERSON et al. 2000). Perhaps the best-known example is the striking association between the development of clear cell adenocarcinoma of the vagina in young women and their mothers' use of diethylstilbestrol in pregnancy (HERBST et al. 1971). Other examples include evidence that an 11q23 abnormality leads to a form of infant leukemia and may be due to exposure in utero to epipodophylotoxins (GREAVES 1997).

II. Genetic Susceptibility

It is hoped that in molecular epidemiological studies, the ability to stratify subjects into subgroups by genotype will reveal environmental risk factors that confer increased risks within one subgroup. For example, the increased risk of lung cancer associated with a GSTM1 deletion polymorphism is present predominantly in smokers, as opposed to nonsmokers (KIHARA and NODA 1994), suggesting that the deletion increases susceptibility only in the presence of smoking (VINEIS et al. 2001).

The more specific goal of assessing interactions between risk factors (e.g., genetic and environmental) has been difficult to achieve for a variety of reasons, including the requirement for large numbers of subjects. A recent study of sample sizes for the proposed UK population cohort showed that the power of a study is critically dependent upon the frequency of the genetic polymorphism, whether it is dominant or recessive, and the magnitude of the interaction (LUAN et al. 2001).

An additional challenge to elucidating gene-environment interactions is the fact that multiple polymorphisms are likely to differentially affect a given gene and the function of the protein encoded by that gene. A lack of consideration of some of these polymorphisms in an epidemiological study may lead to misclassification of subjects with regard to their "risk status." For example, in a study of the epoxide hydrolase gene and acute myeloid leukemia (AML), two common coding sequence polymorphisms at codon 113 and 139 were examined, one of which is associated with increased and one with decreased enzyme activity. It was only by examining a combination of these polymorphisms that the risk associated with disease was delineated (LEBAILLY et al. 2001).

There is a further layer of complexity in that multiple genes may be implicated in any given carcinogenic pathway. HAYASHI et al. (1992) studied polymorphisms in genes coding for two benzo(a)pyrene (B(a)P) metabolizing enzymes, cytochrome P450 1A1 and GSTM1. It was the combination of susceptible genotypes that defined the highest cancer risk. This example with two genes is still a drastic oversimplification in that epoxide hydrolase, CYP1B1, and GSTP1 are also important in B(a)P metabolism.

The above considerations, emphasize the need for both exposure and the complexity of genetic susceptibility to be taken into account when studying gene:environment interactions. Nevertheless, studies where exposure is better defined do provide support for the hypothesis that polymorphisms in genes coding for carcinogen metabolizing enzymes influence cancer risk. One example from our laboratory concerns the risk of developing therapy-related AML (t-AML) (ALLAN et al. 2001). In this study individuals with a polymorphism in the GSTP1 gene were at an increased risk of t-AML, but what was particularly significant was that the increased risk was restricted to those cases who had received chemotherapy, with the highest risk in those exposed to chemotherapeutic agents known to be GSTP1 substrates. This type of information, if confirmed, may be used to optimize treatments for primary malignancies in the future, thus reducing the risk of therapy-related malignancy.

III. Molecular Classification of Cancer

Improved classification of individuals with respect to both environmental and genetic exposures will clearly improve the power of epidemiological studies to detect exposure-disease associations. However, the fact that the molecular alterations occurring in a given tumor type differ between individuals may permit stratification of cancer cases on this basis to allow examination of etiologic risk factors within subgroups. This concept draws support from experimental studies showing that different chemical carcinogens induce different types of genetic change in tumors and from mutation spectra in human tumors associated with different exposures (GREENBLATT et al. 1994). MOORMAN et al. (2001), previously collected cytogenetic reports for cases in a case-control study of acute leukemia in adults. These data were used to select cases whose tumors had different cytogenetic profiles hypothesized to be related to benzene exposure [monosomy 7/deletion 7q and t(8: 21)] or not ("normal" karyotype) (LEBAILLY et al. 2001). The association between tobacco smoke exposure (a major source of benzene), polymorphisms in the microsomal epoxide hydrolase gene (involved in benzene metabolism), and the different subgroups of cases was examined. Associations between leukemia, tobacco smoke and epoxide hydrolase genotype were only present in those cases with benzene-related cytogenetic changes in the malignant cells. This study is interesting in its approach, but also demonstrates one of the weaknesses in that only relatively small numbers of cases were available in each subgroup (24–43) even when drawing from an original study in which cytogenetic reports were obtained from 592 cases. In addition, the rationale for the molecular subgrouping of cases needs to be strong.

IV. Biological Plausibility

By providing opportunities to examine events in the carcinogenic process, biomarkers may contribute to establishing biological plausibility. For example, the interaction between aflatoxin and HBV exposures has been demonstrated in epidemiological studies, but the biological mechanism underlying this interaction is unknown. The availability of biomarkers of aflatoxin exposure has permitted some hypotheses to be tested in human populations, notably the possibility that aflatoxin metabolism is altered in individuals infected with HBV (WILD and HALL 1999), something for which there is support from experimental studies of HBV transgenic mice (KIRBY et al. 1994; CHEMIN et al. 1999). Higher aflatoxin-albumin adduct levels were found in Gambian children (ALLEN et al. 1992; TURNER et al. 2000) and Taiwanese adolescents (CHEN et al. 2001) who were HBsAg positive compared to corresponding uninfected control groups. In adults in The Gambia, HBV infection was not associated with higher adducts (WILD et al. 2000). These results are consistent with a modulation of aflatoxin metabolism in association with HBV infection, particularly in young children. The biological plausibility of the exposure-disease association for aflatoxin and HCC is further emphasized by the observation of the specific mutational fingerprint (codon 249, AGG to AGT) in the *p53* tumor suppressor gene, consistent both with the biochemistry of aflatoxin-induced DNA damage and mutation and with geographical exposure patterns (MONTESANO et al. 1997).

Another example where biomarker data contribute to understanding disease mechanisms and etiology comes from a study of bladder cancer. CASTELAO et al. (2001) showed that the increased risk of this malignancy was significantly greater for women who smoked compared to men who smoked comparable numbers of cigarettes. This observation was consistent with the demonstration that the amount of 3-aminobiphenyl and 4-aminobiphenyl hemoglobin adducts formed for a given number of cigarettes smoked was significantly higher in women than in men.

C. Screening and Surveillance

I. Genetic Markers in Screening

The identification of inherited (germline) mutations in highly penetrant genes provides the potential for screening within families. However, due to the relative rarity of families with high-risk genotypes, this will have little effect on the population burden of cancer (VINEIS et al. 2001). In families at elevated cancer risk, the sociodemographic factors which determine the acceptance of genetic tests and the impact on the subjects with respect to a positive test result are complex areas where research is at an early stage (BOTTORFF et al. 2002; BONADONA et al. 2002).

Even when individuals carry the same inherited germ-line mutations, the timing of disease onset is influenced by other genetic and environmental factors. In individuals with an inherited mutation in the breast cancer susceptibility genes, BRCA1 or 2, age at diagnosis of cancer is not only influenced by the nature of the specific mutation (RISCH et al. 2001), but also by polymorphisms in other genes involved in endocrine signaling (REBBECK et al. 2001) and by hormone-related exposures (JERNSTROM et al. 1999). For the majority of cancers, genetic predisposition involves lower penetrance genes that may be necessary, or highly contributory, but are rarely sufficient to cause the disease. There would therefore seem to be little benefit to screen for genes having low penetrance or those requiring a substantial environmental interaction (VINEIS et al. 2001). A more effective method may be to reduce the level of exposure to the required environmental risk factor(s) if these can be identified.

II. Molecular Markers in Surveillance

Understanding the key genetic alterations occurring early during carcinogenesis may provide biomarkers useful for refining surveillance approaches among high-risk groups. An example is that of Barrett's esophagus, a precancerous condition associated with at least an order of magnitude increased risk of adenocarcinoma of the esophagus and having a number of well-characterized molecular alterations accompanying cancer development (JANKOWSKI et al. 2000). Despite the increased risk in Barrett's patients, the effectiveness of endoscopic surveillance for esophageal adenocarcinoma has been questioned because of the high prevalence of Barrett's esophagus in the population and the relative rarity of adenocarcinoma detection in absolute terms even among Barrett's patients (around one cancer per 100 patient–years). However, in a prospective cohort study of Barrett's patients we found that those with overexpression of cyclin D1 at recruitment had a 6–7-fold increased risk of progression to adenocarcinoma (BANI-HANI et al. 2000). This type of marker may permit the refinement of surveillance to focus on those individuals at highest risk.

The ability to detect tumor DNA in plasma (ANKER et al. 1999) offers promise for the early detection of cancer, particularly if integrated with other available diagnostic approaches. In the majority of studies to date the presence of the genetic alteration in DNA isolated from plasma has been conducted in series of patients with a confirmed clinical diagnosis of cancer. We wanted to examine whether the genetic alterations could be detected during the routine clinical investigations for patients suspected to have lung cancer. We therefore studied a series of patients attending a bronchoscopy clinic who had symptoms suspicious of lung cancer, and examined bronchial mucosa biopsies and plasma DNA for loss of heterozygosity (LOH) at four microsatellite loci. Of the 13 individuals displaying plasma DNA LOH at one or more loci, 12 were eventually diagnosed with lung cancer. These 12 patients represented 41% of the total number of cancer patients identified in this series of patients. Two patients were positive for LOH in plasma samples that predated clinical diagnosis by several months. A similar study of LOH in plasma DNA, but this time in early stage lung cancer patients, showed that alterations were frequently present in those with a stage I tumor, confirming that molecular changes in plasma DNA can be detected in a timeframe of value to clinical diagnosis (SOZZI et al. 2001). These markers, if fully validated, may have utility in the screening of high-risk groups within the population such as heavy smokers.

D. Prognosis

The presence of tumor DNA in the blood of cancer patients may also be valuable in monitoring disease posttherapy, including detection of disease recurrence. For example, in lung cancer patients treated for their primary tumor, SOZZI and colleagues (2001) examined both the amount of DNA in plasma and the occurrence of specific microsatellite alterations identified in the primary tumor. They demonstrated that the mean DNA concentration was more than tenfold higher in cancer patients at the time of surgery than in healthy blood donors. In addition, in 35 patients posttreatment with no evidence of disease, plasma DNA concentration dropped rapidly (in <6 months) to levels similar to healthy subjects. Furthermore, in nine patients with an LOH at a 3p locus detected in plasma DNA, seven patients did not exhibit this marker in plasma collected 4–24 months after surgery when there was no clinical evidence of disease. In two patients with persistent LOH, one had metastasis to the liver and one had a local recurrence of disease.

In a study of bladder cancer cases, *p53* mutations were detected in the urine of patients for whom the same mutation had been detected in the tumor (XU et al. 1996). In those patients where tumor recurrence was subsequently detected by cystoscopy, it was simultaneously possible to detect cells carrying *p53* mutations in DNA extracted from the urine sediment. In an additional six cases, the same *p53* mutation as present in the original tumor was detected in the urine despite a negative cystoscopy result. Four of these patients suffered subsequent recurrences within 4–10 months; the other two patients died of other causes before further cystoscopic examinations took place.

These results suggest that in principle monitoring plasma or urine samples for molecular biomarkers characteristic of the primary tumor could provide an additional clinical tool to monitor patients after treatment for that cancer. This area of research is in addition to considering the molecular characteristics of the tumor when optimizing specific treatment regimens (WEBER 2001), a topic not considered here.

E. Mechanistic Basis for Chemoprevention – The Example of Aflatoxin

Secondary interventions, such as chemoprevention with pharmaceuticals where cancer incidence is the endpoint, are both lengthy and costly, involving large numbers of subjects. Therefore the use of biomarkers as surrogate endpoints for chemoprevention trials is attractive (KELLOFF et al. 2001). These biomarkers include phenotypic and genotypic alterations ranging from molecular changes in specific target genes through to histologically detectable intraepithelial neoplasia. Biomarkers clearly have a potential role as endpoints in trials if their relationship to malignant disease can be established. The reader is referred to a publication arising from an international workshop on this topic (IARC 2001).

Another valuable application of biomarkers in chemoprevention is to examine in shorter-term studies whether the intervention achieves the predicted biological effect which would then be expected to translate to a reduced cancer incidence. This approach also contributes to the need for a strong underlying mechanistic knowledge to maximize the potential benefits and minimize unforeseen risks associated with longer-term treatment. An excellent example is provided by the work of KENSLER and colleagues with aflatoxin (WANG et al. 1999; EGNER et al. 2001). It is important though to emphasize that chemoprevention strategies should be placed within the context of other strategies for prevention of the given disease. Interventions in developing countries to reduce aflatoxin-related disease involve initiatives at the individual level or community level with particular promise relating to primary intervention strategies to reduce aflatoxin exposure at the postharvest level (WILD and HALL 2000). Nevertheless such approaches will not eliminate aflatoxin and cannot be targeted specifically to high-risk individuals, e.g., people with chronic HBV infection. Therefore chemoprevention strategies, using compounds that interfere with the absorption or metabolism of aflatoxins once ingested are also valuable to explore.

In animal models the important role of glutathione S-tranferase (GST) and aflatoxin aldehyde reductase (AFAR) expression in determining aflatoxin-DNA adduct formation and susceptibility to aflatoxin carcinogenicity has been established by modulating these parameters with chemoprevention agents (JUDAH et al. 1993; ROEBUCK et al. 1991; KENSLER et al. 1997; GROOPMAN and KENSLER 1999). This information, combined with an understanding of the specific human cytochrome P450s and GSTs metabolizing aflatoxin, provided a rationale for chemoprevention in humans based on modulating the balance between activation and detoxification.

Oltipraz is one agent which can induce GSTs resulting in increased excretion of the aflatoxin-8,9-epoxide glutathione conjugate as a mercapturic acid (KENSLER et al., 1999). Oltipraz can also inhibit the phase 1 activating enzyme, CYP1A2, resulting in diminished formation of the reactive AFB_1 8,9-epoxide. In Qidong County, China, KENSLER and colleagues (JACOBSON et al. 1997; KENSLER et al. 1998; WANG et al. 1999) have demonstrated, by measuring changes in urinary AFM_1 and aflatoxin-mercapturic acid metabolites and peripheral blood aflatoxin-albumin adducts, that oltipraz can indeed beneficially modulate aflatoxin metabolism in vivo. Similarly, chlorophyllin has been evaluated as a chemopreventive agent in a randomized, double-blind, placebo-controlled trial in Qidong County, China. Chlorophyllin consumption at each meal led to an overall 55% reduction in median urinary levels of aflatoxin N^7-guanine, a marker of DNA damage, compared to those taking placebo (EGNER et al. 2001).

The above clinical trials using biomarkers of aflatoxin metabolites demonstrate that metabolism is modulated in vivo in line with experimental data resulting in a reduction in the level of DNA damage induced. This type of mechanistic information is extremely important to support the rationale for chemoprevention strategies. It is also noteworthy that one entry criterion into the clinical trials was the presence of aflatoxin-albumin adducts in the peripheral blood of study subjects; in this instance biomarkers were therefore also used to select the study population.

Given the multifactorial and multistep nature of HCC, it is unlikely the above biomarkers will be predictive of cancer risk at the individual level or therefore be of value as surrogate endpoints in longer-term intervention trials aimed at evaluating the effects on cancer incidence. The specific codon 249 *p53* mutation related to aflatoxin exposure may be more predictive of individual risk and in this respect the identification of the mutation in plasma is encouraging (KIRK et al. 2000; JACKSON et al. 2001). A far greater understanding of the relationship of this biomarker to the natural history of the disease is required though before it could be considered as surrogate endpoint for disease risk.

F. Conclusion

Molecular epidemiology represents a dynamic field of research where knowledge of mechanisms of carcinogenesis can be translated into biomarkers. Such biomarkers have the potential to contribute to cancer prevention in a number of areas from the identification of etiologic risk factors through to the follow-up of cancer patients posttherapy for disease recurrence. In each case the biomarker approach requires rigorous validation and an application in combination with other available epidemiological and clinical tools. In this context molecular epidemiology can make a growing contribution to reducing the burden of cancer morbidity and mortality.

Acknowledgments. The author would like to thank fruitful discussions with Eve Roman and Graham Law during the preparation of this manuscript, Paul Turner for comments on the final draft and Geraldine Fox for help in finalizing the manuscript. CPW is grateful for financial support from the NIEHS, USA grant no. ES06052.

References

Allan JM, Wild CP, Rollinson S, Willett EV, Moorman AV, Dovey GJ, Roddam PL, Roman E, Cartwright RA, Morgan GJ (2001) Polymorphism in glutathione S-transferase P1 is associated with susceptibility to chemotherapy-induced leukemia, Proc Natl Acad Sci USA 98:11592–11597

Allen SJ, Wild CP, Wheeler JG, Riley EM, Montesano R, Bennett S, Whittle HC, Hall AJ (1992) Aflatoxin exposure malaria and hepatitis B infection in rural Gambian children, Trans R Soc Trop Med Hyg 86:426–430

Anderson LM, Diwan BA, Fear NT, Roman E (2000) Critical windows of exposure for children's health: cancer in human epidemiological studies and neoplasms in experimental animal models, Environ Health Perspect 108 Suppl 3:573–594

Anker P, Mulcahy H, Chen XQ, Stroun M (1999) Detection of circulating tumor DNA in the blood (plasma/serum) of cancer patients, Cancer Metastasis Rev 18:65–73

Bani-Hani K, Martin IG, Hardie LJ, Mapstone N, Briggs JA, Forman D, Wild CP (2000) Prospective study of cyclin D1 overexpression in Barrett's esophagus: association with increased risk of adenocarcinoma, J Natl Cancer Inst 92:1316–1321

Bonadona V, Saltel P, Desseigne F, Mignotte H, Saurin JC, Wang Q, Sinilnikova O, Giraud S, Freyer G, Plauchu H, Puisieux A, Lasset C (2002) Cancer patients who experienced diagnostic genetic testing for cancer susceptibility: reactions and behavior after the disclosure of a positive test result, Cancer Epidemiol Biomarkers Prev 11:97–104

Bonassi S, Hagmar L, Stromberg U, Montagud AH, Tinnerberg H, Forni A, Heikkila P, Wanders S, Wilhardt P, Hansteen IL, Knudsen LE, Norppa H (2000) Chromosomal aberrations in lymphocytes predict human cancer independently of exposure to carcinogens. European Study Group on Cytogenetic Biomarkers and Health, Cancer Res 60:1619–1625

Bottorff JL, Ratner PA, Balneaves LG, Richardson CG, McCullum M, Hack T, Chalmers K, Buxton J (2002) Women's interest in genetic testing for breast cancer risk: the influence of sociodemographics and knowledge, Cancer Epidemiol Biomarkers Prev 11:89–95

Castelao JE, Yuan JM, Skipper PL, Tannenbaum SR, Gago-Dominguez M, Crowder JS, Ross RK, Yu MC (2001) Gender- and smoking-related bladder cancer risk, J Natl Cancer Inst 93:538–545

Chemin I, Ohgaki H, Chisari FV, Wild CP (1999) Altered expression of hepatic carcinogen metabolizing enzymes with liver injury in HBV transgenic mouse lineages expressing various amounts of hepatitis B surface antigen, Liver 19:81–87

Chen SY, Chen CJ, Chou SR, Hsieh LL, Wang LY, Tsai WY, Ahsan H, Santella RM (2001) Association of aflatoxin B(1)-albumin adduct levels with hepatitis B surface antigen status among adolescents in Taiwan, Cancer Epidemiol Biomarkers Prev 10:1223–1226

Egner PA, Wang JB, Zhu YR, Zhang BC, Wu Y, Zhang QN, Qian GS, Kuang SY, Gange SJ, Jacobson LP, Helzlsouer KJ, Bailey GS, Groopman JD, Kensler TW (2001) Chlorophyllin intervention reduces aflatoxin-DNA adducts in individuals at high risk for liver cancer, Proc Natl Acad Sci USA 98:14601–14606

Greaves MF (1997) Aetiology of acute leukaemia, Lancet 349:344–349

Greenblatt MS, Bennett WP, Hollstein M, Harris CC (1994) Mutations in the p53 tumor suppressor gene: clues to cancer etiology and molecular pathogenesis, Cancer Res 54:4855–4878

Groopman JD, Kensler TW (1999) The light at the end of the tunnel for chemical-specific biomarkers: daylight or headlight?, Carcinogenesis 20:1–11

Hall AJ, Wild CP (1992) Aflatoxin Biomarkers. Lancet 339:1413–1414

Hayashi S, Watanabe J, Kawajiri K (1992) High susceptibility to lung cancer analyzed in terms of combined genotypes of P450IA1 and Mu-class glutathione S-transferase genes, Jpn J Cancer Res 83:866–870

Herbst AL, Ulfelder H, Poskanzer DC (1971) Adenocarcinoma of the vagina. Association of maternal stilbestrol therapy with tumor appearance in young women, N Engl J Med 284:878–881

IARC (1990) Cancer: Causes, Occurence and Control Tomatis L, ed. IARC Scientific Publications No 100, IARC, Lyon, France

IARC (2001) Biomarkers in Cancer Chemoprevention Miller AB, Bartsch H, Boffetta P, Dragsted L, Vainio H, eds., IARC Scientific Publications No 154, Lyon, France

Jackson PE, Qian GS, Friesen MD, Zhu YR, Lu P, Wang JB, Wu Y, Kensler TW, Vogelstein B, Groopman JD (2001) Specific p53 mutations detected in plasma and tumors of hepatocellular carcinoma patients by electrospray ionization mass spectrometry, Cancer Res 61:33–35

Jacobson LP, Zhang BC, Zhu YR, Wang JB, Wu Y, Zhang QN, Yu LY, Qian GS, Kuang SY, Li YF, Fang X, Zarba A, Chen B, Enger C, Davidson NE, Gorman MB, Gordon GB, Prochaska HJ, Egner PA, Groopman JD, Munoz A, Helzlsouer KJ, Kensler TW (1997) Oltipraz chemoprevention trial in Qidong, People's Republic of China: study design and clinical outcomes, Cancer Epidemiol Biomarkers Prev 6:257–265

Jankowski JA, Harrison RF, Perry I, Balkwill F, Tselepis C (2000) Barrett's metaplasia, Lancet 356:2079–2085

Jernstrom H, Lerman C, Ghadirian P, Lynch HT, Weber B, Garber J, Daly M, Olopade OI, Foulkes WD, Warner E, Brunet JS, Narod SA (1999) Pregnancy and risk of early breast cancer in carriers of BRCA1 and BRCA2, Lancet 354:1846–1850

Judah DJ, Hayes JD, Yang JC, Lian LY, Roberts GC, Farmer PB, Lamb JH, Neal GE (1993) A novel aldehyde reductase with activity towards a metabolite of aflatoxin B1 is expressed in rat liver during carcinogenesis and following the administration of an antioxidant, Biochem J 292:13–18

Kelloff GJ, Sigman CC, Hawk ET, Johnson KM, Crowell JA, Guyton KZ (2001) Surrogate end-point biomarkers in chemopreventive drug development, in Biomarkers in Cancer Chemoprevention, Miller AB, Bartsch H, Boffetta P, Dragsted L, Vainio H, eds., IARC Scientific Publications No 154, Lyon, France pp 13–26

Kensler TW, Gange SJ, Egner PA, Dolan PM, Munoz A, Groopman JD, Rogers AE, Roebuck BD (1997) Predictive value of molecular dosimetry: individual versus group effects of oltipraz on aflatoxin-albumin adducts and risk of liver cancer, Cancer Epidemiol Biomarkers Prev 6:603–610

Kensler TW, He X, Otieno M, Egner PA, Jacobson LP, Chen B, Wang JS, Zhu YR, Zhang BC, Wang JB, Wu Y, Zhang QN, Qian GS, Kuang SY, Fang X, Li YF, Yu LY, Prochaska HJ, Davidson NE, Gordon GB, Gorman MB, Zarba A, Enger C, Munoz A, Helzlsouer KJ, et al. (1998) Oltipraz chemoprevention trial in Qidong, People's Republic of China: modulation of serum aflatoxin albumin adduct biomarkers, Cancer Epidemiol Biomarkers Prev 7:127–134

Kensler TW, Groopman JD, Sutter TR, Curphey TJ, Roebuck BD (1999) Development of cancer chemopreventive agents: oltipraz as a paradigm, Chem Res Toxicol 12:113–126

Kihara M, Noda K (1994) Lung cancer risk of GSTM1 null genotype is dependent on the extent of tobacco smoke exposure, Carcinogenesis 15:415–418

Kirby GM, Chemin I, Montesano R, Chisari FV, Lang MA, Wild CP (1994) Induction of specific cytochrome P450s involved in aflatoxin B1 metabolism in hepatitis B virus transgenic mice, Mol Carcinog 11:74–80

Kirk GD, Camus-Randon AM, Mendy M, Goedert JJ, Merle P, Trepo C, Brechot C, Hainaut P, Montesano R (2000) Ser-249 p53 mutations in plasma DNA of patients with hepatocellular carcinoma from The Gambia, J Natl Cancer Inst 92:148–153

Lebailly P, Kane EV, Moorman AV, Roman E, Morgan GJ, Wild CP (2002) Genetic polymorphisms in microsomal epoxide hydrolase and CYP2E1 and susceptibility to adult acute myeloid leukaemia with respect to specific cytogenetic abnormalities. Br. J Haem 116, 587–594

Luan JA, Wong MY, Day NE, Wareham NJ (2001) Sample size determination for studies of gene-environment interaction. Int J Epid 30:1035–1040

Maclure M, Bryant MS, Skipper PL, Tannenbaum SR (1990) Decline of the hemoglobin adduct of 4-aminobiphenyl during withdrawal from smoking, Cancer Res 50:181–184

Montesano R, Hainaut P, Wild CP (1997) Hepatocellular carcinoma: from gene to public health, J Natl Cancer Inst 89:1844–1851

Moorman AV, Roman E, Willett EV, Dovey GJ, Cartwright RA, Morgan GJ (2001) Karyotype and age in acute myeloid leukemia. Are they linked?, Cancer Genet Cytogenet 126:155–161

Muller FH (1939) Tabakmissbrauch und lungencarcinom, Zeitschrift fur Krebsforschung 49:57–85

Peluso M, Airoldi L, Magagnotti C, Fiorini L, Munnia A, Hautefeuille A, Malaveille C, Vineis P (2000) White blood cell DNA adducts and fruit and vegetable consumption in bladder cancer, Carcinogenesis 21:183–187

Peto J (2001) Cancer epidemiology in the last century and the next decade, Nature 411:390–395

Qian GS, Ross RK, Yu MC, Yuan JM, Gao YT, Henderson BE, Wogan GN, Groopman JD (1994) A follow-up study of urinary markers of aflatoxin exposure and liver cancer risk in Shanghai, People's Republic of China Cancer Epidemiol Biomarkers Prev 3:3–10

Rebbeck TR, Wang Y, Kantoff PW, Krithivas K, Neuhausen SL, Godwin AK, Daly MB, Narod SA, Brunet JS, Vesprini D, Garber JE, Lynch HT, Weber BL, Brown M (2001) Modification of BRCA1- and BRCA2- associated breast cancer risk by AIB1 genotype and reproductive history, Cancer Res 61:5420–5424

Risch HA, McLaughlin JR, Cole DE, Rosen B, Bradley L, Kwan E, Jack E, Vesprini DJ, Kuperstein G, Abrahamson JL, Fan I, Wong B, Narod SA (2001) Prevalence and penetrance of germline BRCA1 and BRCA2 mutations in a population series of 649 women with ovarian cancer, Am J Hum Genet 68:700–710

Roebuck BD, Liu YL, Rogers AE, Groopman JD, Kensler TW (1991) Protection against aflatoxin B1-induced hepatocarcinogenesis in F344 rats by 5-(2-pyrazinyl)-4-methyl-1,2-dithiole-3-thione (oltipraz): predictive role for short-term molecular dosimetry, Cancer Res 51:5501–5506

Schairer E, Schoniger E (1943) Lungenkrebs und Tabakverbruch, Zeitschrift fur Krebsforschung 261–269

Sozzi G, Conte D, Mariani L, Lo VS, Roz L, Lombardo C, Pierotti MA, Tavecchio L (2001) Analysis of circulating tumor DNA in plasma at diagnosis and during follow-up of lung cancer patients, Cancer Res 61:4675–4678

Stellman SD, Djordjevic MV, Muscat JE, Gong L, Bernstein D, Citron ML, White A, Kemeny M, Busch E, Nafziger AN (1998) Relative abundance of organochlorine pesticides and polychlorinated biphenyls in adipose tissue and serum of women in Long Island, New York, Cancer Epidemiol Biomarkers Prev 7:489–496

Tang D, Warburton D, Tannenbaum SR, Skipper P, Santella RM, Cereijido GS, Crawford FG, Perera FP (1999) Molecular and genetic damage from environmental tobacco smoke in young children, Cancer Epidemiol Biomarkers Prev 8:427–431

Turner PC, Mendy M, Whittle H, Fortuin M, Hall AJ, Wild CP (2000) Hepatitis B infection and aflatoxin biomarker levels in Gambian children, Trop Med Int Health 5:837–841

Vineis P, Schulte P, McMichael AJ (2001) Misconceptions about the use of genetic tests in populations, Lancet 357:709–712

Wang LY, Hatch M, Chen CJ, Levin B, You SL, Lu SN, Wu MH, Wu WP, Wang LW, Wang Q, Huang GT, Yang PM, Lee HS, Santella RM (1996) Aflatoxin exposure and risk of hepatocellular carcinoma in Taiwan. Int J Cancer 67:620–625

Wang JS, Shen X, He X, Zhu YR, Zhang BC, Wang JB, Qian GS, Kuang SY, Zarba A, Egner PA, Jacobson LP, Munoz A, Helzlsouer KJ, Groopman JD, Kensler TW (1999) Protective alterations in phase 1 and 2 metabolism of aflatoxin B1 by oltipraz in residents of Qidong, People's Republic of China, JNCI 91:347–354

Weber WW (2001) Effect of pharmacogenetics on medicine, Environmental and Molecular Mutagenesis 37:179–184

Wild CP, Hall AJ (1999) Hepatitis B virus and liver cancer: Unanswered questions, Cancer Surv 33:35–54

Wild CP, Hall AJ (2000) Primary prevention of hepatocellular carcinoma in developing countries, Mutat Res 462:381–393

Wild CP, Yin F, Turner PC, Chemin I, Chapot B, Mendy M, Whittle H, Kirk GD, Hall AJ (2000) Environmental and genetic determinants of aflatoxin-albumin adducts in The Gambia. Int J Cancer 86:1–7

Xu X, Stower MJ, Reid IN, Garner RC, Burns PA (1996) Molecular screening of multifocal transitional cell carcinoma of the bladder using p53 mutations as biomarkers, Clin Cancer Res 2:1795–1800

Yu MC, Mo CC, Chong WX, Yeh FS, Henderson BE (1988) Preserved Foods and Nasopharyngeal Carcinoma: A Case-Control Study in Guangxi, China, Cancer Res 48:1954–1959

Subject Index

Printing (Computer to Plate): Saladruck Berlin
Binding: Stürtz AG, Würzburg